T0276123

A Computational Perspective on Visual Attention

A Computational Perspective on Visual Attention

John K. Tsotsos

The MIT Press
Cambridge, Massachusetts
London, England

This book was set in Times Roman by Toppan Best-set Premedia Limited.

Library of Congress Cataloging-in-Publication Data

Tsotsos, John K.
A computational perspective on visual attention / John K. Tsotsos.
   p. cm.
Includes bibliographical references and index.
ISBN 978-0-262-01541-7 (hardcover : alk. paper), 978-0-262-54380-4 (pb)
1. Vision. 2. Visual perception–Mathematical models. 3. Computer vision—Mathematical models.
4. Attention—Mathematical models. I. Title.
QP475.T875   2011
612.8′4—dc22
                                                                          2010036050

I dedicate this to my children,
Lia and Konstantine,
who inspire me daily

Contents

Preface

Attention in vision is something that I think has fascinated me since my undergraduate days at the University of Toronto. That is pretty surprising because I went to university wanting to be an aerospace engineer or maybe a physicist. In my first year, I subscribed to *Scientific American*, and in 1971 two papers caught my fancy: "Advances in Pattern Recognition" by R. Casey and G. Nagy and "Eye Movements and Visual Perception" by D. Noton and L. Stark. The first dealt in part with optical character recognition by computer, defining algorithms that might capture the process of vision and allow a computer to see. The second described the possible role of eye movements in vision and how they might define our internal representations of what we see. There had to be a connection! I have been trying to understand vision and what the connection between machine and biological vision might be since about 1974.

All through my graduate research, attention found its way into my work in some way. Back in the mid-1970s, there was a critical need for it in any large computer system: computing power was ridiculously meager by today's standards. I implemented my PhD thesis on a DEC PDP-11/45 with 256 kilobytes of memory! As a result, anything one could do to "focus" resources was a good thing. Similarly, if one looks at the computer vision research of the period (for that matter all of the artificial intelligence research, too), the inclusion of a "focus of attention" mechanism was not questioned.

But then in the early 1980s something happened, and, at least in the computational vision community, attention disappeared. I recall giving a seminar at a major U.S. university (nameless of course) where I spoke on my vision work, which included attention. I was taken aside by a very good friend afterward who apologized that many of the faculty did not attend my talk because, he said, they don't believe in attention at this school. I was surprised and disappointed, determined to "prove" that they were wrong. But how? These were really smart people, researchers for whom I had great respect. Could I really accomplish this? Maybe it was I who was mistaken? Within a couple of years of this event, 1985, as luck would have it, I became part of an amazing organization, the Canadian Institute for Advanced Research. Its president, J. Fraser Mustard, believed that to tackle a difficult problem such as artificial intelligence, one really had to look at it from many perspectives: computation, engineering, neuroscience, psychology, philosophy, robotics, society, and more. It was this connection that appealed to me and that eventually led me to a path for approaching my goal. This superb collection of scientists from all these disciplines pushed me, and in my 10 years as a fellow of the institute, I learned more from them all than I can possibly acknowledge. The lessons were sometimes direct but most often indirect, absorbed simply by observation or through casual conversations. The most important lessons were abstracted from watching how the disciplines interacted with one another. Which was ready to absorb the results of the other? What were the barriers to communication? How does one transform theories from one domain into something useful for another? How could one convince one discipline that another had any utility for it? These, and more questions, made me think about how one might better conduct truly interdisciplinary research. Specifically, the perspectives of multiple disciplines became ingrained in me, and I eagerly embarked on trying to understand those different viewpoints and how they may complement and build on one another. The first papers from which the contents of this volume emerged were directly due to the influence of the Canadian Institute for Advanced Research and its Artificial Intelligence and Robotics program.

Looking at the field of computer vision or computational visual neuroscience today, attention is no longer invisible and seems to be playing an increasingly larger role. The push to develop models and systems that are biologically plausible is prominent. Still, attention is most often thought of as either selection of a region of interest to guide eye movements or as single-neuron modulation. Few seem interested in considering how these two processes might be related, and certainly not many seem interested in an overarching theory of attention.

Such a theory of attention, especially for vision, is what this book proposes, at least with respect to some of its foundations. Whether those foundations are successful in the long term will depend on how well their implications and predictions provide a basis for new insights into how the brain processes visual input and how well the resulting representations and computational constructs contribute to new computational vision systems. As with all scientific endeavors, time will tell.

The audience for which this book is intended is a broad and varied one, mirroring the diversity of research efforts into this domain. The book is intended not only for those embarking on research on visual attention and for its current practitioners but also for those who study vision more broadly, as it is central to the thesis of this volume that without attention, vision as we know it would not be possible. The list of interested disciplines is large: visual neuroscience, visual psychology, cognitive psychology, computational vision, computational neuroscience, engineering, computer science, artificial intelligence, robotics, and more. It would be beyond the scope of any book to provide sufficient background so that anyone would find the book self-contained. To be sure, some background is presented in an abbreviated and certainly incomplete manner. Hopefully, enough pointers to relevant literature are included so the interested reader can track down what he or she might need. Those who have completed senior undergraduate or graduate-level courses in visual perception, computer vision, computational complexity, basic neuroanatomy of the visual system, and computational neuroscience will perhaps find the material more accessible than it will be to those who have not.

To provide a bit of assistance to some readers, the mathematical elements are confined to chapters 2 and 5 and appendixes B and C. Skipping these will of course lead to some gaps, but it shouldn't be too hard to follow the balance—unless you ask questions like "Why is he doing things this way?" In that case, you may have to simply bite the bullet and look at the math. Those who wish to see only the overview of the model can do so by reading chapters 4, 6, 7, and 8 and giving the early chapters less attention. For those who seek background on the main subject—visual attention—chapter 3 (and chapter 1 in a more general manner) is intended to be a comprehensive overview of attention theories and models. This literature is so large that gaps and unintentional omissions—for which I apologize—seem inevitable.

Those readers who identify with computer vision as their "home discipline" will undoubtedly be disappointed. But the current research directions in computer vision are not so compatible with the intent of this book. I am interested in using the language of computation, broadly speaking, to formalize and push forward our understanding of the mechanisms of vision and attention—both biological and artificial. Although I fully acknowledge the strong strides made by the computer vision community on the empirical and practical side of the discipline, that work is not covered in this book. Trust me, I may be more disappointed in this disconnect than you.

Many of the figures are better shown in color or as movies. There is a website associated with this book, <http://mitpress.mit.edu/Visual_Attention>, where one can see all color figures and movies. Where these are available, the citation in the book will be suffixed by "W." For example, if figure 7.3 has a color version, it can be found at the website as figure 7.3W, and it is referred to as such in this book. Movies are referred to as "movie 7.5W," not only pointing out that it is a movie but also that it is only available at the website. Although figures will be referred to with or without the "W" as appropriate, movies are only referred to with the "W" suffix.

Earlier, I wrote that two 1971 papers motivated my studies of vision and attention, but those were not my only motivation. My children played important roles, too, and it is for those roles that this book is dedicated to them. When my daughter, Lia (short for Ioulia), was born in 1985 (the same year that I joined the Canadian

Institute for Advanced Research, as I note in the preface—a fortuitous conjunction!), I was in the delivery room with my wife, Patty. I was the first to hold Lia on her birth and looked into her beautiful eyes—and was surprised! They did not seem to move in a coordinated manner; they gazed around apparently independently! The first thought in my head was, "What is going on in there to cause this? Is she okay?" After I was assured that there was nothing wrong, it occurred to me that I have to figure this out! Well I wound up not quite working on that side of the problem, but I do think this helped push me because the first paper that led to this book was written during the coming year. My son, Konstantine, was born in 1989, and this time I was better prepared for a birth, so no great surprises. However, about a year and a half later, he and I were lazing around at home on a Saturday morning looking for some cartoons on television to watch together. I found a program on robotics instead and was curious. It showed a disabled little boy operating a robotic toy-manipulation system. It was a very tedious system, and the juxtaposition of my healthy son playing on the floor beside me while watching the other little boy on television was actually painful to me. I thought that we should be able to do better, to build better systems to help. That was early 1991. My first paper on active vision was written as a result, appearing in 1992, and led to a robotic wheelchair project I named Playbot, intended to assist disabled children in play. So Lia and Konstantine, you were totally unaware of it at the time, but it is clear to me that if it weren't for you, my path would not be what it is today. And as I really like the research path that I am on, I thank you! You continue to inspire me every day with the wonder of how you are growing and becoming so much more than I will ever be.

My journey as a scientist has always had a modest goal. I have always viewed science as a race to solve a puzzle, a puzzle where the size, shape, and color of the pieces are unknown. Even the number of pieces and the eventual picture are unknown. Yet it is known that a picture exists, so we must discover what those puzzle pieces are and how they may fit together. My goal was always to be lucky enough to discover one or two of those puzzle pieces and to know where they fit within the full landscape that the puzzle represents. I think that every other scientist also has this as a goal. Only time will tell who discovers the right pieces for visual attention at the right time so that the picture is complete.

Acknowledgments

The theory presented in this volume was only possible because of the terrifically good fortune of having many talented people around me all of who contributed to the overall body of work (listed alphabetically). I thank each and every one:

- superb postdoctoral fellows—Neil Bruce, Xin Chen, Florin Cutzu, Daniel Loach, Julio Martinez-Trujillo, Pietro Parodi, Marc Pomplun, and Michael Tombu;

- gifted graduate students and research assistants—Neil Bruce, Sean Culhane, David Dolson, Brian Down, Yuhzong Lai, Randi Lanciwicki, Yueju Liu, Fernando Nuflo, Antonio Rodriguez-Sanchez, Albert Rothenstein, Xun Shi, Ksenia Shubina, Eugene Simine, Ankur Vijh, Winky Wai, David Wilkes, Yiming Ye, Andrei Zaharescu, and Kunhao Zhou;

- talented and generous colleagues and collaborators, some are coauthors, others may have provided a key conversation or pointer at the right time—Ruzena Bajcsy, Nico Boehler, Jochen Braun, Doug Cheyne, Sven Dickinson, Gregory Dudek, Mazyar Fallah, Olivier Faugeras, Fred Hamker, Hans-Joachim Heinze, Jens-Max Hopf, Laurent Itti, Michael Jenkin, Allan Jepson, Pierre Kornprobst, Evangelos Milios, John Mylopoulos (my first and continuing mentor), Zenon Pylyshyn, John Reynolds, Ariel Schoenfeld, Iannis Tourlakis, Anne Treisman, Stefan Treue, Jeremy Wolfe, Richard Wildes, Hugh Wilson, and the one who by far contributed the most, Steven Zucker.

I especially thank Eugene Simine for his programming assistance and for preparing many of the figures.

I also need to thank those who took the time to read drafts of this book and give me feedback and suggestions—Alexander Andreopoulos, Nico Boehler, Neil Bruce, Konstantinos Derpanis, Jens-Max Hopf, Marc Pomplun, Albert Rothenstein, Ehsan Fazl-Ersi, Lia Tsotsos, and Konstantine Tsotsos—and three anonymous referees arranged by The MIT Press. The presentation is much better as a result, but I take full ownership of any remaining errors or problems. Yes, my children did in fact read this and provided terrific feedback. Lia, being a PhD candidate in visual neuroscience, and Konstantine, being a senior engineering undergraduate who has worked on visually guided robotics, are exactly the kinds of people for whom the book is intended and thus were ideal reviewers.

The staff of the MIT Press has been surprisingly easy to work with. I especially thank Susan Buckley, Katherine Almeida, and freelancer Chris Curioli. Finally, I thank Robert Prior for his encouragement, easygoing manner, and, above all, for his patience while I took my snail's pace toward completion. I also thank Sandy Pentland for starting me on this project long ago when he suggested that my 1990 paper in *The Behavioral and Brain Sciences* could form the basis for a good book.

I am grateful to the following main sources of funding that have made my work possible: the Natural Sciences and Engineering Research Council of Canada (NSERC), the Canadian Institute for Advanced Research, the Ontario Centres of Excellence (OCE), and the Canada Research Chairs Program, where I hold the Canada Research Chair in Computational Vision. I also thank my first home base where this research was initiated, the University of Toronto, for their support and the wonderful research environment in the Department of Computer Science. I thank Olivier Faugeras and the France-Canada Research Foundation for providing me with a few quiet weeks in a lovely setting in Provence, France, to focus on my writing. Finally, my current home base, York University, has provided the key elements of research environment and support for the past 10 years while the research program matured and enabled me to write this book. My department, Computer Science and Engineering, the Centre for Vision Research, and the office of the Vice-President of Research and Innovation (special thanks to V.P. Stan Shapson) have provided me with terrific infrastructure, institutional support, funding, and the intellectual playground that allowed me to pursue my research dreams.

As this is my first authored book, I believe the acknowledgments would be incomplete if I did not take the opportunity to thank my parents for the sacrifices of so many kinds, their love, unwavering support, and constant encouragement that formed the foundation for my life. My father taught me the meaning of idealism by his teachings of the ancient Greek ideals and with the romantic poetry he wrote. He always looked through the way the world really was to the way it should be, what he hoped it could become. And as John Polanyi said, idealism is the highest form of reasoning. My mother taught me how to take that idealism and put it into practice. Hard work, perseverance, single-mindedness, focus, and then when you think you have worked hard enough, more hard work. Thomas Edison said that genius is 1% inspiration and 99% perspiration—my mother knew this because I really perspired!

My family has been very supportive while I worked on this book. They realized that while I was focused on this writing, I was at my happiest scientifically! Especially to my wife Patty—the one I celebrate with, the one whose shoulder I cry on, the one with whom I share the trials and joys of raising our beautiful children, my soul mate for over 30 years now—thank you!

1 Attention—We All Know What It Is

But Do We Really?

The title of this chapter is adapted from the classic words of William James (1890), who wrote what has become perhaps the best-known plain language description of attention:

Everyone knows what attention is. It is the taking possession by the mind, in clear and vivid form, of one out of what seem several simultaneously possible objects or trains of thought.

James specified two domains in which these objects occur: sensory and intellectual. He listed three physiologic processes that he believed played a role in the implementation of attention: the accommodation or adjustment of the sensory organs, the anticipatory preparation from within the ideational centers concerned with the object to which attention is paid, and an afflux of blood to the ideational center. With these processes, he set up a good deal of modern attention research including functional magnetic resonance imaging (fMRI) studies. However, since the time of James—and because of the myriad experimental findings exploring each of James' three processes—things have become less and less clear, and it is important to consider the many subsequent points of view.

A book on attention, computational or otherwise, needs to define what it means by attention. It would have been so convenient to end the introduction to attention with James' description. But it is not to be so. Many over a long period of time have written on how difficult it has seemed to pin down this domain of inquiry. Compare James' statement with that of Pillsbury (1908)

[A]ttention is in disarray . . . .

or that of Groos, who wrote in 1896 that

To the question, 'What is Attention,' there is not only no generally recognized answer, but the different attempts at a solution even diverge in the most disturbing manner.

Four decades later, it seemed that little had changed. Spearman (1937) commented on the diversity of meanings associated with the word:

For the word attention quickly came to be associated ... with a diversity of meanings that have the appearance of being more chaotic even than those of the term 'intelligence.'

Almost eleven decades after James, Sutherland (1998) suggested that:

[A]fter many thousands of experiments, we know only marginally more about attention than about the interior of a black hole.

Taken together, these quotes make the situation seem bleak! The field is full of controversy, and it seems that a bit more care is required before moving on. A brief tour through some of the early thinking on the topic helps reveal sources of debate and key issues. A more detailed treatment can be found in Tsotsos, Itti, and Rees (2005). The first scientific reference to attention, even though its etymology is traced to ancient Rome, seems to be due to Descartes (1649), who connected attention to movements of the pineal body that acted on the animal spirit:

Thus when one wishes to arrest one's attention so as to consider one object for a certain length of time, this volition keeps the gland tilted towards one side during that time.

Keeping with the idea that body organs are involved, Hobbes (1655) believed:

While the sense organs are occupied with one object, they cannot simultaneously be moved by another so that an image of both arises. There cannot therefore be two images of two objects but one put together from the action of both.

Leibnitz (1765) first linked attention to consciousness, a possibility that has received much debate recently, and attributed this to inhibition from competing ideas:

In order for the mind to become conscious of perceived objects, and therefore for the act of apperception, attention is required.

Hebart (1824) was the first to develop an elaborate algebraic model of attention using differential calculus and may be considered the first attention modeler. His general view on attention, however, was still rather simple:

He is said to be attentive, whose mind is so disposed that it can receive an addition to its ideas: those who do not perceive obvious things are, on the other hand, lacking in attention.

Since the 1800s, much genius has gone into experimental methods that were hoped to shed some light on the phenomenon of attention. Helmholtz (1860) believed that nervous stimulations are perceived directly, never the objects themselves, and there are mental activities that enable us to form an idea as to the possible causes of the observed actions on the senses. These activities are instantaneous, unconscious, and cannot be corrected by the perceiver by better knowledge—he called this **uncon-scious inference**, and thus he believed that attention is an unconscious phenomenon. On the other hand, Panum (1858) believed that attention is an activity entirely subservient to an observer's conscious will. Attention becomes difficult to hold once interest in an object fades. The greater the disparities between the intensities of two impressions, the harder it is to keep attention on the weaker one. Panum studied this in the specific context of binocular rivalry; but more generally, he observed that we are able to 'see' only a certain number of objects simultaneously. He therefore concluded that it makes sense that the field of view is first filled with the strongest objects. In studying an object, first attention, and then the eye, is directed to those contours that are seen by indirect vision.

Hamilton (1859) wondered about the span of attention:

The doctrine that the mind can attend to, or be conscious of, only a single object at a time would in fact involve the conclusion that all comparison and discrimination are impossible. ... Suppose that the mind is not limited to the simultaneous consideration of a single object, a question arises—how many objects can it embrace at once?

His last question is important even today. Brentano (1874) developed **act psychology,** where an act is a mental activity that affects percepts and images rather than objects. Examples include attending, picking out, laying stress on something, and similar actions. This was the first discussion of the possibility that a subject's actions play a dominant role in perception. Metzger (1974) lists aspects of action that contribute to perception: bringing stimuli to receptors, enlarging the 'accessible area,' **foveation** (the act of centering the central, highest-resolution part of the retina onto an object), optimization of the state of receptors, slowing down of fading and local adaptation, exploratory movement, and finally the search for principles of organization within visual stimuli.

Wundt (1874) further linked attention and consciousness, suggesting that attention, as an inner activity, causes ideas to be present in consciousness to differing degrees. The focus of attention can narrow or widen, reflecting these degrees of consciousness. For Titchener (1908), attention was an intensive attribute of a conscious experience equated with 'sensible clearness.' He compared attention to a wave, but with only one peak (corresponding with one's focus). He argued that the effect of attention is to increase clarity, whereas Kulpe (1902) suggested that attention enhanced not clarity but discriminability. Petermann (1929) argued against the subject being a passive perceiver of stimuli. He proposed an **attention-direction theory**, based on actions, as the mechanism for an active attentive process. As will become apparent, this theme keeps reappearing. These and other ideas were never formalized in any way and remained conceptual, yet interesting, viewpoints on the issue.

Helmholtz (1896) introduced the idea of **covert attention**, independent of eye movements:

The electrical discharge illuminated the printed page for a brief moment during which the image of the sheet became visible and persisted as a positive after-image for a short while. Hence, perception of the image was limited to the duration of the after-image. Eye movements of measurable size could not be performed during the duration of the flash and even those performed during the short persistence of the after-image could not shift its location on the retina. Nonetheless, I found myself able to choose in advance which part of the dark field off to the side of the constantly fixated pinhole I wanted to perceive by indirect vision. Consequently, during the electrical illumination, I in fact perceived several groups of letters in that region of the field. . . . The letters in most of the remaining part of the field, however, had not reached perception, not even those that were close to the point of fixation.

In other words, Helmholtz was able to attend to different portions of an image on his retina without eye movements. Such a demonstration is compelling and represents powerful evidence for the existence of attention independent of gaze change.

Even though experimental evidence supporting a variety of phenomena attributed to attention mounted, the field was not without its nonbelievers. The Gestalt school did not believe in attention. Köhler only barely mentions attention (Köhler, 1947). Gestaltists believed that the patterns of electrochemical activity in the brain are able to sort things out by themselves and to achieve an organization that best represents the visual world, reconciling any conflicts along the way. The resulting internal organization includes portions that seem more prominent than others. Attention, to them, was an emergent property and not a process in its own right. In this sense, Gestaltism was the precursor of the modern Emergent Attention theories that will be described in chapter 3. Figure-ground concerns loomed larger for them, the figure would dominate perceptions within a scene, thus emerging as the focus of attention rather than being explicitly computed as such. Berlyne (1974) tells us that Edgar Rubin, known for his vase/profile illusion of figure-ground perception, actually presented a paper at a meeting in Jena, Germany, in 1926 titled "On the Nonexistence of Attention." More recently, Marr basically discounted the importance of attention by not considering the time intervals of perception where attentive effects appear even though his goal was clearly to propose a theory for full vision. Describing grouping processes and the full primal sketch, he said:

[O]ur approach requires that the discrimination be made quickly—to be safe, in less than 160 ms—and that a clear psychophysical boundary be present. (Marr, 1982, p. 96)

Attention has been viewed as **Early Selection** (Broadbent, 1958), using **Attenuator Theory** (Treisman, 1964), as a **Late Selection** process (Deutsch & Deutsch, 1963; MacKay, 1973; Moray, 1969; Norman, 1968), as a two-part process, **preattentive fol-**

lowed by attentive processing (Neisser, 1967), as a result of **neural synchrony** (Milner, 1974), using the metaphor of a **spotlight** (Shulman, Remington, & McLean, 1979), within **Feature Integration Theory** (Treisman & Gelade, 1980), as an **object-based** phenomenon (Duncan, 1984), as a **shrink-wrap** process (Moran & Desimone, 1985), using the **Zoom Lens** metaphor (Eriksen & St. James, 1986), as a **Premotor Theory** subserving eye movements (Rizzolatti, Riggio, Dascola, & Umilta, 1987), as **Guided Search** (Wolfe, Cave, & Franzel, 1989), as **Biased Competition** (an extension of the shrink-wrap interpretation; Desimone & Duncan, 1995), as **Feature Similarity Gain** (Treue & Martinez-Trujillo, 1999), and more. These are all defined and discussed in later chapters, and they are listed here to show the diversity of opinion on the nature of attention. The field is rich with ideas, but can they all be right?

We have seen how Helmholtz provided a convincing demonstration for the existence of covert attention. Yet eye movements are the most obvious external manifestation of a change of visual attention. Yarbus' classic work (Yarbus, 1979) showed how task requirements affected fixation scan paths for an image. Given the same picture of a family in a Victorian living room scene, Yarbus asked subjects to either freely view the picture or to answer one of the following six questions about the people and situation depicted in the picture:

1. What is their economic status?
2. What were they doing before the visitor arrived?
3. What clothes are they wearing?
4. Where are they?
5. How long is it since the visitor has seen the family?
6. How long has the unexpected visitor been away from the family?

He recorded subject's eye movements while freely viewing and for the period of time before subjects provided a reply to a question. Each recording lasted 3 minutes. The surprise was the large differences among the summary scan paths demonstrating that the reason for looking at a picture plays a strong role in determining what was looked at. In fact, this was a nice extension of the basic Posner cueing paradigm that has played such a large role in experimental work (Posner, Nissen, & Ogden, 1978). Instead of providing a spatial cue that directed attention, Yarbus' questions directed attention. Posner (1980) suggested how overt and covert attentional fixations may be related by proposing that attention had three major functions: (1) providing the ability to process high-priority signals or alerting; (2) permitting orienting and overt foveation of a stimulus; and (3) allowing search to detect targets in cluttered scenes. This is the **Sequential Attention Model:** Eye movements are necessarily preceded by covert attentional fixations. Other views have also appeared. Klein put forth another hypothesis (Klein, 1980), advocating the **Oculomotor Readiness Hypothesis:** Covert and overt attention are independent and co-occur because they are driven by the same visual input. Finally, the afore-mentioned Premotor Theory of Attention also has an opinion: Covert attention is the result of activity of the motor system that prepares eye saccades, and thus attention is a by-product of the motor system (Rizzollati et al., 1987). However, as Klein more recently writes (Klein, 2004), the evidence points to three conclu-sions: that overt orienting is preceded by covert orienting; that overt and covert orienting are exogenously (by external stimuli) activated by similar stimulus condi-tions; and that endogenous (due to internal activity) covert orienting of attention is not mediated by endogenously generated saccadic programming.

What role do stimuli themselves play in attentional behavior? What is the role of the salience of the visual stimuli observed (see Wolfe, 1998a)? Just about everything someone may have studied can be considered a feature or can capture attention. Wolfe presents the kinds of features that humans can detect efficiently and thus might be considered salient within an image: color, orientation, curvature, texture, scale, vernier offset, size, spatial frequency, motion, shape, onset/offset, pictorial depth cues, and stereoscopic depth. For most, subjects can select features or feature values to attend in advance. Saliency has played a key role in many models of atten-tion, most prominently those of Koch and Ullman (1985) and Itti, Koch, and Niebur (1998).

Modern techniques in neurophysiology and brain imaging have led to major advances in the understanding of brain mechanisms of attention through experi-ments in awake, behaving animals and in humans. It is not possible to do justice to the large and impressive body of such research here (but see Itti, Rees, & Tsotsos, 2005). Suffice it to say that evidence abounds for how attention changes perception, and it seems manifested as both enhancement as well as suppression of signals. We also have a better idea about where attentional computations may be taking place in the brain.

How can it be that so many different and sometimes opposing views can be held all for the same "we all know what it is" phenomenon? One possibility is that the nature of a purely experimental discipline lends itself to fragmented theories. Most of the theories and models described earlier are constructed so that they provide explanations for some set of experimental observations with a focus being on the experiments conducted by each researcher. To be sure, each attempts to be as con-sistent with past work as possible so to build upon the past and not to continually reinvent. However, the explanations are almost always stated in natural language, using the ambiguous terminology of attention. In other words, there is no quantita-tive or formal statement of the theory such that it is unambiguous and not open to different interpretations. For many of the main theories of attention, it is easy to find subsequent interpretations that seem rather unjustified. As a result, a large part of the controversy in the field may have two main sources: a vocabulary that has never been defined unambiguously and a theoretical framework that is not formal in a mathematical sense and thus open to interpretation.

Moving Toward a Computational Viewpoint

Although attention is a human ability we all intuitively think we understand, the computational foundations for attentive processes in the brain or in computer systems are not quite as obvious. Notions such as those of capacity limits pervade the attention literature but remain vague. Within all of the different viewpoints and considerations of the previous section, the only real constant—something that everyone seems to believe and thus the only logical substitute for James' original statement—is that attentional phenomena seem to be due to inherent limits in processing capacity in the brain. But if we seek an explanation of attentional processing, even this does not constrain the possible solutions. Even if we all agree that there is a processing limit, what is its nature? How does it lead to the mechanisms in the brain that produce the phenomena observed experimentally?

This presentation, focusing on vision and sensory perception mostly, attempts to make these more concrete and formal. Through mathematical proofs, it is possible to derive the necessity of attentive processes, and through algorithmic approximations and processing optimizations it is possible to discover realizations given either biological or computational resource constraints. Perhaps the most important conclusion is that the brain is not solving some generic perception problem and, by extension, a generic cognition problem. Rather, the generic problem is reshaped—changed—through approximations so that it becomes solvable by the amount of processing power available in the brain.

The human cognitive ability to attend has been widely researched in cognitive and perceptual psychology, neurophysiology, and in computational systems. Regardless of discipline, the core issue has been identified to be **information reduction**. Humans, and many other animals as well, are faced with immense amounts of sensory input, and the size of the brain limits its ability to process all of this input. This is the qualitative statement that has appeared many times in the literature. It is not simply that there is too much input; the problem is that each component of each stimulus can be matched to many different objects and scenes in memory resulting in a combinatorial explosion of potential interpretations, as is caricatured in figure 1.1.

Perhaps the bulk of all perceptual research has focused on how the brain decomposes the visual signal into manageable components. Individual neurons are selective for oriented bars, for binocular disparity, for speed of translational motion, for color opponency, and so on. We know that individual neurons also exist that are

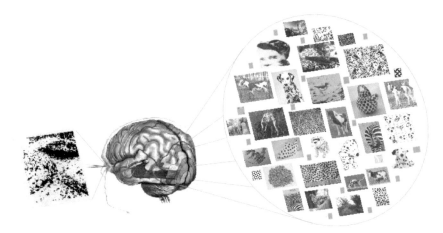

Figure 1.1
The classic "Dalmatian sniffing at leaves" picture (attributed to Richard Gregory) is sufficiently complex
to activate an enormous number of possible interpretations. Each small piece of it has similarities (some
strong, some weaker) to many other possible objects and scenes. The combinatorial explosion of possibilities that results is what any system—brain or machine—must effectively deal with to perceive successfully and act on the world.

tuned to particular faces or other known objects. But how can we deal with unknown
scenes and objects? The neural decomposition of a visual scene gives the brain
many, many pieces of information about a scene. It is in effect a *Humpty-Dumpty*-
like problem—we know how the visual image may be decomposed, but how is it
reassembled into percepts that we can use to guide our day-to-day lives? It is here
where the combinatorial explosion has greatest impact.

This combinatorial view is the one that is central to the theory presented in this
book. However, it is not the only view. For example, Tishby, Pereira, and Bialek
(1999), using information theory, view the relevant information in a signal as being
the information that it provides about some other signal. They formalize this problem
as that of finding a short code that preserves the maximum information about the
other signal, squeezing information through a 'bottleneck' formed by a limited set
of code words (the **information bottleneck method**). Clearly, they address information reduction and do it in a principled and well-defined manner. Although an
interesting and important perspective, it seems difficult to understand how it may
relate to brain processing because it does not address what sort of process may be
responsible for determining what those code words may be; Tishby et al.'s major
concern is the amount of information not its content or how it is processed. The
issues cannot be separated if one wishes to develop a theory of human attention.

The basic idea that humans can be viewed as limited-capacity information processing systems was first proposed by Broadbent (Broadbent, 1958). In computa-

tional systems, attention appears in early artificial intelligence (AI) systems explicitly as a focus of attention mechanism or implicitly as a search-limiting heuristic motivated primarily by practical concerns—computers were not powerful enough, and one had to do whatever possible to limit the amount of processing required so that resources could be allocated to the most relevant tasks. This kind of strategy and its heuristic nature is what Marr objected to. As he wrote:

The general trend in the computer vision community was to believe that recognition was so difficult that it required every possible kind of information. (Marr, 1982, p. 35)

When describing the modular organization of the human visual processor, he added:

[A]lthough some top-down information is sometimes used and necessary it is of only secondary importance . . . . evidence . . . was willfully ignored by the computer vision community. (Marr, 1982, p. 100)

As will become clear, top-down information is hardly secondary, and a heuristic strategy is really the only one possible. But, in contrast with what Marr thought, one *can* execute it in a principled manner.

All search methods that involve ordering or pruning of the search space perform information reduction. Information reduction is needed because the size of the full search space for a problem does not match the computing resources and system performance requirements, and thus a brute-force search scheme is not sufficient.

Motivation from cognitive psychology also made an important impact with the early appearance of a number of systems. The **Adaptive Character of Thought** (ACT) system was intended as a general model of cognition (Anderson, 1976). ACT has a focus of attention that changes as nodes in long-term memory are activated and put in working memory and as other nodes are pushed out of working memory. Focus is implemented with a small working memory (capacity limit), with strategies for determining which productions are applicable at any time. Along a very different application domain, Barstow's automatic programming system PECOS uses intermediate-level grouping to focus attention on the relevant and to ignore detail (Barstow, 1979). LIBRA was a system developed for efficient analysis of computer code (Kant, 1979). LIBRA has explicit attention and resource management rules. Rules determine how LIBRA's own resources are to be allocated on the basis of greatest utility. A landmark in AI, the 1980 HEARSAY-II system for speech understanding (Erman, Hayes-Roth, Lesser, & Reddy, 1980) ranked concepts using goodness-of-fit to focus in on the strongest and those with greatest utility. Several computer vision systems also included attention strategies to limit the region of interest that is processed in an image [the earliest being Kelly (1971) in the context of face outline detection] or even the window in time for video sequence input [the first being Tsotsos (1980) for heart motion analysis]. There are many more examples that help make the point that efficient matching of input, processing methods, and resources has played a major role in the development of computer systems whose performance attempts to match that of humans.

What Is Attention?

The study of attention has a long history, has been examined from many different disciplines, and there is a wealth of ideas, theories, and mechanisms that have been proposed. The bulk of this chapter was devoted to a brief tour through the development of the subject with the goal of searching for a definition. Is there anything within this enormous body of work that may be considered common, basic, or foundational? Perhaps this is the common thread:

Attention is the process by which the brain controls and tunes information processing.

The perspective in this book is that attention seeks to find a satisficing configuration of processes so that at least the minimum requirements of a goal can be achieved. This configuration may approach optimal; but optimality is not the primary objective. Attention adapts the visual system to its dynamic needs that are dictated by current input and task so that it may perform as well as possible within its capacity. But this is not yet a formal definition of attention; it is a qualitative one in the same style as the other proposals mentioned thus far. The remainder of this volume attempts to provide a formal foundation for this statement and to provide particular mechanisms that accomplish this. The overriding goal is to provide a computational explanation for visual attention in the human brain and visual system with the hope that this may also lead to more effective computational vision systems. And this will begin with an investigation of what the brain's visual processing capacity might be.

2 Computational Foundations

Attempting to Understand Visual Processing Capacity

From at least as early as Hamilton (1859), the **span of attention** has been a topic of speculation and inquiry. Span—or how many objects can be attended to at once—has relied on a limited-capacity explanation. This has a significant history and has taken many forms. One common conceptual form is the **bottleneck**, and a great deal of effort has gone into determining exactly where in the processing stream a bottleneck may exist. Interestingly, the early work seems motivated by the **Cocktail Party Effect**; that is, how is it that one can attend to one conversation while ignoring others in a room full of people who are all speaking and with perhaps other ambient sounds (Cherry, 1953)? Broadbent (1958) thought that attentional selection occurred before recognition; that is, the bottleneck due to selecting some stimuli over the rest was early in the processing stream. Deutsch and Deutsch (1963), Norman (1968), Moray (1969), and MacKay (1973) all thought it was late in processing and after the recognition of all stimuli. Treisman (1964) thought it was not a strict bottleneck but an attenuation function, a gradual bottleneck more like a funnel that allowed most stimuli to be processed to some degree and only selected ones to be processed completely. Verghese and Pelli (1992) proposed two successive narrowings of the processing stream, the first called the **span of attention bottleneck** and the second the **categorization bottleneck**. Issues relating to perceptual load are almost as common as those of resource allocation. Lavie (1995) attempted to resolve the early and late selection debate by considering **perceptual load** and suggested that load may determine the locus of selection. That is, when the relevant stimuli do not demand all of the available attentional capacity, there is spare capacity to process irrelevant stimuli. Thus, the perceptual load imposed by the relevant stimuli constitutes a necessary condition for early selection.

Closer to addressing the question asked by Hamilton is the work of Trick and Pylyshyn (1993). They used a subitizing paradigm (enumerating a number of stimulus items in a display) and suggested that their results can only be explained by a limited-capacity mechanism that operates after the spatially parallel processes of feature detection and grouping but before the serial processes of spatial attention. Unfortunately, they did not propose a mechanism that might accomplish this.

Others place the responsibility for the limit elsewhere. Cowan et al. (2005) provide detailed discussion on the possibility that the capacity of attention is tightly tied to that of working memory. Yet another sort of explanation, worthy of consideration because of its attempt to be quantitative and based in information theory, is that of Verghese and Pelli (1992). Verghese and Pelli examine the question: Is visual attention mediated by a small-capacity general-purpose processor? They suggest that this limited capacity corresponds with a fixed amount of information, measured in bits. Studying the tasks of the detection of a stationary dot in a field of moving dots and the detection of a static square in a field of flashing squares, they show that performance of these tasks is perfect up to a critical number of elements (the span of attention) and then falls as the number of elements increases beyond this critical number. The display information required for unimpaired performance in each of these tasks is low; their results indicate that visual attention processes only 30 to 60 bits of display information. Finally, Nakayama (1990) describes his views on an **iconic bottleneck**. For him, early visual processing is built upon a multi-resolution pyramid of features and visual memory consists of many low-resolution scale-invariant icons. He proposes that the limited transmission bandwidth between early vision and visual memory leads to processing strategies that must solve the resulting matching problems: low-resolution matching can be accomplished over the whole image but high-resolution matching only over small portions of the image. This then leads to the iconic bottleneck. He is closest to the overall picture this book will present; he does not present theoretical arguments for his proposal, but Tsotsos (1987) provided exactly what was required, drawing similar conclusions.

In each of these cases, the assumption underlying the research is that there is a physical construct within the visual processing stream (shown schematically in figure 2.1) that is unable to handle the amount of information the visual system receives. The physical construct—except for a small number of notable exceptions such as Verghese and Pelli and Nakayama—is described only metaphorically and thus is very difficult to scrutinize and is open to interpretation. The view in this volume rejects this manner of description and proposes something very different, something more deeply based in the language of computation. This chapter will focus on providing this different perspective—a *computational perspective*—in a formal manner using the tools and language of computational science.

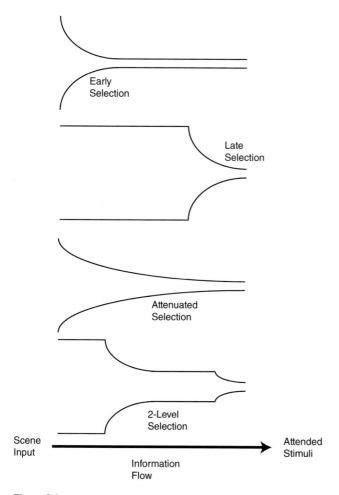

Early
Selection

Late
Selection

Attenuated
Selection

2-Level
Selection

Scene
Input

Attended
Stimuli

Information
Flow

Figure 2.1
Four kinds of bottlenecks proposed to be responsible for attentive behavior. Each makes a particular commitment to when in the information flow attentional selection has its effect.

The Language of Computation

The term *computational model* seems to have many uses. Sometimes it is taken to mean any model that includes mathematical equations. Such equations, at least in the domain of concern here, are usually obtained by fitting functions to data. They form a model because it is possible to make predictions by interpolating or extrapolating the function to obtain values of parameters that reflect the kinds of input presented to subjects. As these equations may be simulated on a computer, the model is thought to be computational. These models are quite useful because they help us understand the relationships among the variables of interest, but they are not computational, they are mathematical. Sometimes the term *computational* seems to refer to any 'in principle' explanation of some phenomenon, as Marr described with the first of his levels of analysis (Marr, 1982). But many 'in principle' solutions, as will become apparent in the following chapters, are in fact not realizable due to their intractability and thus are useless. Only by completing all of the levels of analysis that Marr describes, including achieving a functioning implementation, can 'in principle' solutions be useful (see also Tsotsos, 1987). Another sort of model is created by a data-mining or machine-learning approach. Currently, it is very much in fashion to forego the traditional scientific method and instead follow the data-association approach to solving problems (see Anderson, 2008). This strategy begins with a large database of exemplars and from these discovers or learns the classes of information (and their boundaries) that can partition those exemplars. One might consider this kind of model to be a performance model; that is, a functioning computer program that performs a task with high degree of success, as opposed to a competence model where the goal would be to develop an ideal model that performs all tasks and is formally complete (see Pylyshyn, 1973). However, it is not clear what one has learned, if anything, about the underlying mechanisms from a performance model. An analogy with medicine makes this point clear: It is one thing to say that a diet high in fat is unhealthy because it is associated with higher incidence of heart disease and cancer and a completely different thing to understand the physiologic mechanisms that underlie that association. In the data-association case, one may make very effective predictions about disease incidence given a history of dietary conditions, but one can only suggest that one eliminate fat from the diet as a solution. If one has a deep causal understanding, one might be able to develop medicines or other interventions that target the precise mechanism along the path from dietary intake to disease that is responsible for the problem. If perhaps there are multiple mechanisms on the path, we might be able to target one distinctly from the rest. This is what modern medicine seeks to achieve. Only if such an understanding is not yet available does medicine resort to a data-association kind of recommendation.

Similarly, the data-association approach fails to provide a deep understanding of brain mechanisms.

Although each of the above examples do indeed involve computation, they use only a narrow range of the full power of computational science. Computation is in fact a much broader entity. Computer science, broadly defined, is the theory and practice of representation, processing, and use of information and encompasses a body of knowledge concerning algorithms, communication, languages, software, and information systems (Denning, 2007). As a result, Denning claims that it offers a powerful foundation for modeling complex phenomena such as cognition. The language of computation is the best language we have to date, he claims, for describing how information is encoded, stored, manipulated, and used by natural as well as synthetic systems. It is no longer valid to think of computer science as the study of phenomena surrounding computers. Computing is the study of natural and artificial information processes. Denning defines seven categories along which computing principles can be grouped:

1. *Computation*   (meaning and limits of computation, such as intractability).

2. *Communication*   (reliable data transmission, such as compression).

3. *Coordination*   (cooperation among networked entities, such as choosing).

4. *Recollection*   (storage and retrieval of information, such as locality).

5. *Automation*   (meaning and limits of automation, such as search).

6. *Evaluation*   (performance prediction and capacity planning, such as determining and dealing with bottlenecks).

7. *Design*   (building reliable software systems, such as through the use of hierarchical aggregation).

These form the basis of a language of computation, and although this language cannot be defined syntactically nor semantically as can a natural language, the collection of tools and concepts within these categories forms a powerful and appropriate means for expressing theories of natural information processes.

Interestingly, Zucker argued for the importance of the language of computation in understanding perception many years earlier (Zucker, 1981). Zucker claimed that computational models of perception have two essential components: representational languages for describing information and mechanisms that manipulate those representations. The many diverse kinds of constraints on theories discovered by experimental work, whether psychophysical, neurophysiologic, or theoretical, impact the representations and manipulation mechanisms. Zucker goes on to suggest that all of these different kinds of constraints are needed, or the likelihood of discovering the correct explanation is seriously diminished. Without the computational theories and constraints, one is faced with the problem of inferring what staggering numbers of neurons are doing without a suitable language for describing either them or their scope. Theories can exist at different descriptive levels, and the levels are all instructive, if not necessary, to restrict experimental and theoretical scope at all levels of explanation, whether one is concerned with computer or human perception or both.

For our purposes, and following Zucker and Denning, the language of computation used herein takes this broad form: representations and mechanisms interact, constraints derived from experimental studies shape those representations and mechanisms, levels of representation that match those in the brain matter, causal explanations are required for the model's predictive power, analysis of the properties of the solution provide confidence in the quality of the solution, and the full breadth of computational principles plays an important role.

Capacity Limits and Computational Complexity

One of the most frustrating things about studying attention is the vague discussion of capacity limits, bottlenecks, and resource limits in the published literature. How can these notions be made more concrete? A casual glance at visual psychophysics papers that explore attention, for example, reveals one of the methods experimentalists use to measure human visual performance. For a class of visual search tasks, experimenters relate observed response time (RT) to set size (number of elements in the test display). Graphical plots of RT versus set size are common throughout the literature as are interpretations of them that lead to speculations about the underlying mechanisms that may be responsible for the differences in performance (but this is not at all straightforward—see Wolfe, 1998a,b). But to a computer scientist, this is reminiscent of **time complexity**, a function that gives the amount of processing time required to solve a problem as a function of the size of the input. Could there be a deeper connection?

The area of computer science known as **Computational Complexity** is concerned with the theoretical issues dealing with the cost of achieving solutions to problems in terms of time, memory, and processing power as a function of problem size. Complexity functions can be specific to particular algorithms but also may be developed to apply to the problem as a whole. In the latter case, complexity statements can be made that hold for any algorithm realized on any hardware substrate, biological or silicon or otherwise. It thus provides the necessary theoretical foundation on which to base an answer to the attentional capacity question. A key determination possible using the theoretical tools available is whether or not a problem is tractable in the first place; that is, if the problem may be solved by *any* algorithm using available processors and hardware and in a reasonable amount of time.

It is appropriate to ask whether this theoretical discipline has relevance for real problems. After all, a quick look at the typical sorts of problems considered intractable by theorists reveals very abstract, mathematical issues. Stockmeyer and Chandra (1988) present a compelling argument. The most powerful computer that could conceivably be built could not be larger than the known universe, could not consist of hardware smaller than the proton, and could not transmit information faster than the speed of light. Such a computer could consist of at most 10^{126} pieces of hardware. It can be proved that, regardless of the ingenuity of its design and the sophistication of its program, this ideal computer would take at least 20 billion years to solve certain mathematical problems that are known to be solvable in principle (e.g., the well-known traveling salesman problem with a sufficiently large number of destinations). As the universe is probably less than 20 billion years old, it seems safe to say that such problems defy computer analysis. There exist many real problems for which this argument applies (for a catalog, see Garey & Johnson, 1979; Johnson, 1990), and they form the foundation for the theorems presented here.

Applying complexity theory to problems in science has long been identified as an interesting research direction (Traub, 1990). With respect to neurobiology, several have considered complexity constraints in the past but mostly with coarse, counting arguments of varying kinds. For example, Feldman and Ballard (1982), in laying out the foundations for connectionist models, considered carefully the resource implications of those models when applied to solving problems in vision. They point out that:

• there are not enough neurons or connections to enable obvious solutions to problems;

• there are not enough neurons to provide one to represent each complex object at every position, orientation, and scale of visual space; and

• there are not enough neurons for a separate, dedicated path between all possible pairs of units in two layers.

They concluded that several strategies were possible to help keep the numbers of neurons and connections in a network low enough to be plausible for the brain. These are functional decomposition, limited precision computation, coarse and coarse-fine coding, tuning, and spatial coherence. In important ways, this was the precursor for the work of Tsotsos (1987), who formalized exactly how large a number of neurons and connections the obvious (or 'in principle') solutions in vision required, and then showed how the simple strategies of hierarchical organization, spatiotemporally coherent receptive fields, feature map separation, and pyramidal representations bring those too-large numbers down to brain-size and thus plausible values. This is expanded in the remainder of this chapter; that paper was the starting point for this whole book. Two different but as important kinds of constraints were the concern of Thorpe and Imbert (1989). They argued that the observed speed of human visual processing placed a hard limit on the processing architecture concluding that a single feed-forward pass may be all that is required to account for the bulk of human vision. They further considered learning algorithms in this context and analyzed which sorts of learning schemes may (Hebbian mechanisms) or may not (error-correcting mechanisms) have biological counterparts. Lennie took a different approach attempting to tie computational cost to expenditure of energy required for a single neural spike (Lennie, 2003). For the human cortex, he estimates the cost of individual spikes and then using the known energy consumption of the full cortex estimates how many neurons may be active concurrently. This places a limit on how much of the brain can be working on a given problem as well as the kinds of representations that are being employed. He, consistent with other similar studies, concludes that only a small percentage of neurons in cortex can be active at any one time. He suggests that this limits the range of tasks that can be undertaken simultaneously and, more importantly, necessitates neural machinery that can allocate energy on task demand. Lennie says that this adds a new physiologic perceptive on attention and its need for energy management.

All roads lead to the same conclusions: The resources that the brain has cannot fully process all stimuli in the observed response times. Even though there are hints for what sorts of constraints may be at play to help develop a solution, this is not enough, and this book takes the position that a more formal analysis of vision at the appropriate level of abstraction will help to reveal quantitative constraints on visual architectures and processing. First, however, it is important to address the applicability of this analysis for the neurobiology of the brain.

Human Perception/Cognition and Computation

Can human cognition, intelligence, perception, or vision be expressed in computational form? Zucker certainly believed so in his 1981 invited talk for the International Joint Conference on Artificial Intelligence in Vancouver (Zucker, 1981). Marr, too, takes a similar stand (Marr, 1982). Surely, the discovery of explanatory mechanisms that yield observed performance is central to all experimental studies. In a very real sense, such explanations are presented as algorithms, step-by-step procedures for achieving some result, and algorithms are a central component of the language of computation. They tie together the seven categories of computing principles listed earlier and make the procedure concrete and amenable to further analysis and realization. Marr provided a well-cited conceptualization of this further analysis (Marr, 1982):

Computational Theory   What is the goal of the computation, why is it appropriate, and what is the logic of the strategy by which it can be carried out?

Representation and algorithm   How can the computational theory be implemented? In particular, what is the representation for input and output and what is the algorithm for the transformation?

Hardware implementation   How can the representation and algorithm be realized physically?

As stated, these are quite abbreviated, and many other issues are relevant within each. Tsotsos (1990a) argued that there might even be a fourth level of analysis—the complexity level—that investigates whether or not a particular problem is solvable in principle in the first place [something Feldman and Ballard (1982) also suggested]. Zucker (1981) adds stress on the importance of representation. He points out that computational models have two essential components—representational languages for describing information and mechanisms that manipulate those representations. One important mechanism is clearly the creation of descriptions and the inferential side of perception, first described by Helmholtz (1860) and still very important today. As Zucker (1981) confirms:

One of the strongest arguments for having explicit abstract representations is the fact that they provide explanatory terms for otherwise difficult (if not impossible) notions.

But does the brain actually process signals in an algorithmic manner? This nontrivial issue is important because if it could be proved that human brain processes cannot be modeled computationally (and this is irrespective of current computer hardware), then modeling efforts are futile. A perhaps overwhelming amount of positive support has accumulated beginning with a critical theoretical notion, **decidability**. A proof of decidability is sufficient to guarantee that a problem can be modeled computationally (Davis, 1958, 1965). To show that vision is decidable, it must first be formulated as a **decision problem**. This means the problem must be expressed as follows: We wish to know of each element in a countably infinite set A (elements can be corresponded to the set of non-negative integers) whether or not that element belongs to a certain set B that is a proper subset of A. Such a problem is decidable if there exists a **Turing Machine** that computes 'yes' or 'no' for each element of A in answer to the decision question. A Turing Machine is a hypothetical computing device consisting of a finite state control, a read–write head, and a two-way infinite sequence of labeled tape squares (Turing, 1936). A program then provides input to the machine, is executed by the finite state control, and computations specified by the program read and write symbols on the tape squares. The Turing Machine may be considered the most primitive, yet complete, computation machine. As a result, it forms the foundation of all theory in computer science.

Decidability should not be confused with tractability. A **tractable problem** is one where enough resources can be found and enough time can be allocated so that the problem can be solved. An **undecidable problem** is one that cannot be solved for all cases by any algorithm whatsoever. An **intractable problem** is one for which no algorithm can exist that computes all instances of it in polynomial, as opposed to exponential, time. That is, the mathematical function that relates processing time/space to the size of the input is polynomial as opposed to exponential in that input size. If the input is large, then an exponential function with a large exponent leads to the need for enormous amounts of processing resources, as described in the previous section by the work of Stockmeyer and Chandra.

There are several classes of such problems with differing characteristics, and **NP-Complete** is one of those classes. NP-Complete (NPC) is a subset of NP. NP (Nondeterministic Polynomial time) may be defined as the set of decision problems that can be solved in polynomial time on a nondeterministic Turing Machine (one that includes an oracle to guess at the answer). A problem p in NP is also in NPC if and only if every other problem in NPC can be transformed into p in polynomial time (the processing time required for the transformation can be expressed as a polynomial function of the input size). The reader wishing more background on complexity theory and its use here is referred to appendix A of this volume.

If we look at the perceptual task definitions provided by Macmillan and Creelman (2005), we see that all psychophysical judgments are of one stimulus relative to another—the basic process is comparison. The most basic task is termed **discrimination**, the ability to tell two stimuli apart. The task is a **detection** task if one stimulus class is null (such as in the object on a noise background). If neither stimulus class is null, the task is termed **recognition**. These are all yes–no experiments (i.e., the subject is required to respond to a stimulus with a yes–no answer). This is exactly the decision problem defined above. It is known that this problem is decidable; Yashuhara's **Comparing Turing Machine** (Yashuhara, 1971) proves this. The Visual Match problem, which will be defined below, is an instance of the Comparing Turing Machine, and it provides a formalization of the relevant problem: Does an image contain an instance of a given target?

Showing that one problem is decidable is not a proof that all of human vision can be modeled computationally. If no subproblem of vision could be found to be decidable, then it might be that vision as a whole is undecidable and thus cannot be computationally modeled. There are many vision tasks that are decidable, many of which are described in later sections, so this is not the case. But what if there are other undecidable vision subproblems? Even if some other aspect of vision is determined to be undecidable, this does not mean that all of vision is also undecidable or that other aspects of perception cannot be modeled computationally. Hilbert's 10th problem in mathematics and the Halting Problem for Turing Machines are two examples of famous undecidable problems. The former does not imply that mathematics is not possible, and the latter does not mean that computers are impossible. It seems that most domains feature both decidable as well as undecidable subproblems and these coexist with no insurmountable difficulty. We thus assume the same is true for the computational modeling of human vision.

Once a problem is known to be decidable, it may in fact be an instance of one of the many known problems that have been cataloged with respect to their complexity class (see Johnson, 1990), and proof methods exist for demonstrating the class membership. For problems that are considered intractable, the proofs need to show that for any possible algorithm or implementation, the time complexity function of a solution is exponential in the size of the input. The analysis is asymptotic; that is, the problem becomes intractable only as the input size becomes very large. Small values of an exponent (i.e., small input sizes) often lead to solutions that are quite realizable. Efficient algorithms have polynomial time complexity; that is, complexity is a polynomial function of the input size. In both cases, exponential or polynomial time, the actual size of the input and the power of the processors on which a solution is implemented are the ultimate determinants of whether or not an efficient realization is available.

Some might think that because the brain's neurons operate in parallel, that parallelization of computations makes the overall process tractable. NP-Complete problems are strongly conjectured to not be parallelizable, and showing a problem is NP-Complete is very strong evidence that the problem is not parallelizable (discussed in appendix A). It is important to note that the problem may still be parallelizable on some of the possible inputs, and it might be that all sufficiently small instances may be parallelizable. NP-Completeness is an indication that the problem may be difficult, but it does not rule out efficient algorithms for the search problems the brain must actually compute (because the input is bounded). We are faced with two choices as a result: We can find those algorithms or we can ask if the brain is perhaps not solving the original problem as it was conceptualized. We approach these questions in the context of vision in the next section.

The Computational Complexity of Vision

What is the vision problem? How can we state it in its most general form? Several have tried in the past to provide such a statement. A standard dictionary might say that vision is the act or power of sensing with the eyes. A medical dictionary may be more detailed, saying that vision is the special sense by which the qualities of an object (as color, luminosity, shape, and size) constituting its appearance are perceived and which is mediated by the eye (*Merriam-Webster's Medical Dictionary*, 2002). Helmholtz claimed that vision is the result of some form of unconscious inference: a matter of making assumptions and conclusions from incomplete data, based on previous experiences (Helmholtz, 1896). For Marr, vision proceeds from a two-dimensional visual array (on the retina) to a three-dimensional description of the world as output (Marr, 1982). Noting that vision is not a stand-alone component of intelligent behavior, Aloimonos suggested that vision is the process of deriving purposive space-time descriptions (Aloimonos, 1992); that is, vision is for behavior in the real world. Distilling these, and other similar statements, into their most common basic element, we arrive at the following: Vision is the main sense that allows humans to navigate and manipulate their world, to behave purposefully in the world. And vision answers the question: What object, scene, or event that you know best matches a given set of location/measurement pairs? Extending this to a full understanding of a visual scene: Given a sequence of images, for each pixel determine whether it belongs to some particular object or other spatial construct, localize all objects in space, detect and localize all events in time, determine the identity of all the objects and events in the sequence, determine relationships among objects, and relate all objects and events to the available world and task knowledge.

This section will briefly summarize the steps of an argument that concludes that the generic vision problem as stated above is intractable. The important variables that play a role are the number of image locations P, the number of object/event prototypes in memory N, and the number of measurements made at each image location M. If a vision system needs to search through the set of all possible image locations (pixels) and all possible subsets of locations (there are 2^P of them) and compare them to each element of memory, then without any task guidance or knowledge of the characteristics of the subset it seeks, it cannot know which subset may be more likely than another. Thus, purely **feed-forward** (a single afferent progression of stimulus activation through the visual system—often also known as **data-directed** or **bottom-up**) unguided visual processing has an inherent exponential nature.

We begin by presenting a computational definition of the problem of **Visual Search**, first presented in Tsotsos (1989). The search involves a test image and a target image (as in the decision problem described earlier). The general version of Visual Search seeks to find the subset of a test image that matches some target image, using a specified definition of matching, and in its full generality includes the possibility of noisy or partial matches. The problem is viewed as a pure information-processing task, with no assumptions made about how the data may be presented or organized. The description presented is an abstract one and is not intended as an implementation-level characterization. Further, the problem may be of arbitrary size and may use arbitrary stimulus qualities. Other characterizations of visual search may be possible; however, it is suggested that all useful ones will include the notions of images, measurements over images, and constraints that must be satisfied.

A test image that contains an instance of the target is created by translating, rotating, and/or scaling the target and then placing it in the test image. The test image may also contain confounding information, such as other items, noise, and occluding objects. Other processes may distort or corrupt the images. Because of image discretization, there is a finite but large number of possible two-dimensional (2D) transforms: the target may be translated to anywhere in the test image; the target may be rotated about its center by any angular amount; and the target may be scaled in two directions by arbitrary amounts. As images are discretized, there is only a finite number of possibilities along each of these dimensions that would lead to distinct images. The question posed by Visual Search has two variants: an unbounded and a bounded version. In the unbounded—or task-free—case, the targets are either not known in advance or even if they are, they are not used, except to determine when the search terminates. Of course, it is assumed that even in free viewing without a task, some sort of interpretation process is taking place perhaps setting up target hypotheses in some manner that gives the viewer pleasure without also solving some visual problem. The bounded—or task-directed—case uses the target explicitly to assist in optimizing the solution to the problem. Both will be addressed by the following analysis. The solution to Visual Search involves solving a subproblem, which we call **Visual Match**. Given a 2D spatial transformation of the target, the Visual Match procedure determines if that target appears in the image. Therefore, an algorithm for Visual Search for a single target may be the following:

> For each possible object/event prototype
> > For each possible 2D spatial transformation of the prototype
> > > Apply transform to hypothesize location, orientation, and scale of
> > > > target in test image
> > > Execute the Visual Match procedure
> > > If Visual Match returns 'yes' exit and return 'yes'
> return 'no'

So, the input to the Visual Match procedure is two images (test and target after a transformation) and a method of measuring goodness of fit. In many psychophysical experiments, no scale or rotation is present, so in such cases the only parameter to hypothesize is location.

Similarly as for Visual Search, Visual Match can be further broken down into two variants. **Unbounded Visual Match** is intended to model recognition where no task guidance to optimize search is available or permitted. It corresponds to recognition with all top-down connections in the visual processing hierarchy removed or disabled. In other words, this is pure data-directed vision. More precisely, Unbounded Visual Match determines if there exists a subset of pixels in an image that matches a particular target. Recall that N represents the number of objects in memory. Unbounded Visual Match assumes $N = 1$, whereas Visual Search is for any positive integer N. The formal statement of the unbounded problem follows.

Given a test image (I, the image, is a set of P pixels), a target image G (whose size is not greater than P pixels), a difference function *diff* (an L_1 error measure), and a correlation function *corr* (a cross-correlation measure), is there a subset of pixels of the test image such that the value of *diff* between that subset and the corresponding subset of pixels in the target image is less than a given threshold and such that the value of *corr* between the two is at least as large as another specified threshold? The error and correlation measures are computed with respect to a target image; however, importantly, the target is not allowed to affect processing in any way. The two functions could be set up as table lookup; this way the target image does not explicitly enter the computation. In other words, is there a set $I' \subseteq I$ such that it simultaneously satisfies

$$\sum_{a \in I'} diff(a) \le \theta \text{ and } \sum_{a \in I'} corr(a) \ge \phi \, ?$$

The two separate criteria here require a solution to satisfy an error bound and also to be the maximal set (or rather, a large enough set) that satisfies that bound. In this way, trivial solutions are eliminated.

The second problem is **Bounded Visual Match**. This is recognition with knowledge of a target and task in advance, such that the knowledge is used to optimize the process. The bounded problem changes the definition slightly to reflect the addition of task knowledge, given in the form of an explicit target image G. The subsets a are constrained to be only those of the same size and extent as G. The basic theorems, proved in Tsotsos (1989, 1990a) (see appendix B), are the following:

Theorem 2.1   *Unbounded (Bottom-up) Visual Match (UVM) is NP-Complete, with time complexity an exponential function of P [the worst-case time complexity is $O(P^2 2^P)$; see appendix B].*

The notation $O(\cdot)$, known as Big-O notation, signifies the order of the time complexity function; that is, its dominating terms asymptotically.

Theorem 2.2   *Bounded (Task-directed) Visual Match (BVM) has linear time complexity [the worst-case time complexity is $O(\|G\| \|M_g\|)$; see appendix B].*

$\|A\|$ represents the cardinality of the set A. As Visual Match is a component of the Visual Search algorithm given earlier, then:

Theorem 2.3   *Unbounded Visual Search (UVS) is NP-Complete.*

The manner in which Visual Match is included in the Visual Search algorithm leads to the obvious conclusion that if Bounded Visual Match has linear time complexity, then:

Theorem 2.4   *Bounded Visual Search (BVS) has linear time complexity.*

The results have important implications. They first tell us that the pure data-directed approach to vision (and in fact to perception in any sensory modality—nothing about the proofs is specific to vision) is computationally intractable in the general case. They also tell us that bounded visual search takes time linearly dependent on the size of the input, something that has been observed in a huge number of experiments (for an overview, see Wolfe, 1998a). Even small amounts of task guidance can turn an exponential problem into one with linear time complexity.

Although this formalization of visual match can be immediately criticized because it lacks the realism of real vision—it does not capture any variability in appearance at all—it is clear that is it hard enough to show that pure data-directed processing is not a viable solution. Any further realism would only make it harder. However, perhaps biological vision systems are designed around average or best-case assumptions and not worst-case assumptions as are the bases of the above theorems (Lowe, 1990). Lowe suggested that perhaps expected case analysis more correctly reflects biological systems. Addressing such a question, however, is not straightforward. To proceed in a purely theoretical manner would require a formal definition of the expected image (i.e., a characterization of what our vision systems expect to see). Such a characterization does not exist and seems impossible to determine. As a result, an empirical strategy seems the only route. Even for this, one would need to consider some image domain for which one can determine an expected or average image result, and the domain must be known to have worst-case complexity that is also NP-Complete in order to compare with our previous results. Fortunately, such a domain does exist, and Parodi, Lanciwicki, Vijh, and Tsotsos (1996, 1998) addressed this issue in the context of line drawing interpretation.

It may appear at first glance that the brain is very efficient at reconstructing the three-dimensional (3D) structure of a scene from a single-image line drawing with no texture, color, or shading. Marr's view was exactly this. In fact, we all do this all the time, and even children have little difficulty with this. One might be led to conclude that there is an efficient (i.e., polynomial-time) algorithm that interprets line drawings, at least qualitatively labeling their segments as being one of a number of types: convex, concave, occluding boundary, and so on, following the classic work of Huffman (1971), Clowes (1971), and of Waltz (1975). Kirousis and Papadimitriou, however, proved that this is unlikely to be the case by showing that both the labeling problem and the realizability problem (does a given line drawing correspond with the 2D projection of an actual polyhedral scene?) are NP-Complete even for the simple case of trihedral, solid scenes (Kirousis & Papadimitriou, 1988). This was an unexpected result and stimulated research to find special cases for which the labeling problem was polynomially solvable. Further, Kirousis and Papadimitriou proved that the labeling problem has polynomial complexity for line drawings of Legoland scenes (i.e., scenes made of objects whose 3D edges can only have one of three possible orthogonal directions). This suggests that the brain may exploit geometrical regularities often found in natural scenes. Another possible explanation, which was offered by Kirousis and Papadimitriou themselves, is that the distribution of natural scenes might be such that the average-case complexity for the set of line drawings extracted from real scenes is polynomial, unlike the complexity for general line drawings.

Parodi et al. (1996, 1998) took on Lowe's challenge and analyzed the complexity of labeling line drawings empirically. The choice of domain takes advantage of the fact that worst-case results are known to be the same as for the Unbounded Visual Search problem; the problem is NP-Complete as described in the previous section. To tackle this issue, they needed to devise a method to generate random instances of polyhedral scenes. Such a method enabled them to generate random line drawings that are guaranteed to be the projection of an actual scene (see figure 2.2). They then tested several different search methods to label the constructed line drawings. The labeling problem in this case is not the problem of deciding whether a labeling exists, but that of finding a particular labeling. This problem resembles more closely that which the brain solves well, namely the extraction of 3D information from a drawing.

The experimental portion of the work proceeded as follows. Random scenes were generated, and the number of trihedral junctions they contained were counted. For numbers of junctions in increments of 5, bins of 100 scenes each were created. Each scene was labeled using standard algorithms and the number of labeling steps counted. The median number of steps for each bin was determined. The labeling algorithms tested were the following:

A. *Simple depth-first search with backtracking*   This achieves arc-consistency by the relaxation algorithm AC-1 (Mackworth & Freuder, 1985) and then performs a depth-first search on the constraint network. AC-1 performs relaxation in the following way. For each pair of adjacent junctions J1 and J2, remove all labelings of J1 for which there is no labeling in J2 that is compatible with it, and vice versa. Repeat the operation for all pairs of junctions until we have gone through all the pairs of junctions once without deleting a single labeling. Time for the search stage is computed as the number of times that the depth-first-search stack containing all nodes that have been visited (touched at least once) but not explored (i.e., such that

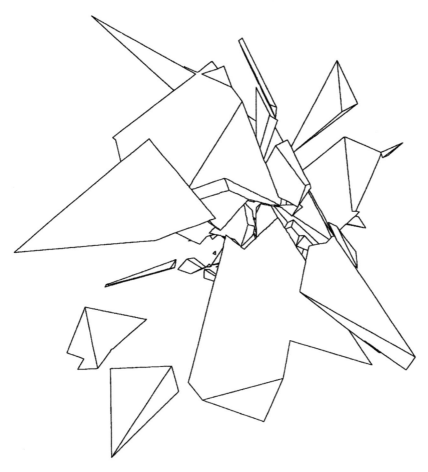

Figure 2.2
An example of a random trihedral scene (from Parodi et al., 1998, © 1998, with permission from Elsevier).

all the nodes adjacent to them have not been visited) is updated. In this experiment, 8 bins of 100 scenes each were used to compute the points shown in figure 2.3.

B. *Best-first search with backtracking*   In the depth-first search method with simple backtrack, junctions are chosen blindly as deeper layers of the depth-first search tree are explored. A more refined search method is the so-called *best-first search*, which exploits the fact that it is more efficient to label the junctions that have the smallest possible set of permissible labelings and try them first. Furthermore, the search is guided by the *a priori* knowledge about the structure of the problem, and labelings that are more likely for certain junctions are tried first. Specifically, this is *a priori* knowledge of the relative frequency of different types of junctions. T-junctions have

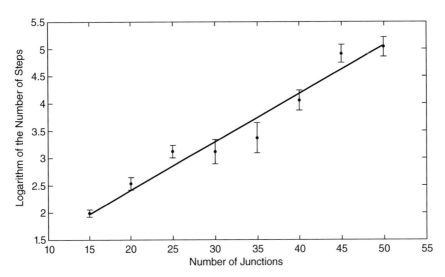

Figure 2.3
The base-10 logarithm of the median-case complexity of labeling line drawings of random trihedral scenes as a function of the number of junctions. The error bars give error on the median estimated by the bootstrap procedure. Labeling is performed by simple depth-first search (from Parodi et al., 1998, © 1998, with permission from Elsevier).

six possible labelings. Four of them are common to the basic and the extended trihedral world; the other two only appear in the extended trihedral world, and they appear more seldom. Therefore, it is convenient to try first the common labelings and only successively the remaining two labelings. For E-junctions, first try the labeling with the middle-segment labeled as a convex segment and the remaining segments labeled as arrows. These were empirically determined. In this experiment, 24 bins of 100 scenes each were used to compute the points in figure 2.4.

The experiments revealed that the computational complexity of labeling line drawings is, in the median case, exponential in its complexity for the blind, simple depth-first labeling method (figure 2.3). On the other hand, it is linear in the number of junctions when using an informed search method, where the information allows knowledge of the task domain to guide processing (figure 2.4b). The informed search was tested on a much larger set of scenes. Interestingly, there is increasing variability in computational time needed as the number of junctions increases (figure 2.4a). This is probably due to the highly constrained nature of the labeling problem for trihedral scenes. Although it is possible to construct line drawings containing components that are difficult to label, randomization in the construction of scenes makes these components unlikely to appear.

This empirical evidence suggests that, in response to the question raised earlier, both worst-case and median-case analysis lead to the same conclusion: The applica-

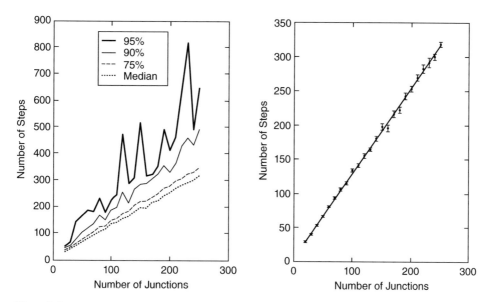

Figure 2.4
(a) The curves show the best-first search results, from top to bottom giving the 95% (median), 90%, 75%, and 50% percentiles of the distribution of the computational time. (b) Time (median number of steps) versus the number of junctions for the best-first search (from Parodi et al., 1998, © 1998, with permission from Elsevier). Both plots use linear scales.

tion of task knowledge guides the processing and converts an exponential complexity problem into a linear one. The shaping or modulation of processing using task-specific knowledge is a major attentive mechanism.

Extending to Active Vision

In 1985, Bajcsy presented a view of perception to the computer vision community that she termed **active perception** (Bajcsy, 1985) following in the footsteps of Brentano (1874), Petermann (1929), and Barrow and Popplestone (1971). She proposed that a passive sensor be used in an active fashion, purposefully changing the sensor's state parameters according to sensing strategies. Basically, it is a problem of intelligent control applied to the data acquisition process that depends on the current state of data interpretation including recognition. It is interesting to note that this use of the term *active* in vision appeared in the dissertation of Freuder in 1976. He used what he called **active knowledge** to assist in determining where to look next in an image based on the current state of interpretation (Freuder, 1976). He did not include considerations of camera movements, but the general idea is the same.

Here, a broad view of active vision is taken, and the term is not restricted to strategies that move cameras only. Active vision includes sampling a scene over time, which in the trivial case with fixed cameras is simply processing image sequences. Any hypothesize-and-test strategy is included as well if the choice of next image sample is determined by the state of the hypothesis space. A critical feature of active approaches is that time is required, that is, a sequence of perceptual signals over time, where the active strategy controls what signals are to be acquired and how they are to be processed.

The visual search problem from the previous section—qualified further as the passive version of the problem—can now be extended to cover time-varying input, leading to the **Active Unbounded Visual Match** and **Active Bounded Visual Match** problems defined now. Given a test image sequence in time I_t, is there a sequence of sets $\mathcal{I}_t$ for t = 1 to τ, where $\mathcal{I}_t$ is the union of all sets $I'_t \subseteq I_t$, such that each I'_t satisfies

$$\sum_{a \in I'_t} diff(a) \le \theta_t \ \text{ and } \ \sum_{a \in I'_t} corr(a) \ge \phi_t$$

and $\theta_1 \ge \theta_2 \ge \theta_3 \cdots \ge \theta_\tau$ and $\phi_1 \le \phi_2 \le \phi_3 \cdots \le \phi_\tau$?

The thresholds, θ_1 and ϕ_1 are both positive integers set as for the UVM problem. The sequence of thresholds may be trivially set to $\theta_{t+1} = \theta_t - 1$ and $\phi_{t+1} = \phi_t + 1$ or may be determined from task requirements. The thresholds act as hypothesis pruning filters tuned more and more tightly as time progresses. The idea is that as more and more data over time is acquired, the match to a target improves steadily. Therefore, this strategy and formalism works equally well for the general case of hypothesize-and-test with or without sensor motions and for static or time-varying images. The distinction between unbounded and bounded versions is the same as presented earlier for Visual Match as is the embedding of the problem within a Visual Search algorithm. As result, the main theorem can be stated.

Theorem 2.5 *Active Unbounded Visual Search is NP-Complete.*

Proof The active problem consists of a sequence of UVS problems. Earlier, it was shown that the UVS problem is NP-Complete. Thus, the active version is also NP-Complete.

The complexity of the unbounded version of this problem is still exponential, because it has the passive problem described earlier as a subproblem. Its worst-case time complexity would be $O\left(\sum_{t=1}^{\tau} \|I_t\|^2 2^{\|I_t\|} \right)$ because all viable hypotheses must be carried over from one image to the next, and only if all image subsets are considered will all viable hypotheses be found.   ∎

Theorem 2.6 *Active Bounded Visual Search has linear time complexity.*

Proof The active bounded problem is a sequence of BVS problems, and therefore it, too, has behavior linear in the number of pixels of the image.   ∎

This formulation is guaranteed to work correctly, if a solution exists, because the solution subset(s) are not discarded during the iterations. The thresholds are set up in such a way so that the correct solutions that would satisfy thresholds defined for the passive case will satisfy the thresholds for each iteration up to the last in the active case. In essence, this formulation describes a hypothesize-and-test search framework, where at each time interval a number of hypotheses are discarded. This formulation enables partial solutions to be inspected midstream through an image sequence for the active strategy. Conditions to determine if an active or a passive approach is more efficient are analyzed in Tsotsos (1992a), where the above theorems and proofs first appeared.

Why is this active vision idea related to attention? The obvious answer is that active vision implies, by definition, camera fixation changes. Eye movements are perhaps the most obvious external manifestations of attentive changes. But it goes beyond the obvious. Metzger (1974) summarizes aspects of action, first described by Brentano, that contribute to perception: bringing stimuli to receptors, enlarging the accessible area, foveation, optimization of the state of receptors, slowing down of fading and local adaptation, exploratory movement, and finally the search for principles of organization within visual stimuli. All of these actions may be considered ways that attention exerts control on the visual processing machinery of what information the system considers. In Bajcsy's terms, these are all also aspects of controlling the sensing apparatus of a system based on the state of interpretation.

Metzger's list can be expanded. **Active vision** is necessary for behavior that:

- moves the fixation point or depth plane or to track motion;
- seeks to see a portion of the visual field otherwise hidden due to occlusion;
- manipulates objects in the scene to achieve better viewpoints;
- seeks to change its viewpoint;
- seeks to see a larger portion of the surrounding visual world;
- explores a scene to understand the scene;
- compensates for any spatial nonuniformity of processing;
- foveates;
- moves to increase spatial resolution or to focus;
- moves viewpoint to disambiguate or to eliminate degenerate views;

- induces motion (kinetic depth);
- completes a task requiring multiple fixations.

Attention and active vision are intimately connected, but as shown by Tsotsos (1992a), attention is an even broader concept than active vision.

Extending to Cognition and Action

Much of human cognition is action based, and actions need sensory input for their guidance. Simple stimulus-action human behavior may be conceptualized as:

1. Localize and recognize a stimulus (with or without a prespecified target).
2. Link the stimulus to applicable actions.
3. Decide among all possible actions.
4. Generate actuator commands.

The first step is exactly the visual match problem; as a result, the complexity of the overall problem is at least as great as that of visual match. The second step can be solved by table lookup, the table size being the number of possible stimuli times the number of possible behaviors and where the table entries code strength of applicability, perhaps dependent on stimulus characteristics (thus, each stimulus may be associated with more than one behavior). The third step can be done by choosing the largest applicability strength from among all the entries, and the fourth would involve a function call or table lookup again.

The problems are formalized in Tsotsos (1995a) with proofs for:

Theorem 2.7   *Unbounded Stimulus-Behavior Search is NP-hard.*

Theorem 2.8   *Bounded Stimulus-Behavior Search has linear time complexity.*

If sensory perception is an integral component of intelligence, sensory search problems are integral subproblems of intelligent behavior. The kind of visual search described above seems ubiquitous within intelligent behavior.

Extending to Sensor Planning

The extension described earlier to active vision deals only with the interpretation problem and not with any issue regarding the determination of what part of the scene to view or from where. How a system chooses the viewpoint and scene to inspect is called the **Sensor-Planning Problem**. Extensions to the Sensor-Planning Problem for visual search mirror the above results (Ye & Tsotsos, 1996). How an agent, human or otherwise, might search a given 3D space for a given object is called the **Object Search Problem** and is an example of sensor planning for recognition. Object Search is defined as the selection of a sequence of actions that will maximize the probability that a mobile agent with active sensing capabilities will find a given object in a partially unknown 3D environment with a given set of resources. Let F be the ordered set of actions applied in the search, Ω be a 3D region (union of space elements), O_Ω represent all possible actions that can be applied to Ω, $T(F)$ be the total time required to apply F, $P[F]$ be the probability of finding the target with F, and K be a constant representing the maximum acceptable time for the search. Then formally, the problem is to find $F \subset O_\Omega$ that satisfies $T(F) \leq K$ and maximizes $P[F]$. The proof for the following theorem appears in Ye and Tsotsos (1996, 2001):

Theorem 2.9   *Object Search is NP-hard.*

Visual Match is one of the actions possible in the set O_Ω. It must be executed each time an image is inspected for the object that is being sought. It is not the source of the NP-hardness, however; the determination of the subset F is sufficient. When combined, the complexity for the problem of object search becomes even worse. Nevertheless, knowledge of why, how, and where the difficulties of these problems arise has led to very successful algorithms and real implementations of robotic visual object search tasks (Dickinson, Christensen, Tsotsos, & Olofsson, 1997; Shubina & Tsotsos, 2010; Wilkes & Tsotsos, 1992; Ye & Tsotsos, 1999).

As the Visual Match problem, in both unbounded and bounded forms, seems to play an important role in all of the vision problems just described, it seems reasonable to believe that it is central to all perceptual tasks. Macmillan and Creelman (2005) provide extensive definitions of general perceptual tasks, and they point out that all psychophysical judgments are of one stimulus relative to another—the basic process is comparison. The most basic task is discrimination, the ability to tell two stimuli apart. This is exactly what Visual Match formalizes, and thus its centrality in perception is justified. As a result, we may suggest that any visual processing task (and extending to any perception task) has at least this same complexity characterization.

Complexity Constrains Visual Processing Architecture

The major conclusion of the previous sections is this: The computational complexity of the vision problem as defined earlier in this chapter has an exponential character if not directed by task requirements. This result is independent of algorithm or implementation. Because the time complexity function includes the number of image elements P as part of the exponent—one might use retinal photoreceptors, so $P \approx 125,000,000$, or one might use the number of axons from each eye, so $P \approx 1,000,000$—its value is enormous when compared with the time human vision requires for a visual response. Even if parallelized, the number of neurons—or synapses if they perform sufficient computation—required would be impossibly large (for more on this, see Tsotsos, 1990a). Natural vision is not always task directed, so somehow this exponential character is overcome. One quickly then concludes that there is a huge mismatch between the definition of the general vision problem, its computational complexity, and the realization of vision in humans (and indeed any animal with sight).

How does one deal with an intractable problem in practice? A direct understanding of the size of the problems of interest and the size of the processing machinery helps to determine appropriate approximations. Garey and Johnson (1979) provide a number of guidelines:

1. Develop an algorithm that is fast enough for small problems but that would take too long with larger problems (good if anticipated problems are small).

2. Develop a fast algorithm that solves a special case of the problem but does not solve the general problem (assumes special cases have practical importance).

3. Develop algorithms that quickly solve a large proportion of the cases that come up in practice but in the worst case may run for a long time.

4. For an optimization problem, develop an algorithm that always runs quickly but produces an answer that is not necessarily optimal.

5. Use natural parameters to guide the search for approximate algorithms. There are a number of ways a problem can be exponential. Consider the natural parameters of a problem rather than a constructed problem length and attempt to reduce the exponential effect of the largest-valued parameters.

The relevant guidelines for the analysis presented here are items (4) and (5): develop an algorithm that always runs quickly but produces an answer that is not necessarily optimal, and guide the development of the approximations used by that algorithm using the problem's natural parameters. The key is to use them with the goal of finding approximations that are biologically justified. The full analysis was presented in Tsotsos (1987, 1988a, 1990a, 1990b, 1991a) and is expanded here. In Tsotsos (1991a), a detailed discussion of the various previously presented approximation algorithms appears with arguments as to why they may not be biologically relevant.

The natural parameters of the computation for unbounded visual match are N (the number of object/event prototypes in one's knowledge base), P (the number of input locations or pixels), and M (the number of measurements or features computed at each pixel). Recall the worst-case time complexity of UVM is $O(P^2 2^P)$; extending this to the visual search problem and adding in the fact that not only is the correct image subset unknown a priori but so is the feature subset, the worst-case complexity is $O(NP^2 2^{PM})$ assuming the size of each model is the same, a constant, and thus ignorable. Consider now how the values of these three parameters affect the overall result and how they may be modified to improve time complexity.

1. Hierarchical organization takes search of the model space from $O(N)$ to $O(\log_2 N)$. Rather than a linear, blind search through the number of models, a hierarchical organization reduces this to a logarithmic search as long as the criteria for deciding choice points are known. For example, in a game of "20 Questions," one may navigate a hierarchy containing $2^{20} = 1,048,576$ items. Biederman (1987) has used his Recognition by Components (RBC) strategy to derive the possible number of categories that humans recognize, and he arrived at the figure of 30,000 categories. The Visual Dictionary (Corbeil, 1986) contains more than 3000 images portraying more than 25,000 generic objects in all (cars, stadiums, forks, etc.). These images do not include variations in object context that could lead to very different behaviors (picking up a fork at the dinner table while seated is very different from picking up the fork your child dropped behind the living room couch); variations due to object type or brand (the act of sitting on a chair is virtually identical to the act of sitting on a sofa even though the images are very different); variations due to color (the human eye is sensitive to about 500 different hues, 20 steps of saturation for each and 500 levels of brightness for each hue-saturation pair); variations due to lighting (the eye is sensitive to luminance spans of 10,000,000,000 to 1); or time-varying events. Seeing an object from one viewpoint may cause a shift to another viewpoint to recognize it fully. Depending on the resolution of the sensing system and on the method of perceptual processing, up to 30% of the viewing sphere around a single object may contain degenerate viewpoints that require sensor motion for disambiguation (Dickinson, Wilkes & Tsotsos, 1999). The point is that the depth of a category hierarchy—using Biederman's figure of 30,000 would lead to $\log_2 30,000$, or about 15 levels of a binary decision tree—is not large, but the variability in appearance of any of the instances of a category is quite large.

2. A pyramid representation of the image is a layered representation, each layer with decreasing spatial resolution and with bidirectional connections between locations in adjacent layers (for a review, see Jolion & Rosenfeld, 1994). Introduced by Uhr (1972), they permit an image to be abstracted so that a smaller number of locations at the top level, in a data-directed strategy, may be the only ones over which some algorithm needs to search. At least, they may provide the starting point for a coarse-to-fine search strategy from top to bottom of the pyramid. Such a representation would reduce the size of the variable P. Figure 2.5 shows a hypothetical pyramid of four layers. The number of locations represented in the lowest layer (layer 1) is p_1; $p_1 > p_2 > p_3 > p_4$. In most pyramid definitions, the value at

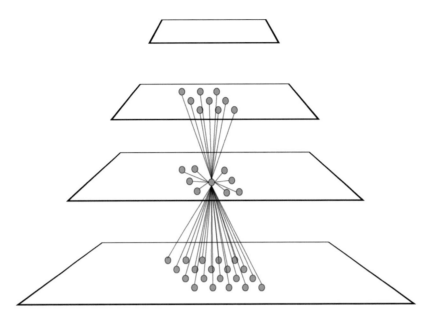

Figure 2.5
A hypothetical pyramid representation.

each location in each layer is determined by a computation based on a subset of the other layer values. Each element is not only connected to others in the adjacent layers but may also be connected to elements within the same layer. Again, this pattern of connectivity requires a definition when creating a particular pyramid representation.

Hubel and Wiesel (1962, 1965) are responsible for the original concept of hierarchical processing in the visual cortex. They sought to explain the progressive increase in the complexity of receptive field properties in the cat visual cortex and suggested that a serial, feed-forward scheme could account for the processing of simple cells from lateral geniculate nucleus (LGN) inputs. Complex cells could similarly be formed from simple cells, and neurons further along, such as hypercomplex cells and beyond, exhibit processing that can be accounted for by considering only their immediate input from the previous layer. In essence, this exactly corresponds with the simplest kind of pyramid architecture. Since then, however, the complexity of processing has been seen to be not so straightforward.

3. The objects and events of the visual world are mostly spatially and temporally confined to some region; however, we can also recognize scattered items as well (such as star constellations, or collections of animals as flocks or herds, or group motion say as in a rugby play, etc.). Spatiotemporally localized receptive fields

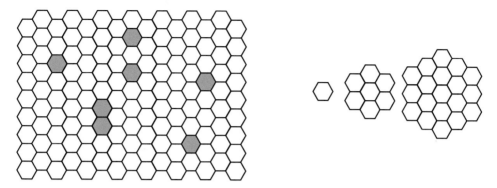

Figure 2.6
Arbitrary RFs (left) compared with spatially localized RFs (right).

reduce the number of possible receptive fields from 2^P to $O(P^{1.5})$ (this assumes contiguous receptive fields of all possible sizes centered at all locations in the image array and is derived in Tsotsos, 1987). The leftmost diagram in figure 2.6 shows a hexagonal tiling of an image. The set of solid hexagons represents an arbitrary receptive field such as the most general case should handle. If receptive fields are spatially localized, then the number of them is dramatically smaller. More importantly, the possible combinations of locations is also smaller, and the generality of the receptive field definition is restricted as the diagrams on the right-hand side of the figure show.

After applying these three constraints, $O(P^{3.5}\, 2^M \log_2 N)$ is the worst-case time complexity. The next three strategies reduce the variables further to bring the expression down to perhaps its lowest value. These last three are all manifestations of attentive processing.

4. Selection of a single or group of receptive fields to consider can further reduce the $P^{1.5}$ term of point 3 above to $P' < P^{1.5}$. This may be not only a selection of location but also a selection of a local region or size. As such, it also impacts the P^2 portion of that term since a smaller set of pixels $q, 1 \leq q < P$, is involved in the search (similarly to Bounded Visual Match).

5. Feature selectivity can further reduce the M term to $M' < M$; that is, the subset M' of all possible features actually present in the image or important for the task at hand. If indexing into a representation of image features organized by location only—as has been assumed to this point—all features at the indexed location are necessarily indexed whether or not they are necessary for a given computation. A reorganization of features into separate representations, one for each feature, permits a processing mechanism to involve only the required features into a computation and leave the irrelevant ones outside the computation.

6. Selection of model space can further reduce the N term to $N' < N$, reflecting task-specific information. Not all of the objects or events in the model base may be relevant for a given image or task.

These additional three attentive manipulations bring the time complexity down to $O(P'M'N')$, that is, the product of the number of receptive fields, features, and models to be considered. The details in terms of numbers of pixels (linear terms) have been left out for simplicity here. But how do these actions affect the generic problem described above? Hierarchical organization does not affect the nature of the vision problem. However, the other mechanisms have the following effects:

• Pyramidal abstraction affects the problem through the loss of location information and signal combination (further detailed later).

• Spatiotemporally localized receptive fields force the system to look at features across a receptive field instead of finer-grain combinations, and thus arbitrary combinations of locations must be handled by some other strategy.

• Attentional selection further limits what is processed in the location, feature, and object domains. The knowledge that task-related attentive processes use to accomplish the selection can be as generic as statistical regularities.

As a result of these, the generic problem as defined earlier has been altered. Unfortunately, it is not easy to characterize formally this altered problem. But it is clear that certain aspects of the problem are lost with these approximations, and this may be the source of many of the obvious failings on the visual system, such as illusions, or incorrect judgments.

The Problems with Pyramids

That pyramid representations offer distinct advantages for reducing search times has been clear since they were introduced by Uhr in 1972. But does this representation have relevance for the visual cortex? There, too, it is clear that the same representational strategy is used. As proposed in a classic paper (Felleman & Van Essen, 1991), the visual areas of the macaque monkey cortex can be placed into levels. Twenty-five areas that are predominately or exclusively visual in function are identified, and an additional seven areas are considered as visual-association areas on the basis of their extensive visual inputs. Regarding their interconnectivity, a total of 305 connections were reported; of these there are 121 reciprocal pairs (the remainder seem to not have been tested). The average number of pathways per visual area is 19 with the highest number being 39. Most pathways are over one or two layers but some cross up to seven levels. There are also extensive connections with cortical areas outside the visual system. Based on the laminar patterns of connections between areas, Felleman and Van Essen proposed a hierarchy of visual areas including 10 levels of cortical processing. If the retina and lateral geniculate nucleus are included at the bottom and the entorhinal cortex and hippocampus at the top, there are 14 levels. Within this hierarchy, there are multiple, intertwined processing streams. The size of receptive fields of neurons in each level increases from lower to higher levels. Connectivity between levels is also defined in the same manner as in a pyramid. More on this will be presented in a subsequent chapter. For now, this suffices to show that the pyramid representation is exactly the right building block for both computational and biological vision systems.

Although pyramids may provide a nice solution to part of the complexity problem, the remaining problems are now joined by a set of new ones due directly to the nature of pyramidal representations and how information might flow within them (see also Nakayama, 1990). There are top-down, bottom-up, and lateral flow problems to deal with. The bottom-up ones are termed the Blurring, Cross-talk, Context, Boundary, Sampling, and Routing Problems. The Sampling Problem was first mentioned in Tsotsos (1987), where the mismatch between the need for high-resolution recognition was contrasted with the low-resolution nature of pyramid processes. The Context and Boundary Problems were first described in Culhane (1992), the first implementation of Selective Tuning. They and the Blurring and Cross-talk Problems were subsequently detailed in Tsotsos et al. (1995). The bottom-up ones are presented next, beginning with the Boundary Problem, and the top-down and lateral problems will follow.

Boundary Problem

Suppose we consider a simple hierarchical, layered representation where each layer represents the same number of locations of the full visual field; this is not a pyramid by definition. Let's say that at each position of this uniform hierarchy a neuron exists selective for some feature; this hierarchy may represent some abstraction of features layer to layer. Due to the nature of convolutions—the basic mathematical counterpart of the implementation of neural tuning that takes one function, the image, and another, the kernel that models the tuning properties of a neuron to create the response of those tuning properties across the image—at each layer a kernel half-width at the edge of the visual field is left unprocessed because the kernel does not have full data for its convolution (see figure 2.7). This is compounded layer by layer because the half-widths are additive layer to layer. The result is that a sizeable annulus at the top layer is left undefined, and thus the number of locations that represent true results of neural selectivity from the preceding layer is smaller. In essence, this forces a pyramidal representation. Tsotsos et al. (1995) and van der Wal and Burt (1992) point out that this is an inherent

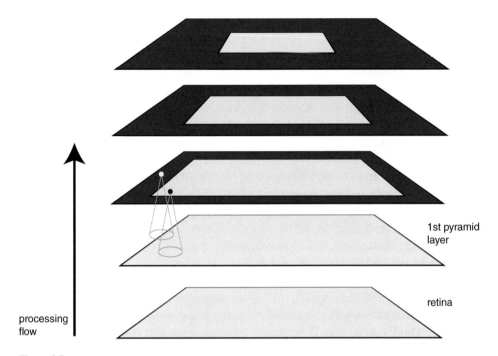

Figure 2.7
The Boundary Problem. The two units depicted in the second layer from the bottom illustrate how the extent of the black unit's receptive field is entirely within the input layer whereas only half of the receptive field of the gray unit is within the input layer.

issue with all such hierarchical, layered representations, and figure 2.7 depicts this. In the figure, the black regions are those where the additive, nonveridical convolution results are present. There is only a small central area in the top layer whose processing is unaffected. The extent is determined by the sum of kernel half-widths of the processes in each layer.

As if this were not enough of a problem, given that we wish to consider the impact of this mathematical abstraction on real neural processing, we must consider the actual distribution of receptors in the retina. Østerberg (1935) provided the classically accepted picture of human rod and cone distribution as a function of eccentricity. More recently, Curcio, Sloan, Kalina, and Hendrickson (1990) provided the 2D view, and this discussion follows their data. The human retina contains cones that are sensitive to color and rods that are sensitive to luminance. There are on average 4.6 million cones (4.08 million to 5.29 million).

Peak foveal cone density averages 199,000 cones/mm^2 and is highly variable between individuals (100,000–324,000 cones/mm^2). The point of highest density may be found in an area as large as 0.032 deg^2. Cone density falls steeply from this point with increasing eccentricity and is an order of magnitude lower 1 mm away from the foveal center, decreasing until about 10° eccentricity where it plateaus to about 3000–5000 cones/mm^2. The isodensity contours of the distribution of human cones form rough concentric circles across the retina centered at the fovea. The human retina contains on average 92 million rods (77.9 million to 107.3 million). In the fovea, the average horizontal diameter of the rod-free zone is 0.350 mm (1.25°). Rod density is zero at the fovea and peaks at about 20° eccentricity and then slowly decays through the periphery to a value of about 40,000/mm^2. What is the implication of such a distribution on our representation? This means that if the peripheral representation is eroded by the nature of layered neural convolutions, but the central representation is not, the overall result at the top layer of the representation will mostly represent the central portion of the visual field and thus mostly represent the input from retinal cones.

The average human retina contains 1,070,000 ganglion cells with approximately 50% of cells within 16° of visual angle from the foveal center (see Curcio & Allen, 1990). There are at least two ganglion cells per cone in the central region up to about 3.5° eccentricity, and this decreases further out toward the periphery. Curcio and Allen show that their findings are consistent with the notion that the cortical magnification (Daniel & Whitteridge, 1961) observed in area V1 seems proportional to the functional gradient of human ganglion cell density throughout the visual field. Daniel and Whitteridge, looking at macaque monkey and at baboon, measured the millimeters of cortex concerned with each degree of visual field and called this the magnification factor. The exact mathematical fit of the data is not important here. The overall result, that the central regions of the visual field have a far greater representation than the peripheral region, is what matters. Near the fovea, there is about 6.5 mm^2 of cortex devoted to each degree of visual angle, and this drops rapidly to 1 mm^2/deg by 10° of eccentricity and continues to decline at greater eccentricities.

Human visual area V1 has an area of 1500–3700 mm^2 (Stensaas, Eddington, & Dobelle, 1974). Following Wandell and Silverstein (1995), half of area V1 represents the central 10° (2% of the visual field) with the width of a human ocular dominance column 0.5–1.0 mm. There is much variability in all of these characteristics among individuals as well as in terms of topography, cell types, and more. These differences are ignored for our purposes.

These general points impact our pyramid representation. The overall Boundary Problem is depicted in figure 2.8. This illustrates that a pyramid representation not only helps with computational complexity, but it is forced to play this role by the nature of hierarchical convolution processing. This resulting structure has similar qualitative properties to what is found in subsequent layers of the visual cortex. Moving to higher levels of visual processing, Gross, Bruce, Desimone, Fleming, and

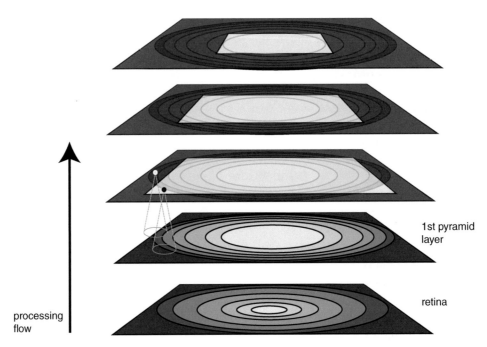

1st pyramid
layer

retina

processing
flow

Figure 2.8
The Boundary Problem. The bottom layer represents the retina and the concentric circles characterize
the isodensity contours of cone distribution. The next layer of the pyramid (say area V1) represents the
spatial dimension of the viewing field in a manner that gives more cortical area to central regions than
peripheral. Then, the boundary problem forces more and more of the periphery to be unrepresented in
higher layers of the pyramid.

Gattass (1981) were the first to detail properties of inferotemporal (IT) neurons in
the macaque monkey and showed that the median receptive field size was about
23° diameter and that the center of gaze or fovea fell within or on the border of the
receptive field of each neuron they examined. Geometric centers of these receptive
fields were within 12° of the center of gaze implying that the coverage of the visual
field is about 24° at best from center of gaze. Gattass, Sousa, and Gross (1988) look
at areas V3 and V4 of macaque. Following the Felleman and van Essen hierarchy,
V3 feeds V4, and V4 feeds IT. V3 contains a systematic representation of the central
35° to 40° of the visual field; V4 contains a coarse, but systematic, representation of
approximately the central 35° to 40° of the visual field. In both V3 and V4, the
representation of the central visual field is magnified with respect to dedicated
neural machinery relative to that of the periphery. In both areas, the size of receptive fields increases with increasing eccentricity; however, at a given eccentricity, the
receptive fields of V4 are larger than those of V3. V3 receptive field sizes range from
a few degrees of visual angle at the center of gaze to about 6° at an eccentricity of

about 25°; for V4, the range is from a few degrees at center of gaze to about 9° at 25° eccentricity. V4 has a very poor representation greater than 15° or 20° eccentricity, with the majority of representation less than 10°.

All of this supports the general structure derived thus far. In a very real sense, this representation is a physical bottleneck at least with respect to its clear physical bias for central versus peripheral input. Now that the pyramid structure is established computationally and neurobiologically, we can continue to see what other issues arise from pyramid representations.

Sampling Problem

If sampling is linked to spatial resolution, then we may say that the pyramid represents the visual field at a coarse spatial scale at the top and at a fine spatial scale at the bottom. If the higher levels of processing are associated with more abstract computations, then those computations are represented at a coarse spatial resolution. A key paradox is posed as a result: The top layer is composed of units with very large receptive fields, which therefore represent space coarsely and do not provide for the detail seemingly required for high-resolution vision [see Moran and Desimone (1985) and Nakayama (1990) for the biological and Tsotsos (1987, 1990a) for the computational arguments]. The Sampling Problem, then, is to achieve an overall high-resolution percept even though the neurons that perhaps may be the last in the recognition path have the least detailed spatial representations.

Blurring Problem

A single event at the input will affect a subpyramid of units. Signals from it connect to a diverging pattern of neurons. Thus, although a single event may be well localized at the input layer, location specificity is lost because a spatially large portion of the output layer is affected by it. Neural connectivity works against localization, and the Blurring Problem and the loss of location information is the result (figure 2.9).

Cross-talk Problem

Two separate visual events in the visual field will activate two subpyramids (diverging neural connectivity patterns) that overlap. The region of overlap will contain units whose activity is a function of both events. Thus, each event interferes with the interpretation of other events in the visual field. The Blurring and Cross-talk Problems negatively impact one another, creating greater interference than each alone. In figure 2.10, two input elements will each activate a feed-forward diverging pattern of locations, and depending on their spacing, those patterns may overlap, often significantly. Any neurons in the overlap areas will thus 'see' both elements in their receptive fields, and one will interfere with the interpretation of the other. Of course,

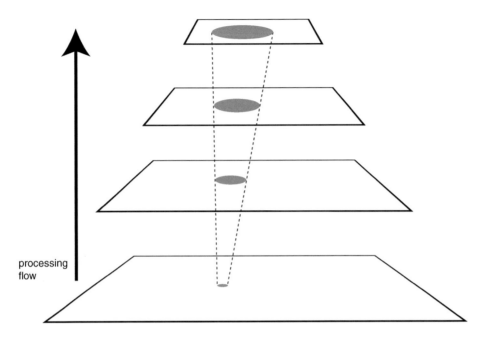

Figure 2.9
The Blurring Problem. An input element in the lowest layer will affect, via its feed-forward connections, a diverging pattern of locations in the later layers of the pyramid.

the larger the number of input elements, the greater and more widespread the interference.

Context Problem

A single unit at the top of the pyramid receives input from a large subpyramid and thus from a large portion of the visual field (i.e., its receptive field; RF). Unless an object is alone in the visual field, the response of neurons whose receptive fields contain the object will necessarily be affected not only by the object but also by any other image event in that receptive field. These other image events may be termed the context in which the object is found. Thus, the response of those neurons is confounded by the object's context. In figure 2.11, any neuron in a higher layer of the pyramid will necessarily have a receptive field that is large in the input layer due to the connectivity pattern within the network. In real scenes, most stimuli will never appear without surrounding stimuli nearby.

It is important to distinguish this use of the term *context* with that of Oliva, Torralba, Casthelano, and Henderson (2003) or Torralba (2003). There, they consider the relationships among objects in a scene, such as relative position in the scene, spatial relationships between objects, general scene statistics, and so on. These

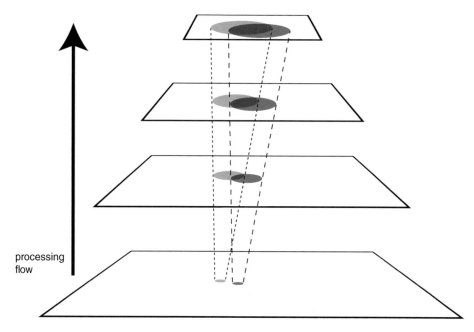

processing
flow

Figure 2.10
The Cross-talk Problem. Two input stimuli activate feed-forward projections that overlap, with the regions of overlap containing neurons that are affected by both. Those might exhibit unexpected responses with respect to their tuning profiles.

are important to be sure, and such prior knowledge has shown its utility in computer vision systems since the early 1970s. What Culhane (1992) and Tsotsos et al. (1995) described and what is presented here is a different, more local, version of context. Here, the context is the relationship between figure and background within a single neuron's receptive field. The global version of context, perhaps more related to domain knowledge, plays an attentional role in setting up top-down guidance (see the section "Peripheral Priority Map Computation" in chapter 5 for more on this).

Routing Problem

Let there be L layers in the pyramid representation, $L > 1$, and R_i neurons in layer i. Layer 1 is the input layer, and $R_n < R_k$ for $1 \leq n < k \leq L$. Assume that the feed-forward and feedback connectivity is C and for all i, $R_i > C$. There are therefore $R_1 C^{L-1}$ possible single-node feed-forward paths and $R_L C^{L-1}$ possible single-node feedback paths. These exponential expressions illustrate the magnitude of the routing problem. If we use $L = 14$ following Felleman and Van Essen (1991) and $C = 1000$, a common average neural connectivity, $C^{L-1} = 10^{39}$! It is clear that straightforward solutions are not possible. This problem is not so much one of determining

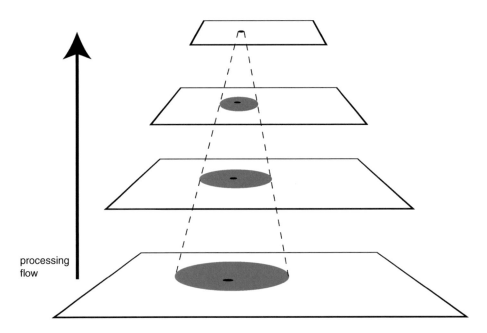

processing
flow

Figure 2.11
The Context Problem. A stimulus (black dot) within the receptive field of the higher layer neuron—its
spatial context.

which path a particular signal takes; hard-wired connectivity takes care of this. The
problem arises for whatever decision process must operate using this representation.
Which neurons and which pathways represent the best interpretation of the stimulus? Figure 2.12 illustrates the extent of spatial constraints that may be used by a
decision process in its search through the pyramid for the best interpretation (the
case for any feature dimension is similar). If the search is bottom-up—from stimulus
to highest-layer neuron—then the search is constrained to the feed-forward cone
outlined by the dotted lines. If the decisions are based on locally maximal neural
responses, then there is nothing to prevent a bottom-up search losing its way and
missing the globally maximum response at the top layer. It is clear that to be successful, the correct path must always go through the overlap regions shown in dark
ovals. But nothing guarantees that the local maximum must lie within those overlap
regions. If the search is top-down—from the globally maximum responding neuron
to the stimulus—the search is constrained by the dashed lines. Only top-down search
is guaranteed to correctly connect the best responding neuron at the top with its
stimulus.

There is one exception to this. Suppose that the size of all receptive fields was
fixed—all of one size—and that they do not overlap. A purely feed-forward scheme
would be able to find the value of the largest input with local computations for each

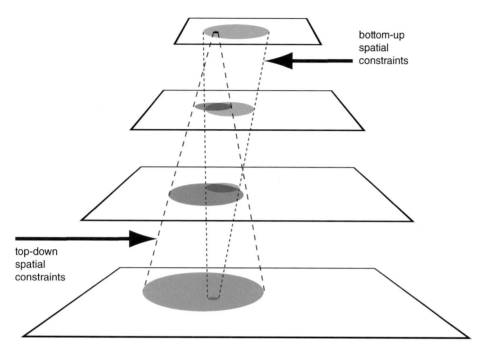

Figure 2.12
The Routing Problem. Interacting top-down and bottom-up spatial search constraints are shown with the areas of overlap representing the viable search regions for best neural pathway.

receptive field. However, location and spatial extent cannot be recovered. This might be useful for certain computer vision detection tasks only, but it cannot be considered as a reasonable proposal for biological vision.

As information flow is not only feed-forward, top-down flow must also be considered, and as mentioned, pyramid representations present a number of problems there, too. The problems, termed the Multiple Foci, Convergent Recurrence, Spatial Interpolation, and Spatial Spread Problems, are now described.

Multiple Foci Problem

Can the visual system attend to more than one item at a time? Experimentalists call this **divided attention** (Braun, 1998b; Sperling & Dosher, 1986; Sperling & Melchner, 1978). Most assume that attention can only be focused on one item at a time (e.g., Posner, Snyder, & Davidson, 1980). Others suggest that under certain conditions attention can be allocated to two items or even a ring of items (e.g., Egly & Homa, 1984). Our everyday experience makes us believe that we certainly can—we can chew gum and pat our tummy at the same time! But these are not two visual tasks. In the pyramid examined here, if there are two neurons in the top layer that are to be attended, each of those has a receptive field in the input, and most neurons in

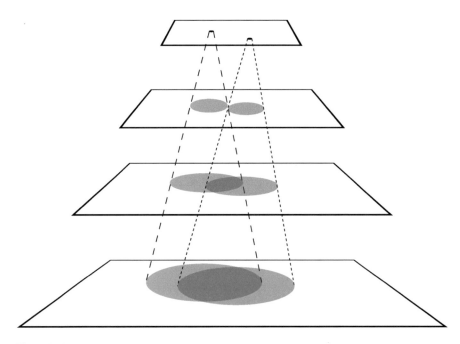

Figure 2.13
The Multiple Foci Problem. Attending to two items at the top leads to interfering fields of influence throughout the pyramid.

the top layer will have overlapping receptive fields. This overlap is undefined in the general case; it may be small or large in both space and feature dimensions. Only if stimuli are sufficiently separated in space may a mechanism that selects pathways that connect those neurons to their stimuli operate correctly without causing interference to the other. Figure 2.13 illustrates this; two attended neurons in the top have potentially damaging interactions within the pathways to the stimuli that they represent. Finally, because virtually all neurons in area IT of the visual cortex have large receptive fields including the fovea, it seems unlikely that it is possible to have sufficient separation to avoid any interference between sets of pathways. This position has recently received support from Scalf and Beck (2010), who concluded, after imaging experiments that focused on area V4, that competition might prevent attention from processing multiple items as well as it might for single-stimulus items. This is exactly the point here.

Convergent Recurrence Problem

When a top-down signal makes its way to a lower layer of the pyramid, it follows a set of diverging connections. That is, if it originates with one neuron, it is com-

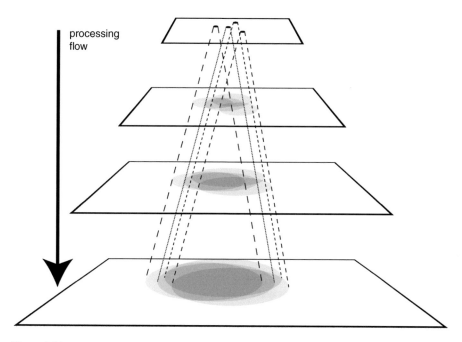

Figure 2.14
The Convergent Recurrence Problem. Regions of overlap show the extent of how recurrent signals from multiple sources might converge onto single neurons.

municated to many—a one-to-many mapping. As any number of neurons at one level may send recurrent signals to lower layers of the representation, many neurons will experience a convergence of recurrent signals, as shown in figure 2.14. Even if only four neurons as are shown in the figure generate recurrent signals, the resulting extent of affected neurons throughout the pyramid is quite large, and the overlap of signals is complex. Further, these signals may not be necessarily mutually consistent, and as a result a convergence rule or policy is required to eliminate the ambiguity. The problem is how to resolve the convergence of these signals.

Spatial Interpolation Problem

In the feed-forward direction, it is clear that spatial resolution is sacrificed to gain on efficiency of search. Conversely, in the feedback direction, spatial detail must be added back as a top-down signal traverses to lower layers. This is the inverse of the Sampling Problem. This may be accomplished by interpolation of the signal, and this interpolation may be trivial (uniform) or more complex (perhaps following feature types).

Spatial Spread Problem

This is the inverse of the Context Problem described earlier. Here, it is due to top-down information flow. The top-down signal may affect unintended neurons because of the top-down spread due to divergence of neural connectivity. The extent of the spread is defined by the size of receptive fields of the neurons from which the top-down signal originates. The diagram of figure 2.10 is not repeated here; but with a change in direction of information flow, it is as applicable.

Lateral Spread Problem

Each neuron in a particular layer may be connected to others within the layer. This requires specification, such as immediate neighbors only or all other neurons within a given radius. However, given the nature of overall lateral connectivity and the interrelationships of the computations performed laterally, there is the issue of Lateral Spread to contend with. This problem is due to the fact that although a single connection between two neurons has a limited effect—one neuron on the other—the effect ripples through to others along the lateral connections over time. This is shown in figure 2.15.

If the computation of the effect of lateral connections for a single neuron, as shown in the left half of figure 2.15, requires a time step T, and if that computation is allowed to continue for $2T$, the effects of the next annulus of neighbors will also make its way to that neuron, and so on, for each T time allowed. There may be situ-

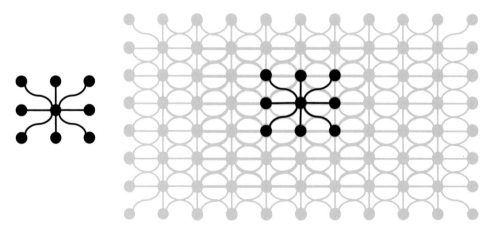

Figure 2.15
Lateral Spread Problem. A single neuron and its lateral connections is shown on the left, and that neuron embedded within the full array of neurons is shown on the right to highlight how lateral influences spread over time.

ations where this is acceptable and perhaps even required. But there will also be situations where this spread must be controlled.

All of these flow problems are inherent to single pyramid representations. They are worsened when more biologically realistic representations are considered in chapter 5. The realization of their nature provides strong constraint on how they may be solved as will be elaborated in chapters 4 and 5.

Attention Is . . . .

This chapter presented a particular viewpoint on the problem of visual attention, a computational perspective (see also Tsotsos & Bruce, 2008). In particular, the tools of the theory of computational complexity were brought to bear because it is this area of computer science that addresses the key rationale for attention—that attention is needed because the brain's size in terms of memory, processing speed and number of processors is too small for the combinatorial nature of extracting and then appropriately reuniting the elements present in the input that human sense organs receive. Several other elements of the language of computation as defined by Denning also played important roles. Various vision problems were defined, and their computational complexity was proved. We have shown that visual search, and by extension any other intelligent behavior that requires some sensory perception as an integral component, has exponential time complexity where the exponents are too large to enable it to be tractably solved in any realization. By reshaping the problem—through optimizations and approximations—the problem can be solvable with very low complexity. In a very real sense, those optimizations and approximations are all different kinds of attention in that they start from the general and thus largest possible problem definition and then focus in and scale down the problem to more manageable sizes, losing some generality along the way. We thus arrive at a more specific definition than we could present at the end of chapter 1:

Attention is a set of mechanisms that help tune and control the search processes inherent in perception and cognition.

This chapter dealt with what Marr (1982) called the computational level of the problem—what are the *in principle* problems that must be solved—independent of how they are solved and in what sort of being or agent these solutions are realized. This kind of analysis is largely missing from the attention literature, where one sees a dominating interest in the phenomena one can observe as a result of attention, quite removed (removed at least by choice of mechanisms and their implementation) from the *in principle* problems that must be solved. The next chapters will move to the strategies and algorithms that might be used to deal with these problems.

At the beginning of this chapter, the capacity of attention was identified as a long-standing problem. Have we made any progress on this here? Perhaps not as much as we might have hoped, but to be sure, there is real progress. The best that a single feed-forward pass of any visual processing architecture can accomplish is to process one subset of pixels. Parallelism permits that subset to be of any size, from the output of a single photoreceptor to the full visual field. If that chosen subset happens to suffice for the task at hand, then the single feed-forward pass is enough. If not—for any reason—then visual processing must resort to a more complex strategy, necessarily longer in time than a single feed-forward pass. The roots of that more complex strategy were first described in Tsotsos (1987), where the suggestion that attention is a top-down process that deals with some basic representational and processing issues in pyramid representations was made.

Although many have suggested attentional bottlenecks of one kind or another, in this chapter we have actually shown that one exists, albeit not of a form previously identified or suggested. The complexity analysis points to the utility of a pyramid representation, which in turn leads to the boundary problem. Once the anisotropy of the retina and the isotropy of cortical processes are included, it is easy to see how the overall architecture has an inherent, structural priority for central stimuli and a minimal representation for peripheral stimuli.

The capacity of the system, therefore, is not limited by numbers of bits or other measures. It is limited by the location of the stimuli in retinotopic terms, by the degree of ambiguity in the image being considered, and by the task requirements.

3 Theories and Models of Visual Attention

The variety of theories and models of visual attention and the number of relevant experimental papers that have been presented over the course of the past few decades are numbing to say the least. One of the implications is that throughout this book, and especially in this chapter, any attempt at complete and fair acknowledgment of all this research is doomed to failure, if for no other reason than space limits. It is almost just as difficult to determine priority for the important ideas; however, we will attempt to cite papers where an idea first appears and perhaps a small number of key publications. No matter how careful and diligent, this strategy will surely be insufficient, and apologies are extended in advance for its shortcomings.

The previous chapter detailed the computational—or *in principle*—problems that must be solved. These problems were not specific to attention; rather, they arose as part of the overall task of visual perception, and it was implied that attention is likely to play a role in their solution. However, the road from computational problem to strategies and mechanisms for attention is not sufficiently constrained by only that discussion, recalling that the nature of the problem as observed through experiment also plays an important role (Zucker, 1981). This chapter examines the characteristics of attentive visual behavior and neurobiology. The elements that might be considered important for inclusion in a complete model or theory of visual attention are introduced and defined; the reader is referred to the several in-depth treatments of the topic for further discussion and detail (e.g., Itti, Rees, & Tsotsos, 2005; Pashler, 1998a,b; Rothenstein & Tsotsos, 2008). Then, what is meant here by the terms 'model' and 'computational model' is clarified. Model classes are placed within a taxonomy and briefly characterized; there are many different kinds of models, and not all theories and models are designed for the same purpose. As a result, evaluations and comparisons are difficult and not entirely useful. Still, useful constraints do emerge from such an organization and review, and the chapter will conclude with these.

The Elements of Visual Attention

What are the elements of attention that a complete theory must include? This is a difficult question, and there have been several previous papers that attempt to address it. Posner (1980) was among the earliest and strongest influences in this regard, arguing that attention played three major roles: alerting, orienting, and search. These are fully defined later, along with several other such terms appearing in this section. Palmer (1995) was interested in the roles of attentional elements in the set-size effect (response time and accuracy change with the number of stimulus elements). He concluded that each of the preselection, selection, postselection, and decision-making elements, in a purely feed-forward organization, played roles in the set-size effect to differing degrees. Rather than delineating elements of attention, Tsotsos et al. (1995) presented a list of reasons for attention in vision systems. The needs for attention were to select a region of interest, to select features of interest, to control information flow and solve the context, blurring, cross-talk, and boundary problems, to shift attention in time solving the order of selection, reselection, and selection for time-varying scenes, and to balance data-directed and task-directed processing. Mozer and Sitton (1998) had a similar view and chose to define the uses of attention as controlling the order of readout, reduction of cross-talk, recovery of location information, and coordination of processing by independent modules. Itti and Koch (2001) review the state of attentional modeling, but from the point of view that assumes attention is primarily a bottom-up process based largely on their notion of saliency maps. Knudsen (2007) provides a more recent review; his perspective favors an early selection model as well. He provides a number of functional components fundamental to attention: working memory, competitive selection, top-down sensitivity control, and filtering for stimuli that are likely to be behaviorally important (salience filters). In his model, the world is first filtered by the salience filters in a purely bottom-up manner, creating the various neural representations on which competitive selection is based. The role of top-down information and control is to compute sensitivity control affecting the neural representations by incorporating the results of selection, working memory, and gaze. Another functional structure is that of Hamker (2000, 2005) whose work is an excellent example of the neurodynamical approach. Neurons are pooled into excitatory and inhibitory neural collections. High-level cognitive processes are directed from the top down and modulate stimulus signals. Prior knowledge is combined with feed-forward image responses by a population-based inference to update dynamically the conspicuity of each feature. Decisions, such as object detection, are based on these distributed saliencies. Finally, Shipp (2004) provides yet another useful overview where he compares several different models along the dimension of how they map onto system-level circuits in the brain. He presents his Real Neural Architecture (RNA) model for attention, integrating several different modes of operation—parallel or serial, bottom-up or top-down, preattentive or attentive—found in cognitive models of attention for visual search.

All of these examples, and additional ones, provide useful perspectives into potential solutions to the problem of attentive processing, using a variety of elements of attentional processes. The main difference among these overviews is that they are not at the same level of abstraction nor are they designed with the same purpose. Many focus strongly on connecting function with specific brain areas, and all present the functional components of attention in a manner biased by the particular model they propose. In this chapter, a view that is orthogonal to the neural correlates of function, independent of model and modeling strategy, is adopted.

It is far from a straightforward task to detail in a manageable manner the elements that comprise attention without missing anything important. Figure 3.1 and the explanations that accompany it were developed with this goal; there are likely other interpretations of these elements and their organization. Not all of these elements are of the same kind. There seem to be three major categories: representational elements, control elements, and observed characteristics. An executive controller is responsible for the integration of representation with control elements, which together result in the behavior that can be observed.

The point of this organization is to begin to bring some order to this difficult area (recall the quotes in chapter 1 regarding its chaotic nature). This taxonomy is certainly not complete (although it was a goal to be as complete as possible) and not necessarily optimal. For each item, the seminal paper(s) that first identified it are cited as well as one or more good survey papers where they are available. As noted in the first paragraph of this chapter, the sheer volume of literature and space limits make a fair and comprehensive set of citations virtually impossible, and we hope readers can accept our apologies for this in advance.

Alerting   The ability to process, identify, and move attention to priority signals (Posner, 1980).

Attentional Footprint   Optical metaphors describe the 'footprint' of attentional fixation in image space, and the main ones are **Spotlight** (Shulman et al., 1979), **Zoom Lens** (Ericksen & St. James, 1986), **Gradient** (LaBerge & Brown, 1989), and **Suppressive Surround** (Tsotsos, 1990a).

Binding   The process by which visual features are correctly combined to provide a unified representation of an object (Rosenblatt, 1961).

Covert Attention   Attention to a stimulus in the visual field without eye movements (Helmholtz, 1896)

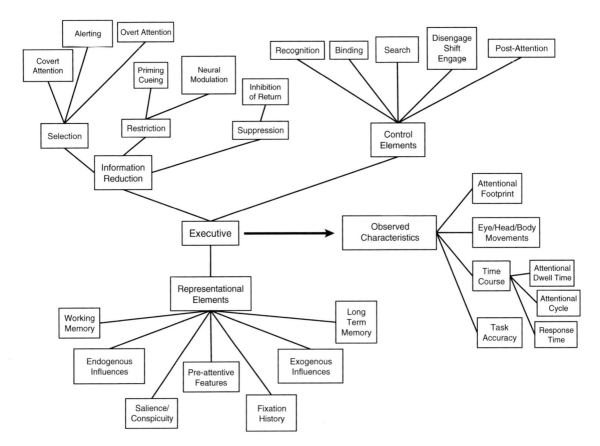

Figure 3.1
A taxonomy of the elements of visual attention. The overall system involving Executive, Control, and
Representational elements leads to the characteristics observed experimentally.

Disengage Attention   The generation of the signals that release attention from
one focus and prepare for a shift in attention (Posner, Petersen, Fox, & Raichle,
1988).

Endogenous Influences   Endogenous influence is an internally generated signal
(Posner, 1980) used for directing attention. This includes domain knowledge or task
instructions (Yarbus, 1967).

Engage Attention   The actions needed to fixate a stimulus whether covertly or
overtly (Posner et al., 1988).

Exccutive Control   The system that coordinates the elements into a coherent unit
that responds correctly to task and environmental demands (Egeth & Yantis, 1997;
Norman & Shallice, 1980; Posner & Petersen, 1990; Posner & Snyder, 1975; Shallice,
1988; Shiffrin & Schneider, 1977; Yantis & Serences, 2003).

Exogenous Influences   Exogenous influence is due to an external stimulus and contributes to control of gaze direction in a reflexive manner (Posner, 1980). Most common is perhaps the influence of abrupt onsets (Yantis & Jonides, 1984).

Inhibition of Return   A bias against returning attention to previously attended location (Posner, Rafal, Choate, & Vaughan, 1985) or object (Jordan & Tipper, 1998).

Neural Modulation   Attention changes baseline firing rates as well as firing patterns of neurons for attended stimuli (Fallah, Stoner, & Reynolds, 2007; Hernández-Peón et al., 1956; Moran & Desimone, 1985; O'Connor et al., 2002 Reynolds & Chelazzi, 2004).

Overt Attention   Also known as **Orienting**—the action of orienting the body, head, and eyes to foveate a stimulus in the 3D world (Hayhoe & Ballard, 2005; Posner, 1980; Schall & Thompson, 1999). Overt fixation trajectories may be influenced by covert fixations (Sheliga, Riggio, Craighero, & Rizzolatti, 1995).

Postattention   The process that creates the representation of an attended item that persists after attention is moved away from it (Wolfe, Klempen, & Dahlen, 2000).

Preattentive Features   The extraction of visual features from stimulus patterns perhaps biased by task demands (Neisser, 1967; Wolfe, 1998a).

Priming   Priming is the general process by which task instructions or world knowledge prepares the visual system for input. **Cueing** is an instance of priming; perception is speeded with a correct cue, whether by location, feature, or complete stimulus (Posner et al., 1978). Purposefully ignoring has relevance here also and is termed **Negative Priming**. If one ignores a stimulus, processing of that ignored stimulus shortly afterwards is impaired (Tipper, 1985).

Recognition   The process of interpreting an attended stimulus, facilitated by attention (Milner, 1974).

Salience/Conspicuity   The overall contrast of the stimulus at a particular location with respect to its surround (Fecteau & Munoz, 2006 Koch & Ullman, 1985; Treisman & Gelade, 1980).

Search   The process that scans the candidate stimuli for detection or other tasks among the many possible locations and features in cluttered scenes (Neisser, 1964; Posner, 1980; Wolfe, 1998a,b).

Selection   The process of choosing one element of the stimulus over the remainder. Selection can be over locations (Posner, 1980), over features (Martinez-Trujillo & Treue, 2004), for objects (Duncan, 1984), over time (Coull & Nobre, 1998), and for behavioral responses (Boussaoud & Wise, 1993), or even combinations of these.

Shift Attention   The actions involved in moving an attentional fixation from its current to its new point of fixation (Posner et al., 1988).

Time Course   The effects of attention take time to appear, and this is observed in the firing rate patterns of neurons and in behavioral experiments, showing delays as well as cyclic patterns (Duncan, Ward, & Shapiro, 1994; Mehta, Ulbert, & Schroeder, 2000; Van Rullen & Thorpe, 2001; Van Rullen, Carlson, & Cavanaugh, 2007).

Update Fixation History   The process by which the system keeps track of what has been seen and processed, and how that representation is maintained and updated that then participates in decisions of what to fixate and when (Colby & Goldberg, 1999; Duhamel, Colby, & Goldberg, 1992).

One particularly ingrained concept requires some additional discussion. The words 'serial' and 'parallel' did not appear in the above list of attentional elements, yet they may be the most used in the literature. The separation of visual processing into parallel and serial components has a history that includes Neisser (1967), Treisman and Gelade (1980), and Marr (1982), at least. At the time, it was a promising concept and provided for a nice separation of strategies. As time moved on and more and more experimental data mounted, the separation no longer seemed so clear. If there was ever any doubt, a nice analysis by Wolfe (1998b) really has laid the question to rest. He examined 2500 experimental sessions from the literature representing more than 1,000,000 trials of visual search in a variety of tasks. The most clear conclusion was that the distribution of search slopes was unimodal; that is, there was no clear separation into serial or parallel processes. Further, the most commonly accepted strategy of a serial, self-terminating search is also not supported by the data. His analysis presents several other insights, but at this point, it provides the justification to not tie experimental results too closely with potential underlying computations.

It is interesting to note that through the history of attention research, and even though it is almost universally agreed that attention is due to information load and processing capacity limits, there is very little discussion of how to reduce information to some manageable level (but see an important exception in Tishby et al., 1999). Yet, it is not so difficult to rethink many of the above into the kind of information reduction mechanisms they lead to. Clearly, Alerting, Inhibition of Return, Priming, Salience/Conspicuity, Selection, and Shift Attention are all elements that lead to information reduction. Selection has Overt and Covert Attention as subclasses. Considered together and adding some additional detail, there seem to be three classes of information reduction mechanisms: **Selection** (e.g., choice of next fixation), **Restriction** (such as priming), and **Suppression** (inhibition of return is one example). Bringing to bear the list of behaviors discussed in the "Extending to Active Vision" section of the previous chapter, one may add to and enhance each of these classes and develop the following set of mechanisms:

- Selection mechanisms include selection of
  - spatiotemporal region of interest;
  - features of interest;
  - world, task, object, or event model;
  - gaze and viewpoint;
  - best interpretation or response.
- Restriction mechanisms are those dealing with
  - task relevant search space pruning;
  - location cues;
  - fixation points;
  - search depth control during task satisfaction;
  - modulating neural tuning profiles.
- Suppression applies in a number of ways, among them
  - spatial and feature surround inhibition;
  - inhibition of return;
  - suppression of task-irrelevant computations.

All models include at least a subset of these mechanisms used to address some subset of the above attentional elements.

A Taxonomy of Models

A **Model of Visual Attention** is a description of the observed and/or predicted behavior of human (or animal) visual attention. Models can use natural language, system block diagrams, mathematics, algorithms, or computations as their embodiment and attempt to mimic, explain, and/or predict some or all of visual attentive behavior. Of importance are the accompanying assumptions, the set of statements or principles devised to provide the explanation, and the extent of the facts or phenomena that are explained. Models must be tested by experiments, and such experiments replicated, both with respect to their explanations of existing phenomena but also to test their predictive validity.

A **Computational Model of Visual Attention** is a particular kind of model of visual attention and not only includes a formal description for how attention is computed but also can be tested by providing image inputs, similar to those an experimenter might present to a subject, and then seeing how the model performs by comparison. It should be pointed out that this definition differs from the usual, almost casual, use of the term 'computational' in the area of neurobiological modeling. It has come to mean almost any model that includes a mathematical formulation of some kind. Mathematical equations can be solved and/or simulated on a computer, and thus the term *computational* has seemed appropriate to many authors. Marr's levels of analysis (Marr, 1982) provide a different view (see chapter 1). The use of the term 'computational model' in this book is intended to capture models that specify all three of Marr's levels in a testable manner, and not just his first level. This view is a bit more narrow than that of Mozer and Sitton (1998); however, both agree on the need to explain the experimental data and offer predictions for future experimental testing.

The terms *descriptive*, *data-fitting*, and *algorithmic* as used here describe three different methodologies for specifying Marr's algorithmic level of analysis. Models of attention are complex; they need to provide mechanisms and explanations for a number of functions all tied together within a system. Because of their complexity, model evaluation is not a simple matter, and objective conclusions are still elusive. The point of the next section is to create a context for such models; this enables one to see their scientific heritage, to distinguish models on the basis of their modeling strategy, and to situate new models appropriately to enable comparisons and evaluations.

In figure 3.2, a taxonomy of models is laid out with computational models clearly lying in the intersection of how the biological community and how the computer vision community view attentive processes. There are two main roots in this lattice—

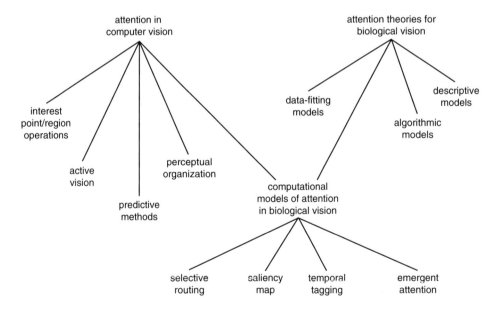

Figure 3.2
A taxonomy of attention models across disciplines and modeling strategies.

one due to the uses of attentive methods in computer vision and one due to the development of attention models in the biological vision community. Although both have proceeded independently, and indeed, the use of attention appears in the computer vision literature well before most biological models, the major point of intersection is the class of computational models.

The models and theories in these classes can also be grouped according to a different organizational principle. Models may address attentional effects for single neurons or small neural assemblies, for networks of neurons, or for the visual system as a whole [see Wilson (1999) or Churchland, Koch, & Sejnowski (1990) on levels of abstraction in computational neuroscience]. Model scope will be mentioned in the descriptions that follow where possible for the biological and computational branches of the taxonomy. One must take care when comparing models to compare only those whose scope is the same.

It is quite clear that the motivations for all the modeling efforts come from two sources. The first is the deep interest to understand the perceptual capability that has been observed for centuries; that is, the ability to select, process, and act upon parts of one's sensory experience differentially from the rest. The second is the need to reduce the quantity of sensory information entering any system, biological or otherwise, by selecting or ignoring parts of the sensory input. Although the motivations seem distinct, the conclusion is the same, and in reality the motivation for attention in any system is to reduce the quantity of information to process in order to complete some task as detailed in chapter 2.

But depending on one's interest, modeling efforts do not always have the same goals. That is, one may be trying to model a particular set of experimental observations, one may be trying to build a robotic vision system and attention is used to select landmarks for navigation, one may have interest in eye movements, or in the executive control function, or any one or more of the elements seen in figure 3.1. As a result, comparing models is not straightforward, fair, or useful. What follows tries to avoid judgment, opting for an exposition that might be useful for its breadth and organizational structure.

The effectiveness of any theory, regardless of type, is determined by how well it provides explanations for what is known about as many of the above elements as possible. Just as importantly, theories underlying models must be falsifiable; that is, they must make testable predictions regarding new behaviors or functions not yet observed—behaviors that are counterintuitive (i.e., not easily deduced from current knowledge)—that would enable one to support or reject the theory.

The Computer Vision Branch

The use of attentive methods has pervaded the computer vision literature recently demonstrating the importance for reducing the amount of information to be processed. Several early analyses of the extent of the information load issue have appeared (Feldman & Ballard, 1982; Grimson, 1990; Tsotsos, 1987; Uhr, 1972) with converging suggestions for its solution appearing in a number of the models below (particularly Burt, 1988; Tsotsos, 1990a). The scope of the many ways information reduction methods have been used in computer vision is far too broad and beyond the intent of this book. Almost all authors, if they consider computational complexity, look at the complexity of their specific algorithms and try to show the properties of their implemented solutions operating on some particular task domain. Problem complexity is only rarely considered. However, problem complexity is the focus of this book and in particular how it relates to human visual processes. As a result, the computer vision branch of this taxonomy may seem somewhat abbreviated. Specifically, the methods can be grouped into four categories. For each, only pointers to the earliest description of the basic idea are given. All subsequent methods within each group are direct descendants of the idea.

Interest Point Operations   One way to reduce the amount of an image to be processed is to concentrate on the points or regions that are most interesting or relevant for the next stage of processing (such as for recognition or action). The idea is that perhaps 'interestingness' can be computed in parallel across the whole image and then those interesting points or regions can be processed in more depth serially. The first of these interest operators is due to Moravec (1981). A feature is conceptually a point in the three-dimensional world and is found by examining collections of one or more points. A feature is good if it can be located unambiguously in different views of a scene. Regions such as corners, with high contrast in orthogonal directions, are best. Moravec's **interest operator** tries to select a relatively uniform scattering of good features to maximize the probability that a few features will be picked on every visible object by returning regions that are local maxima of a directional variance measure. Featureless areas and simple edges, which have no variance in the direction of the edge, are avoided. Since then, a large number of different kinds of computations have been used. This may be considered the antecedent to the Saliency Map Model.

Perceptual Grouping   The computational load is not only due to the large number of image locations but also due to the nature of combinations of positions or regions. In perceptual psychology, how the brain might group items is a major concern, pioneered by the Gestaltists (Köhler, 1929). Thus, computer vision has used grouping strategies following Gestalt principles, such as proximity, similarity, collinearity, symmetry, familiarity, and so on, to limit the possible subsets of combinatorially defined items to consider. The first such use appeared in Muerle and Allen (1968) in the context of object segmentation where they began with a very fine partition and simplified it by progressively merging adjacent elements together that are found to be similar according to certain statistical criteria. An important distinction, mostly ignored by the computational community, is that the Gestalt principles were not strict laws, but rather *tendencies*. That is, humans tend to group items by proximity, for example, and do so as a kind of default in the absence of any other grouping method. Task requirements, for instance, can overrule this tendency. Further, if more than one of these principles is applicable, there is an interaction among them, and this interaction has not been fully explored.

Active Vision Human eyes move, and humans move around their world to acquire visual information; in chapter 1, the act psychology framework of Brentano and the attention-direction theory of Petermann were briefly described. In computer vision, these ideas first appear in a Barrow and Popplestone (1971) paper where they say:

[C]onsider the object recognition program in its proper perspective, as a part of an integrated cognitive system. One of the simplest ways that such a system might interact with the environment is simply to shift its viewpoint, to walk round an object. In this way, more information may be gathered and ambiguities resolved. A further, more rewarding operation is to prod the object, thus measuring its range, detecting holes and concavities. Such activities involve planning, inductive generalization, and indeed, most of the capacities required by an intelligent machine.

Active vision in computer vision uses intelligent control strategies applied to the data acquisition process that depend on the current state of data interpretation (Bajcsy, 1985). A variety of methods have appeared, perhaps the earliest one most relevant to this discussion is the robotic binocular camera system of Clark and Ferrier (1988), featuring a salience-based fixation control mechanism. They used a control system paradigm and implemented shifts in attention by altering feedback gains in the position and velocity control loops for the binocular camera system. In this way, they performed feature selection by enhancing saliency of selected features while reducing that of nonselected features. Particular instances of active object recognition strategies that use attention include Wilkes and Tsotsos (1992) and Dickinson et al. (1997).

Predictive Methods The application of domain and task knowledge to guide or predict processing is a powerful tool for limiting processing, a fact formally proved in Tsotsos (1989). The first use in a vision system was for oriented line location in a face-recognition task (Kelly, 1971). Edges in reduced resolution images were found first, then mapped onto the full image to provide face outline predictions. Kelly called this process 'planning,' an idea he credits to Kirsch, Cahn, Ray, and Urban (1957). The idea was also used for temporal window prediction in a motion recognition task (Tsotsos, Mylopoulos, Covvey, & Zucker, 1980) where speed and direction of motion was used to extrapolate possible next positions for segments of the left ventricle to limit the region of the X-ray image to search as well as to predict the pose of the segment in the hypothesized window.

Within modern computer vision, there are many, many variations and combinations of these themes because regardless of the impressive rapid increases in power in modern computers, the inherent difficulty of processing images demands attentional processes. Even so, purely feed-forward architectures with no attention remain popular, and many expect them to provide sufficient performance. If you think about it, all efforts try to limit the size of the variables P and M (from chapter 2), using regions of interest computed every which way, by using pyramid representations to scale down the image, by using impoverished feature spaces (such as orientation quantized into only four values), and so forth. As computers become faster, the sizes of P and M that can be handled grow, giving the appearance that the theory does not matter. But this does not scale, and as the problem size increases (increases in image size or feature number), solutions do not follow. They rely on computing speed to increase correspondingly. In other words, the computational complexity of such feed-forward approaches to vision in the general case remain exponential, as shown in chapter 2, and outside the range of any improvements in computing power.

The computer vision literature also includes a large number of more engineering applications that effectively use attention as part of their solutions to a wide variety of tasks. They are important because they show the value of the key concepts; but they are too many to be included here. Fortunately, there is an excellent recent survey covering these (Frintrop, Rome, & Christensen, 2010).

The Biological Vision Branch

Clearly, in this class, the major motivation has always been to provide explanations for the characteristics of biological, especially human, vision. Typically, these have been developed to explain a particular body of experimental observations. This is a strength; the authors usually are the ones who have done some or all of the experiments and thus completely understand the experimental methods and conclusions. Simultaneously, however, this is also a weakness because the models are often difficult to extend to a broader class of observations. Along the biological vision branch, the four classes identified follow.

Descriptive Models   These models are described primarily using natural language and/or block diagrams. Classic models, even though they were motivated by experiments in auditory attention, have been very influential. **Early Selection** (Broadbent, 1958), **Late Selection** (Deutsch & Deutsch, 1963; Moray, 1969; Norman, 1968; MacKay, 1973), and **Attenuator Theory** (Treisman, 1964) and Kahneman's **General Purpose Limited Resource** model (Kahneman, 1973) are all early descriptive models. Their value lies in the explanation they provide of certain attentional processes; the abstractness of explanation is also their major problem because it is typically open to interpretation. For example, a model of late selection does not specify exactly where in the processing stream selection occurs, only that it is later than in the early selection model. As such, one might choose any of a variety of intermediate processing steps to label as late.

Broadbent suggested a model of sensory processing that included the following components: a short-term store to act to extend the duration of a stimulus; a partitioning of stimuli into channels (modalities); a selective filter that selects among channels; and a limited capacity channel to process the selected channel. This is the prototypical early selection model of attention. Deutsch and Deutsch (1963), Norman (1968), Moray (1969), and MacKay (1973) proposed late selection models. Late selection theories propose that all information is completely processed and recognized before it receives the attention of a limited-capacity processor. Recognition can occur in parallel, and stimulus relevance determines what is attended. Treisman (1964) included a filter that attenuates (in a graded fashion) unattended signals, leaving them incompletely analyzed. Importantly, this filter can operate at different stages of information processing. Treisman thus introduced the notion that the effects of attention may be hierarchically described.

Kahneman (1973) argued that attention is a general-purpose limited resource whose total available processing capacity may be increased or decreased by other factors such as arousal. Rules or strategies exist that determine allocation of resources to various activities and to various stages of processing. Kahneman thus believed in the existence of a central processor that operates a central allocation policy, constantly evaluating the demands made by each task and adjusting attention accordingly. Notions of resource allocation persist in the literature even though there is no evidence whatsoever for any physical counterpart; no neurons can be physically moved around, no connections can be physically moved dynamically (although strong modulations of neurons or connections may show some, but not all, of the characteristics or such a physical reallocation), and no visual areas can, in a dynamic real-time fashion, change to become auditory and then change back again.

Other models such as **Feature Integration Theory** (Treisman & Gelade, 1980), **Guided Search** (Wolfe, 1994, 2007; Wolfe & Gancarz, 1996; Wolfe et al., 1989), and **Animate Vision** (Ballard, 1991) are conceptual frameworks, ways of thinking about the problem of attention. Many have played important, indeed foundational, roles in how the field has developed.

Feature Integration Theory (FIT) suggests that we become aware of objects in two different ways—through focal attention or through top-down processing. The first route to object identification depends on focal attention, directed serially to different locations, to integrate the features registered within the same spatiotemporal spotlight into a unitary percept. Top-down processing can provide predictions about objects in a familiar context. Their presence is checked by matching the disjunctive features to those in the display, without also checking how they are spatially conjoined.

The Guided Search (GS) model addressed a problem with the original Feature Integration Theory. FIT had proposed a division between parallel, preattentive searches and serial, attentive searches. This dichotomy does not, however, appear in the data. In particular, FIT proposed that searches for conjunctions of two (or more) features require serial processing. However, often they proved to be more efficient than serial search, sometimes as efficient as preattentive searches (see Wolfe, 1998a). GS kept the basic structure but proposed that preattentive processes could guide the deployment of the serial, attentive stage. The guidance can be bottom-up, stimulus-driven but may be tempered by task demands. Alternatively, top-down guidance can be a response to explicit task demands.

Animate Vision claims that the central asset of animate vision is gaze control (Ballard, 1991). Animate vision systems can use physical search, make approximate camera movements, use exocentric coordinate frames, use qualitative algorithms, segment areas of interest precategorically, exploit environmental context, and employ learning. The important claim is that in comparison with passive systems (without gaze control), animate systems show that visual computation can be much less expensive when considered in the context of behavior because the control of gaze provides additional constraints on computation. In addition, the environment plays an important role because animate systems, under real-time constraints, can use environmental cues to further constrain computations.

The number of other such conceptual models is large, and the following list presents many more (in chronological order) along with the key ideas behind each.

Premotor Theory of Attention (Rizzolatti et al., 1987)   Covert attention is strictly linked to programming of explicit ocular movements. Attention is allocated when the oculomotor program for moving the eyes to the new fixation is ready to be executed. Attentional cost is the time required to erase one ocular program and prepare the next one.

Multiple Object Adaptive Grouping of Image Components (MAGIC) (Mozer, Zemel, Behrmann & Williams, 1992)   Object-based attention is based on a mechanism that groups features using internal representations developed with perceptual experience and preferentially gates these features for later selective processing.

Sequence Seeking and Counter Streams (Ullman, 1995)   Information flow is solved by a parallel and bidirectional process that searches for a sequence of transformations linking source and target patterns.

Resolution Theory of Visual Attention (Tsal, Meiran, & Lamy, 1995)   Directing attention to a location improves resolution of features by computing relative activation of relatively coarse resolution, overlapping detectors.

Ambiguity Resolution Theory of Visual Selective Attention (Luck, Girelli, McDermott, & Ford, 1997b)   The role of attention is to resolve ambiguity and the attention-related Event-Related Potential (ERP) wave N2pc seems to be a manifestation. Neural coding can be ambiguous for the reasons given earlier. Using Event-Related Potentials (ERPs are measured with electroencephalography; EEG), one observes the resulting waveforms and attempts to connect wave characteristics to behavior. A particular signal, the N2pc wave, typically arises at post-stimulus latencies of 180–300 milliseconds and is interpreted as a distractor suppression mechanism.

FeatureGate (Cave, 1999)   The model includes a hierarchy of spatial maps within which attentional gates control the flow of information from each level of the hierarchy to the next. The gates are jointly controlled by a bottom-up system favoring locations with unique features and a top-down system favoring locations with features designated as target features.

Real Neural Architecture (RNA; Shipp, 2004)   RNA proposes that the pulvinar combines both bottom-up and top-down influences within a single salience computation. RNA includes the frontal eye field (FEF), parietal eye field (PEF) and superior colliculus (SC), being active in shifts of gaze, to account for the close ties between overt and covert shifts of attention.

Four-Process Model (Knudsen, 2007)   Four processes are fundamental: working memory, top-down sensitivity control, competitive selection, and automatic, early, bottom-up filtering for salient stimuli. Voluntary control of attention involves the first three processes operating in a recurrent loop.

Data-Fitting Models   These models are mathematical and are developed to capture parameter variations in experimental data in as compact and parsimonious a form as possible. Their value lies primarily in how well they provide a fit to experimental data and in interpolation of parameter values or in extrapolation to other experimental scenarios. Good examples are the **Theory of Visual Attention** (Bundesen, 1990), **Biased Competition** (Desimone & Duncan, 1995; Reynolds, Chelazzi, & Desimone, 1999), and two different models based on normalization, the **Normalization Model of Attention** (Reynolds & Heeger, 2009) and the **Normalization Model of Attentional Modulation** (Lee & Maunsell, 2009). The Biased Competition Model has garnered many followers mostly due to the conceptual aspect of it combining competition with top-down bias, concepts that actually appeared in earlier models [such as Grossberg (1982) or Tsotsos (1990a)].

An issue of interest, particularly to those developing single-neuron models, is whether attention modulates contrast or response (for an overview, see Reynolds, Pasternak, & Desimone, 2000). The **Contrast Gain Model** suggests that attention modulates the effective contrast of stimuli at attended locations. The contrast–response function is plotted as a function of the logarithm of contrast. A lateral shift in the function corresponds with a multiplication of the contrast necessary to reach a given level of response. The **Response Gain Model** differs and proposes that attention causes the neuronal response (above baseline) to be multiplied by a constant gain factor, resulting in increases in firing rate with attention that grow larger with contrast. The debate on which best represents attentional function continues (Palmer & Moore, 2009; Reynolds et al., 2000; and more). Recently, however, Khayat, Niebergall, and Martinez-Trujillo (2010), testing macaque area MT (middle temporal), found that their results were incompatible with models proposing that attention was a scaling or additive modulation of neural responses. They concluded that their data supports models where both spatial and feature-based attention modulates input signals of neurons. The main models are now summarized.

Theory of Visual Attention (TVA; Bundesen, 1990)   TVA unifies visual recognition and attentional selection by integrating the biased-choice model for single-stimulus recognition with a choice model for selection from multielement displays in a race model framework.

Contour Detector (CODE)–Theory of Visual Attention (Logan, 1996)   CODE provides input to TVA. It clusters nearby items into perceptual groups and integrates spatial and object-based processes; the attentional capacity is the same as that of TVA.

Biased Competition (Desimone & Duncan, 1995; Reynolds et al., 1999)   This model has its roots in the shrink-wrap interpretation resulting from the observations of Moran and Desimone (1985). The Desimone and Duncan (1995) version is purely descriptive. Reynolds et al. (1999) later brought in the quantitative counterpart. This is a single-neuron model where representation in the visual system is competitive, where both top-down and bottom-up biasing mechanisms influence the ongoing competition, and where competition is integrated across brain systems. Attention is modeled as an integer gain multiplier in a dynamical equation and its source is left unspecified.

Feature Similarity Gain Model (Boynton, 2005; Treue & Martinez-Trujillo, 1999) Treue and Martinez-Trujillo observed nonspatial, feature-based attentional modulation of visual motion processing and showed that attention increases the gain of direction-selective neurons in visual cortical area MT without narrowing the direction-tuning curves. Their model is an attempt to unify the effects of spatial location, direction of motion, and other features of the attended stimuli. Boynton later mathematically formalized the model.

Instance Theory of Attention and Memory (ITAM; Logan, 2002)   Performance depends on a choice process that is modeled as a race between competing alternatives; attention, categorization, and memory are different aspects of the same choice process.

Feedback Model of Visual Attention (Spratling & Johnson, 2004)   In this more detailed version of Biased Competition, feedback stimulation is integrated in the apical dendrite, and feed-forward information is separately integrated in the basal dendrite. The total strength of the top-down activation multiplicatively modulates the total strength of feed-forward activation to determine final response.

Normalization Model of Attention (Reynolds & Heeger, 2009)   This single neural layer model suggests that stimulus drive is multiplied by the attention field (region in the visual field where attention is allocated) and divided by the suppression drive to yield output firing. This model combines Heeger's normalization model of visual response (Heeger, 1992), Treue and Martinez-Trujillo's feature-similarity gain idea (Treue & Martinez-Trujillo, 1999), and Reynolds' version of Biased Competition (Reynolds et al., 1999).

Normalization Model of Attentional Modulation (Lee & Maunsell, 2009)   Attention only works through the same mechanism that adjusts responses to multiple stimuli (normalization) to achieve single-cell attentional modulation. The model explains how attention changes the gain of responses to individual stimuli and why attentional modulation is more than a gain change when multiple stimuli are present in a receptive field.

Algorithmic Models   These models provide mathematics and algorithms that govern their performance and as a result present a process by which attention might be computed and deployed. They, however, do not provide sufficient detail or methodology so that the model might be tested on real stimuli. These models often provide simulations to demonstrate their actions. In a real sense they are a combination of descriptive and data-fitting models; they provide more detail on descriptions so they may be simulated while showing good comparison with experimental data at qualitative levels (and perhaps also quantitative). The best known of these models is the **Saliency Map Model** (Koch & Ullman, 1985); it has given rise to many subsequent models. It is interesting to note that the Saliency Map Model is strongly related to the Interest Point Operations on the other side of this taxonomy. Other algorithmic models include **Adaptive Resonance Theory** (Grossberg, 1975, 1982), **Temporal Tagging** (Niebur, Koch, & Rosin, 1993; Niebur & Koch, 1994; Usher & Niebur, 1996), **Shifter Circuits** (Anderson & Van Essen, 1987), **Visual Routines**

(Ullman, 1984), the phase oscillators model of Wu & Guo (1999), **CODAM** (Taylor & Rogers, 2002), and a SOAR-based model (Wiesmeyer & Laird, 1990). Some models are very briefly described below.

Adaptive Resonance Theory (ART; Grossberg, 1975, 1982)   ART is a neural unsupervised learning model. It includes a processing framework where attentional and orienting subsystems have a complementary relationship to control the adaptive self-organization of internal representations. Attention establishes precise internal representations, responses to expected cues, and learned expectations.

Saliency Map Model (Koch & Ullman, 1985)   This model features a topographic saliency map combining properties across all feature maps for each location into a conspicuity measure. A Winner-Take-All method selects the most salient location, and it is inhibited to enable selection of the next fixation.

Shifter Circuits (Anderson & Van Essen, 1987)   Shifter circuits realize dynamic shifts in the relative alignment of input and output arrays without loss of spatial relationships. The shifts are produced in increments along a succession of relay stages that are linked by diverging excitatory inputs. The direction of shift is controlled at each stage by inhibitory neurons that selectively suppress appropriate sets of ascending inputs.

Not Overt Visual Attention (NOVA; Wiesmeyer & Laird, 1990)   Within the SOAR (State, Operator, and Result) cognitive architecture, attention is claimed to precede identification, is a deliberate act mediated by an ATTEND operator, and functions as a gradient-based, zoom lens of oval shape that separates figure from ground. Attended features move on to recognition.

Temporal Tagging Model (Niebur et al., 1993)   The firing rate of neurons, whose receptive fields overlap with the "focus of attention," is modulated with a periodic function in the 40-Hz range of unspecified origin. This modulation is detected by inhibitory interneurons in V4 and is used to suppress the response of V4 cells associated with nonattended visual stimuli.

Visual Routines (Ullman, 1984)   Visual routines are composed of sequences of elemental operations, assembled by the visual system to operate on early representations and realize shifts of focus, indexing operations, boundary tracing, and more.

Corollary Discharge of Attention Movement (CODAM; Taylor & Rogers, 2002)   CODAM is an engineering control model of primary and associative cortices acting as the 'plant' modulated by the attention control signal. A forward model or predictor of the future state of the system, created by an efference copy or corollary discharge of the attentional control signal, is used to generate speed-up in the access of content by earlier entry to the relevant buffer working memory.

Among the above models, those that focus on single neurons or small assemblies include the Temporal Tagging, Biased Competition, and Normalization Models. Models that include hierarchical networks of neurons are Shifter Circuits, Saliency Map Model, Adaptive Resonance Theory, and FeatureGate. Finally, system-level models are Visual Routines, the SOAR-based model, Theory of Visual Attention, Feature Integration Theory, Guided Search, Animate Vision, and Real Neural Architecture.

The Computational Hypotheses

As mentioned earlier, the point of intersection between the computer vision and biological vision communities is represented by the set of computational models in the taxonomy. **Computational Models** not only include a process description for how attention is computed but also can be tested by providing image inputs, similar to those an experimenter might present a subject, and then seeing how the model performs by comparison. The biological connection is key, and pure computer vision efforts are not included here. Under this definition, computational models generally provide more complete specifications and permit more objective evaluations as well. This greater level of detail is a strength but is also risky because there are more details that require experimental validation.

Many models have elements from more than one class so the separation is not a strict one. Computational Models necessarily are Algorithmic Models. Algorithmic Models often include Data-Fitting elements as well. Nevertheless, in recent years four major schools of thought have emerged, schools that will be termed *hypotheses* here as each has both supporting and detracting evidence. In what follows, an attempt is made to provide the intellectual antecedents for each of these major hypotheses.

The Selective Routing Hypothesis   This hypothesis focuses on how attention solves the problems associated with stimulus selection and then transmission through the visual cortex. The issues of how signals in the brain are transmitted to ensure correct perception appear, in part, in a number of works. Milner (1974), for example, mentions that attention acts in part to activate the feedback pathways from the cell assembly to the early visual cortex for precise localization, implying a pathway search problem. The complexity of the brain's network of feed-forward and feedback connectivity highlights the physical problems of search, transmission, and finding the right path between input and output (see Felleman & Van Essen, 1991). Anderson and Van Essen's Shifter Circuits proposal (Anderson & Van Essen, 1987) was presented primarily to solve these physical routing and transmission problems using control signals to each layer of processing that shift selected inputs from one path to another. A number of routing problems arise as a result of the architecture, and these were described in chapter 2.

Models that fall into the Selective Routing class include **NeoCognitron** (Fukushima, 1986), **Pyramid Vision** (Burt, 1988), **Selective Tuning** (Rodriguez-Sanchez, Simine, & Tsotsos, 2007; Rothenstein, Rodriguez-Sanchez, Simine, & Tsotsos, 2008; Tsotsos, 1990a; Tsotsos et al., 1995, 2005; Zaharescu et al., 2005), **MORSEL** (Mozer, 1991), the model of Olshausen, Anderson, and Van Essen (1993), and **SCAN** (Postma et al., 1997). The work of Olshausen et al. was the first attempt to realize the Shifter Circuits ideas and included the selection mechanisms of Koch and Ullman (1985) that provided the location of the items to be attended and thus routed using the shifting scheme. Of these, perhaps most impressive is the practical performance of the Pyramid Vision system in motion-tracking tasks. All of the models address one or more of the routing problems described in chapter 2, and all provide some level of realization and empirical evidence of a working mechanism. NeoCognitron presents a top-down strategy for localizing an attended stimulus, tracing back connections through the hierarchy of representations. Fukushima's model included a maximum detector at the top layer to select the highest responding cell, and all other cells were set to their rest state. Only afferent paths to this cell are facilitated by action from efferent signals from this cell. The NeoCognitron competitive mechanism is lateral inhibition, performed at the highest and intermediate levels, to find strongest single neurons, implicitly assuming that all spatial scales are represented explicitly. Burt describes three elements of attention: foveation, to examine selected regions of the visual world at high resolution; tracking, to stabilize the images of moving objects within the eye; and high-level interpretation, to anticipate where salient information will occur in a scene. Further, he states that attention includes mechanisms for directing the allocation of processing and mechanisms for rapidly interpreting the information as it is gathered. As such, Burt was really the first to implement multiple mechanisms in a computational attention system. He also first used pyramid representations for this purpose, specifically a Laplacian pyramid (Burt & Adelson, 1983).

MORSEL (Multiple Object Recognition and attentional Selection) is a connectionist model of spatial attention and object recognition that builds location invariant representations of letters and words. It includes a pull-out net and an attentional mechanism to limit processing. The pull-out net uses semantic and lexical knowledge to select best interpretation, and attention selects location guided bottom-up by locations of stimuli and by top-down task bias (as in controlling temporal order in reading). Interestingly, it demonstrated failures of reading, such as dyslexia. SCAN stands for Signal Channeling Attentional Network and is a scalable neural network model for covert attention only. SCAN involves a gating lattice, a sparsely connected neural network, through which selected patterns are channeled and mapped onto an output window. SCAN furthers incorporates an expectation-generating classifier network to allow selection to be driven by expectation. The Selective Tuning models are the focus of chapters 4–8.

The Saliency Map Hypothesis   This hypothesis has its roots in Feature Integration Theory (Treisman & Gelade, 1980), Moravec's interest operator (Moravec, 1981), and appears first in the class of algorithmic models above (Koch & Ullman, 1985). It includes the following elements:

1. an early representation—feature maps—computed in parallel, permitting separate representations of several stimulus characteristics;

2. a topographic saliency map where each location contains the properties across all feature maps for that single location combined as a conspicuity measure;

3. a selective mapping into a central non-topographic representation through the topographic saliency map of the properties of a single visual location;

4. a Winner-Take-All (WTA) network implementing the selection process based on one major rule: conspicuity of location (minor rules of proximity or similarity preference are also suggested); and

5. an Inhibition of Return mechanism that inhibits the selected location to cause an automatic shift to the next most conspicuous location.

Feature maps code conspicuity within a particular feature dimension. The saliency map combines information from each of the feature maps into a global measure where points corresponding with one location in a feature map project to single units in the saliency map. Saliency at a given location is determined by the degree of difference between that location and its surround. The models of Clark and Ferrier (1988), Sandon (1990), Itti et al. (1998), Itti and Koch (2000), Walther et al. (2002), Navalpakkam and Itti (2005), Itti and Baldi (2006), **SERR** (Humphreys & Muller, 1993), Gao, Mahadevan, and Vasconcelos (2008), Zhang, Tong, Marks, Shan, and Cottrell (2008), and **AIM** (Attention via Information Maximization; Bruce & Tsotsos, 2005, 2009) are all in this class.

The drive to discover the best representation of saliency or conspicuity is a major current activity. Whether or not a single such representation exists in the brain remains an open question with evidence supporting many potential loci: superior colliculus (Horwitz & Newsome, 1999; Kustov & Robinson, 1996; McPeek & Keller, 2002); LGN (Koch, 1984; Sherman & Koch, 1986); V1 (Li, 2002); V1 and V2 (Lee, Itti, Koch, & Braun, 1999); pulvinar (Petersen, Robinson, & Morris, 1987, Posner & Petersen, 1990; Robinson & Petersen, 1992); FEF (Thompson, Bichot, & Schall, 1997); parietal areas (Gottlieb, Kusunoki, & Goldberg, 1998). In each of these, the connection to a saliency representation is made because maxima of response that are found within a neural population correspond with the attended location. Each of the examined areas has such correlated maxima; could it be that they all do simultaneously? Perhaps this is why evidence has been found in so many areas for the neural correlate to the saliency map. Maybe saliency is a distributed computation, and, like attention itself, evidence reflecting these computations can be found in many, if not all, neural populations.

Related and worth mentioning is the approach of Amit and Geman (1998) because it learns to determine what sort of input patterns are salient. That is, what groupings of basic features are rare in the background of an image yet likely to appear as part of objects. This learning approach has shown its utility in subsequent work, notably the AIM model of Bruce and Tsotsos (2005, 2009).

The Temporal Tagging Hypothesis   The earliest conceptualization of this idea seems to be due to Grossberg, who between 1973 and 1980 presented ideas and theoretical arguments regarding the relationship among neural oscillations, visual perception, and attention (e.g., Grossberg 1980), leading to the **ART** model that provided details on how neurons may reach stable states given both top-down and bottom-up signals and play roles in attention and learning (Grossberg, 1982). Milner also suggested that the unity of a figure at the neuronal level is defined by synchronized firing activity (Milner, 1974). Von der Malsburg (1981) wrote that neural modulation is governed by correlations in temporal structure of signals and that timing correlations signal objects. He defined a detailed model of how this might be accomplished, including neurons with dynamically modifiable synaptic strengths that became known as **von der Malsburg synapses**. Crick and Koch (1990) later proposed that an attentional mechanism binds together all those neurons whose activity relates to the relevant features of a single visual object. This is done by generating coherent semisynchronous oscillations in the 40- to 70-Hz range. These oscillations then activate a transient short-term memory. Singer and Gray's Temporal Correlation Hypothesis is summarized in (Singer & Gray, 1995), where supporting evidence is detailed. Models subscribing to this hypothesis typically consist of pools of excitatory and inhibitory neurons whose actions are governed by sets of differential equations; it is a dynamical system. Strong support for this view appears in a nice summary by Sejnowski and Paulsen (2006). The models of Hummel and Biederman (1992), Deco and Zihl (2001), Corchs and Deco (2001), and Deco, Pollatos, and Zihl (2002) are within this class. This hypothesis remains controversial (see Shadlen & Movshon, 1999).

The Emergent Attention Hypothesis   The emergent attention hypothesis proposes that attention is a property of large assemblies of neurons involved in competitive interactions (of the kind mediated by lateral connections), and selection is the combined result of local dynamics and top-down biases. In other words, there is no explicit selection process of any kind. Duncan (1979) provided an early discussion of properties of attention having an emergent quality in the context of divided attention. Grossberg's 1982 **ART** model also played a formative role here. Such an emergent view took further root with work on the role of emergent features in attention by Pomerantz and Pristach (1989) and Treisman and Paterson (1984). Later, Styles (1997) suggested that attentional behavior emerges as a result of the complex underlying processing in the brain. Shipp's (2004) review concludes that this is the most likely hypothesis. The models of Hamker (1999, 2000, 2005), Deco and Zihl (2001), and Corchs and Deco (2001) and Heinke and Humphreys Selective Attention for Identification Model (**SAIM**) (1997) belong in this class among others. Desimone and Duncan (1995) seem to suggest that their biased competition model is a member of this class, writing "attention is an emergent property of slow, competitive interactions that work in parallel across the visual field." In turn, many of the models in this class are also strongly based on Biased Competition. Finally from chapter 1, recall how the Gestaltists also thought of attention as an emergent phenomenon; they might be considered the roots of this hypothesis.

It seems as if at least some aspect of each of the four hypotheses may play an important role in our overall understanding of attention, yet few theories have emerged that successfully combine hypotheses. There are many possible combinations, and these are illustrated in figure 3.3. Example models within each of the four major ovals of the diagram were presented above. At the intersections there are a few examples: The Olshausen et al. (1993) model and the AIM model of Bruce and Tsotsos (2005, 2009) are really combinations of the Saliency Map and Selective Routing hypotheses; a nice combination of Emergent Attention and Temporal Tagging can be found in Grossberg's ART family of models and the Deco group models (Corchs & Deco, 2001; Deco & Zihl, 2001); Saliency Maps and Emergent Attention are components of the model of Lanyon and Denham (2004); finally, Hamker's model exhibits elements of the Emergent Attention, Saliency Maps and Selective Routing Hypotheses (Hamker 2005). Future research on the eight unexplored combinations may prove fruitful.

Other Relevant Ideas

It is important to stress that the text discussion above, no matter how extensive it might appear, does not really capture the full breadth of experiment and theory that has been published. A few examples of major results can demonstrate this, while recognizing that this will still not be complete.

Although this book will not deal with attention and memory at all, important studies on this relationship have appeared, beginning with a classic one. How atten-

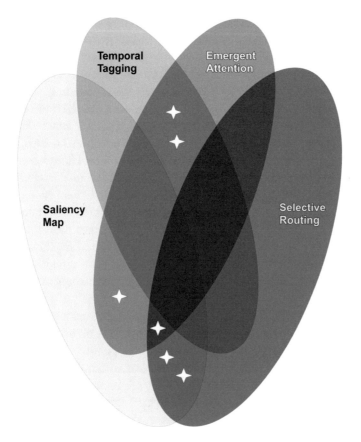

Figure 3.3
A Venn diagram of the four major theoretical hypotheses described in this chapter and their combinations, a total of 15 possibilities. The stars represent existing models that combine hypotheses as described in the text.

tion may interact with perceptual memory was first investigated by Sperling (1960), who observed that cues that follow a visual display by a short fraction of a second can be used to select information from a brief sensory memory system that seems to hold much more than the subject was able to report (the **partial report task**).

How one might learn to attend, computationally or developmentally, will also not be considered in this book, although it is clear that it might have important impact on theories of attention. Good examples for the interested reader can be found in the Grossberg papers cited earlier (perhaps the earliest works on this topic), Olson and Sherman (1983), Shiffrin and Schneider (1977), Whitehead and Ballard (1990), Mozer, Zemel, Behrmann, and Williams (1992), Triesch, Ballard, Hayhoe, and Sullivan (2003), among others.

A number of authors have suggested a variety of mechanisms that may play a role in attention. Hillyard, Vogel, and Luck (1998) suggest that sensory gain amplification operates in early stages of extrastriate processing looking at ERP (event-related potential) population measures in humans. Ghose and Maunsell (2008) propose that spatial summation suffices to account for neural modulations in monkey area V4 during an attentive task. Maunsell and Treue (2006) and Martinez-Trujillo and Treue (2004) argue for feature-based attention (as opposed to location- or object-based strategies) and give evidence for this using single-cell studies in monkey area MT. Roelfsema, Lamme, and Spekreijse (1998) and Valdes-Sosa, Bobes, Rodriquez, and Pinilla (1998) argue for object-based mechanisms, something that has not made its way into the models as much as one might hope.

These are all concepts tied to single-neuron characteristics. A proposal that is at the system level in the sense that it addresses properties of more than one visual area is that of Buschman and Miller (2007). Recording from monkey, they found prefrontal neurons reflected the target location first during top-down attention, whereas parietal neurons signaled it earlier during bottom-up attention. Synchrony between frontal and parietal areas was stronger in lower frequencies during top-down attention and in higher frequencies during bottom-up attention. They conclude that top-down signals arise from frontal cortex and bottom-up signals arise from the sensory cortex, respectively, and different modes of attention may emphasize synchrony at different frequencies. This study followed on another that showed that monkey V4 neurons activated by an attended stimulus showed increased gamma frequency synchronization and reduced lower frequency synchronization in comparison with other V4 neurons (Fries, Reynolds, Rorie, & Desimone, 2001).

Moore and Fallah (2004) tested the hypothesis that saccade preparation biases visual detection at the location to which the saccade is prepared. The authors found that when they stimulated sites within the FEF (using currents too weak to evoke a movement), it led to improved detection of visual events at the location represented by neurons at the stimulation site. Thompson, Biscoe, and Sato (2005) demonstrated attentional modulation of FEF neurons in a task that does not involve a saccadic eye movement. The authors find that of the three major classes of neurons—visual, visuomovement, and movement—defined in a standard memory-guided saccade task, it is the visual and visuomovement neurons that are modulated by attention. The movement neurons appeared to be suppressed, thus demonstrating that the functional divergence of covert and overt signals occurs in FEF.

More on the modeling side, Salinas and Abbott (1997) present the idea of an **attentional gain field**, a mathematical realization of single-neuron gain modulation in translation invariant receptive fields. They demonstrate how, using a model of V4 neurons feeding a single IT neuron, the attentional gain field might be used to transform images from a retinal representation to a more object-centered form that may be used for invariant recognition

More generally, Schall (2001) reviews neural mechanisms of choice, decision making, and action. He concludes that their neural correlates are not too complex to identify or even manipulate. In some experimental domains, an agent's choice appears to rely on the activation of a small number of neurons in discrete brain areas. By monitoring those signals, an experimenter can predict and even influence what monkeys will choose, even though we do not yet know how these signals are produced by the circuits of the brain. This deterministic, algorithmic perspective is consistent with the overall perspective in this book.

This is only a beginning, and there is much more that is not possible to include here. An excellent set of papers on the full breadth of attention can be found in Itti et al. (2005).

Summary

The main conclusion here is that one chapter can hardly do justice to the literature on attention and theories suggested to explain it. Nevertheless, it seems that there is too great an emphasis on finding explanations or models of the phenomenology rather than on seeking an explanation of the underlying causes of the phenomenon. Further, the view that attention is some monolithic mechanism is not justifiable. In many models, this seems to be the prevailing view. Even though the breadth and diversity of theories and models is enormous, there seems to be much room for future investigations as the Venn diagram of figure 3.3 shows. The reality seems to be that there are elements of each of the four major proposals within the observed performance of human attentive vision. The question then is which are the relevant ideas, how to combine them, and how to examine the space of what we might not yet know so that we may arrive at an overall theory of vision and attention? Here, it is argued that attention is a *set* of mechanisms (such as the list given in the earlier section "The Elements of Visual Attention") the goal of which is to tune the search processes inherent in perception and cognition. The list of attentional elements also in that section provides a starting point for any theory, and the list of mechanisms is proposed as a first-order mechanistic counterpart to those elements. In other words, there is no single mechanism of attention.

The argument is not without its controversy (see Pastukhov, Fischer, & Braun, 2009). The reason that we suggest it is a set is due to its cause. As mentioned earlier, the goal here is to search for the cause of attention and not focus on only its manifestations. At the first principles level, the cause is the mismatch between the computational complexity of vision and the brain's neural machinery. This has been formalized in chapter 2, and no *single* solution exists save for the evolution of a

much larger brain. The reason that no single solution exists has to do with the mul-
tivariate nature of the problem. Although earlier, two variables of relevance were
described (pixels and features), there are many more ranging from neural packag-
ing, heat management, and nutrient and waste transport to more computational
issues such as memory, connectivity, transmission speed, and more. No single mechanism could possibly optimize all of this effectively. In any case, as is well known in
all engineering tasks, simultaneously optimizing many interrelated variables can
only be dealt with by defining sufficient criteria for a solution. Optimizing one variable often leads to suboptimal values for another, and as a result a globally satisficing solution is what is sought in practice. Even if we restrict consideration to visual
processes, it is very difficult to be precise about the nature of the objective function
for this optimization, although it is clear that minimizing processing time, minimizing neural cost, and maximizing correctness of perception are primary ingredients.

The elements of attention presented provide a set of very tough constraints for
any theory. There is no denying that experimental observations exhibit characteristics of emergence, saliency, selective routing, and synchrony. Similarly, there is no
denying that the decomposition of attentional mechanisms or elements, such as
appears in this chapter (likely incomplete), is complex. The difficulty is not how to
provide an explanation for each of them—the very abbreviated listing of proposed
mechanisms of the previous section shows some of this. Rather, the problem is how
to define a theory that covers *all* of those elements without it being simply a sum
of separate solutions. Add in the constraints that arose in chapter 2, namely, the
ones arising from the complexity analysis and those due to information flow in the
main data structure, and the challenge is great. The next chapter takes on that challenge and outlines a candidate proposal.

4 Selective Tuning: Overview

The previous chapter ended with the suggestion that most theories and models of visual attention emphasize explanations for the observed characteristics of attention rather than the causes of attention. In chapter 2, we tried to show from 'first principles' that the primary reason for attention is the mismatch between the computational complexity of general visual information processing and the processing capacity of the brain. The 'first principles' arise because vision is formulated as a decision problem (a problem requiring a decision on the success of a search task) and analyzed using methods from complexity theory, which is concerned with the cost of achieving solutions to such problems. The discussion featured nine theorems and their proofs that one might consider as part of the theoretical foundation for vision science as a whole. The key aspect is that with the general definition of vision, there can be no physical realization of any kind. There would then be two possible solutions: Make the brain larger and more powerful (the fixed size of input could make this possible) or make the problem it needs to solve easier and less costly. Assuming the former is not an option at this time (although evolution might be on that path anyway!), the latter option is the one examined in this book. The question then becomes how to make the smallest changes to the problem so that it becomes sufficiently less costly to solve but also retains the essential character of the original problem definition. In other words, how can the original problem of vision be reshaped so that the brain can solve a good approximation to it with the available processing power? This is where an examination of the problem complexity in a deeper sense comes in, and the latter parts of chapter 2 detailed the kinds of architectural optimizations and approximations that might help. These in turn revealed additional issues to be addressed. Taken together, it is clear that the brain is not solving the general problem of vision as first stated—that it can never solve it—and that what the brain must be solving is a sufficiently close approximation so that in the visual world where we exist, the solution gives the illusion of general vision.

The result of that analysis is the **Selective Tuning** model of visual attention—indeed, perhaps more broadly of visual processing as a whole—and its overview is the subject of this chapter. The Selective Tuning (ST) model was first described in Tsotsos (1990a) with its theoretical foundations in Tsotsos (1987, 1988a, 1989). The first papers to describe the mechanisms that realize ST appeared in Tsotsos (1991b), Culhane and Tsotsos (1992), and Tsotsos (1993), and the first implementations were described in Culhane and Tsotsos (1992), Tsotsos (1995b) and Tsotsos et al. (1995) where the name *Selective Tuning* also first appeared. Extensions of the model can be found in Lai (1992), Wai and Tsotsos (1994), Dolson (1997), Liu (2002), Zhou (2004), Zaharescu et al. (2005), Simine (2006), Tsotsos et al. (2005), Tsotsos, Rodriguez-Sanchez, Rothenstein, and Simine (2008), Bruce and Tsotsos (2005, 2009), Rodriguez-Sanchez, Simine and Tsotsos (2007), and Rothenstein, Rodriguez-Sanchez, Simine and Tsotsos (2008). Selective Tuning incorporates many of the strategies described in the previous section and makes important predictions that, since their presentation, have been strongly supported experimentally.

This chapter will give a broad overview of the model and theory without any mathematics. Chapter 5 will provide mathematical and algorithmic details. Chapter 6 will extend the model to show how attention, recognition, and binding are interrelated. Examples of the operation and performance of ST will follow in chapter 7, and details about the biological relevance of the model will be provided in chapter 8.

The Basic Model

The visual processing architecture is pyramidal in structure: layers of neurons with decreasing spatial resolution, but increasing abstraction and complexity of selectivity in higher layers. A hypothetical pyramid is caricatured in figure 2.5. The connections shown are based on the same observations and conclusions that Salin and Bullier (1995), Lamme and Roelsfema (2000), and Bullier (2001) describe. There are both feedback (recurrent) and feed-forward connections for each neuron, and the spatial extent of connectivity is reciprocal. Each neuron has diverging connections to the next highest layer and receives converging input from neurons in the previous layer. Similarly, each neuron provides diverging feedback signals to lower layers and receives converging feedback from higher layers. Finally, each neuron has lateral connections to its neighbors. There is no assumption that there is only one 'processing stream' (such as dorsal or ventral), and the model allows complex lattices of processing layers.

Decisions on the perceived stimulus are based on the level where the information appropriate for the task is computed. This may be at the topmost layer if the task is categorization, for example, or in one of the middle layers if the task is identification. In ST, decisions are made in a competitive manner as first described in Tsotsos (1990a) using the task-modulated (or biased) responses of neurons throughout the processing network. The main goal is to determine which neurons and pathways best represent the input, given a task to be performed. This is a key characteristic of the theory and distinguishes ST from other theories. The full representation of a scene, object, or event includes the full set of neurons and connecting pathways that are determined to best respond to it. This differs from the classic population representation; here all neurons and pathways play a representational role, from category of an object, for example, down to all the details of its appearance and location.

The selection strategy of ST relies on a hierarchical process. Recall the Routing Problem analysis of the section "Complexity Constrains Visual Processing Architecture" of chapter 2. There, the search problem of finding the pathway of neurons that best represent the input was quantified, and top-down search was identified as the more appropriate strategy. If the search starts at the top, the search for best response(s) at that layer must consider R_L neurons. Once the top-layer best response is determined, the next search is only over the afferents to that best response, and so on recursively downward. In this way, the process breaks up the search into $L - 1$ consecutive searches over C connections. The resulting time complexity is $O(LC)$, a tractable function in comparison with the exponential one of the chapter 2 section "Complexity Constrains Visual Processing Architecture." This expression is valid only for single-neuron pathways; if pathways involve more than one neuron (say for an object that is represented by many neurons over a contiguous spatial extent), then the function degrades in terms of its complexity. Say that some subset of the connections s_λ at each level λ of the pyramid represents the number of connections for an object's contiguous spatial extent. Then the search complexity would become

$$O\left(\sum_{\lambda=1}^{L-1} C s_\lambda \right),$$

larger but still a tractable polynomial function. This general algorithm is an instance of **Branch-and-Bound**, a classic mechanism that is used for such a task in optimization problems (Lawler & Wood, 1966). Recursive pruning within the branch-and-bound strategy is especially useful for a hierarchical system.

Fuster reached a rather similar conclusion but without any mathematical formalization:

[I]f the relevance of a stimulus feature depends on its context, any influences that attention may have on cells that respond to that feature will arrive to those cells after analysis of the context that signals the relevance of the feature. The time taken by that analysis will be reflected by a relatively long latency of attention-modulated cell responses to the relevant feature. (Fuster, 1990, p. 682)

Interestingly, the hierarchical, top-down, recursive pruning strategy of ST not only has good complexity characteristics, but it also in one stroke provides solutions to the Routing, Context, Blurring, Cross-talk, and Sampling Problems of chapter 2 (the

Boundary Problem requires a different mechanism to be presented later in this chapter). The result of the top-down search yields the set of pathways that connect the stimulus in the input layer to the neurons that best represent it at each layer of the hierarchy; that is, a solution to the Routing Problem. This structure is the key output of attention because all of the information extracted by the visual system about its attended stimulus is unified, and thus, details in terms of location, extent, features, composition are also within that structure. Contextual interference has been ameliorated or eliminated by the pruning process yielding a suppressive region surrounding the attended stimulus, the loss of localization exemplified by the Blurring Problem no longer is an issue, and there is no Cross-talk as the attended stimulus has been isolated throughout the processing hierarchy.

We are now ready to provide an overview of the basic Selective Tuning algorithm. It is important that the basic algorithm function appropriately under both task-direction and free-viewing conditions. If a task is given, then at the beginning of any task—say, for example, a visual search task—subjects are provided with information about the task. This may include what the stimuli will be, where will they appear, what is the goal, how to respond, and so forth. A free-viewing situation would have no such additional specific starting point; however, the body of knowledge and experience we all have learned certainly plays a role in setting up the default values for task requirements. If we are walking, enjoying a nice sunny day along a seashore, our world model has little to do with driving on a snow- and ice-covered road in a blizzard! These expectations clearly play a role; imagine our shock if as we breathe in a lung-full of salty sea breeze, we immediately find ourselves behind the wheel of a car in an uncontrollable skid on an icy road! Task information affects processing as has been shown by Yarbus (1967) and in all experimental work since the Posner cueing paradigm was first presented (Posner et al., 1978), if not earlier. There is no reason to believe that our world model, due to our knowledge and experience, does not also play a similar role even though it may be only an implicit one or a have limited impact.

Let us begin with a pyramid of neurons, as described in chapter 2, all in their rest state. Task information—explicit or implicit—affects such a blank processing pyramid, as shown in figure 4.1a by inhibition of task-irrelevant computations [Melcher, Papathomas, and Vidnyánsky (2005) have observed the same effect with attention to one feature and its modulation of all task-irrelevant computations in the visual field]. Figure 4.1b shows this top-down pass through the pyramid, and the subsequent coloring of the pyramid is meant to represent the fact that the whole pyramid is affected by this inhibition. For the sake of this description, let us say that the task leads to a subject's expectation of a centrally located stimulus, and as a result, the noncentral region (in this example, the extent is hypothetical) is inhibited (darker shading means greater suppression) throughout the pyramid and remains so through the several stages of processing; it thus continues to reduce the extent of the pyramid that is active in any competitive process.

When a stimulus is presented to the input layer of the pyramid (figure 4.1c), it activates in a feed-forward manner all of the units within the pyramid with receptive fields (RFs) that include the stimulus location; the result is a diverging cone of activity within the processing pyramid. It is assumed that response strength of units in the network is a measure of goodness-of-match of the stimulus within the RF to the model that determines the selectivity of that unit. We term the portion of each layer that is affected the neuron's **projective field** [similar to Lehky and Sejnowski's (1988) use of the term but with the difference that we limit the projection to feed-forward connections].

The basic decision-making process that will be used is the same as in most other models—search for maximum response over a set of neurons. Winner-Take-All is a parallel algorithm for finding the maximum value in a set. ST uses a unique formulation that is detailed in the next chapter [Valiant (1975) provides optimality conditions for all parallel comparison algorithms; discussion on how the ST algorithm approaches the optimal values described by Valiant appears in Tsotsos et al. 1995]. First, a WTA process operates across the entire visual field at the top layer where it computes the global winner; that is, the unit(s) with largest response (see figure 4.1d). The global winner activates a WTA that operates only over its direct inputs to select the strongest responding region within its RF. Next, all of the feed-forward connections in the visual pyramid that do not contribute to the winner are pruned (inhibited). This strategy of finding the winners within successively smaller RFs, layer by layer, in the pyramid and then pruning away irrelevant connections through inhibition is applied recursively through the pyramid. As a result, the input to the higher-level unit changes, and thus its output changes. The projective field shrinks in each layer as the pruning process proceeds down the pyramid. We suggest that this is the source of the well-observed attentional modulation of single-neuron responses. This refinement of unit responses is important; it provides a solution to the signal interference problem described earlier. By the end of this refinement process, the output of the attended units at the top layer will be the same as if the attended stimulus appeared on a blank field. The paths remaining may be considered the pass zone of the attended stimulus, and the pruned paths form the inhibitory zone of an attentional beam (figure 4.1d). A final feed-forward pass, if the task requires it, permits reinterpretation of the stimulus by all neurons within the pass zone with context reduced or removed. However, this final pass is not strictly ordered as shown in figure 4.1e, and the feed-forward changes arise while the recurrent pass is in progress.

An executive controller is responsible for implementing the sequence of operations depicted in figure 4.1, and for this level of description the following algorithm plays the executive role:

Algorithm 4.1

1. Acquire any explicit task information, store in working memory.

2. Apply top-down biases based on explicit task information or any applicable implicit knowledge, inhibiting units that compute task-irrelevant quantities; set up task-completion criteria.

3. See the stimulus activating feature pyramids in a feed-forward manner.

4. Activate top-down WTA process at top layers of the pyramid representation.

5. Implement a layer-by-layer top-down search using the layer-by-layer results of the WTA, suppressing connections from losing neurons (branch-and-bound).

6. After completion, permit time for refined stimulus computation to complete a second feed-forward pass, if needed. Note that this feed-forward refinement does not begin with the completion of the lowermost WTA process; rather, it occurs simultaneously with completing WTA processes (step 5) as they proceed downward in the hierarchy. On completion of the lowermost WTA, some additional time is required for the completion of the feed-forward refinement.

7. Extract items selected by the attentional beam within the task-relevant layers and place in working memory for task verification.

8. Inhibit pass zone connections to permit the next most salient item to be processed.

This multipass process may not appear to reflect the reality of biological processes that seem very fast. However, it is not claimed that all of these steps are needed for all tasks; this issue will be reexamined in a later chapter.

Saliency and Its Role in ST

At first blush, it might appear as if ST uses a hierarchical version of a data-driven saliency map, that the top layer of the processing network is in fact the same as the saliency map as used by others, with a winner-take-all algorithm to make next fixation decisions. But this is not the case. The early demonstrations of ST may have appeared to be this (Culhane & Tsotsos, 1992; Tsotsos et al., 1995) but were intended to show how the hierarchical attentional mechanism performs and made no statement about the representations over which the algorithm operates. In fact, the whole point was to show that the algorithm performs correctly regardless of

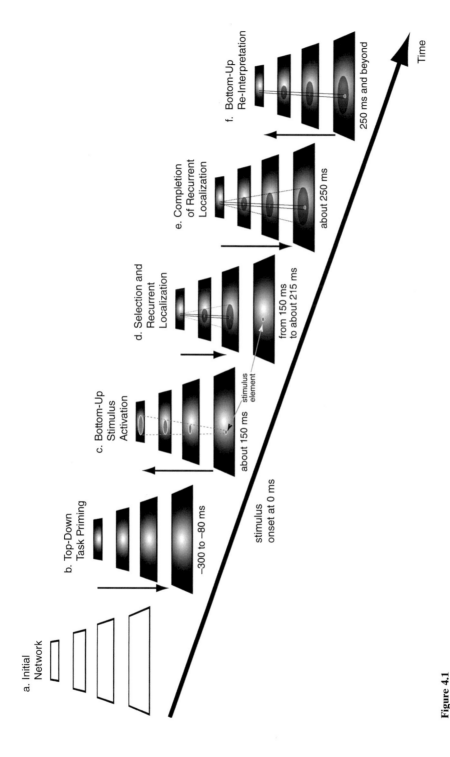

Figure 4.1
The stages of Selective Tuning processing. The processing pyramid shows six different stages of computation from its initial, blank state (white means unaffected) to priming, then stimulus activation, and so on. Dark shading means those spatial portions of the representation are suppressed. Lighter shading means less or no suppression.

representation. To be sure, a kind of saliency was implied, but this is not the kind of global conspicuity proposed by Koch and Ullman (1985) and by Itti et al. (1998). In ST, neural response as a measure of goodness-of-fit to the neuron's tuning profile is the corresponding input to the winner-take-all algorithm. The peak across a population of like-tuned neurons across the visual field is what our WTA seeks. This is not related to saliency or conspicuity mathematically because it is not a measure that is comparative [with relation to its surround as computed in Itti et al. (1998)] nor is it a measure that combines all feature maps on a point-by-point basis into a new representation.

In ST, the notion of saliency as a global measure is used in the fixation mechanism, to be described in the next section, and only there. It is part of the solution to the Boundary Problem of chapter 2; as such, the fact that it is applied only to the periphery of the visual field is yet another characteristic that distinguishes it from saliency map models.

Selective Tuning with Fixation Control

The earlier sections of this chapter show how ST deals with the Routing, Cross-talk, Context, Blurring, and Sampling Problems; the Boundary Problem remains. Previous solutions for the Boundary Problem have concentrated on extending the edges of the input images in a variety of ways (van der Wal & Burt, 1992) to enable convolutions at the edges to have full, albeit fake, input for their computation. These methods included simple extension of the image using blank elements or repeated elements from the image, mirror images, wraparound images, and attempts to discover compensatory weighting functions. If a multilevel representation was used, they ensured that the hierarchy has few layers with little change in resolution between layers to reduce the size of boundary affected. However, a different and more biologically plausible solution exists if one simply remembers that the eyes can move. Suppose that instead of artificially altering the input layer size and contents, an independent mechanism is provided that can detect peripheral salient items separately and saccade to fixate them, thus bringing them to the central region and allowing veridical processing. To detect the most salient item in the input layer peripheral annulus, an independent selection mechanism is required whose inputs are representations of early layers before the Boundary Problem becomes significant. This idea first appeared in Tsotsos et al. (1995). What is needed here is a true representation of saliency in the periphery of the visual field, where the extent of that periphery is defined by the extent of the Boundary Problem. If the spatial width of the filters at each level of the pyramid is known, call the width of the filter at layer i z_i, and the first layer of the pyramid, layer 1, is the image, then the width of the annulus around the edge of the visual field where such a saliency computation is required can be defined as $\sum_{i=1}^{L} 0.5z_i$ for a pyramid with L layers. In fact, because task requirements tune processing throughout, the actual information represented is more like that discussed by Fecteau and Munoz (2006). As result, here it is named the **Peripheral Priority Map** (PPM). A simple algorithm emerges:

Algorithm 4.2

1. Compute both the overall strongest response at the top (call this the **Next Central Focus**; NCF) and in the PPM.

2. Combine the two representations to create a full field priority representation.

3. Choose the location or region with the highest priority; that is, with the largest neural response. If a peripheral item is stronger than the central item, move the eye to fixate it; otherwise the central item is the one attended covertly.

Saccades have been previously described that appear to have similar function (Hallett, 1978; Whittaker & Cummings, 1990). These saccades are elicited in response to a visual stimulus in the periphery (differences most apparent with ≥10° eccentricity) where the exact location of the stimulus is unpredictable. The saccade results in the approximate foveation of the stimulus. Those authors hypothesized that a separate mechanism must be present to drive these special saccades. In monkey, parieto-occipital area (PO) seems to have the connectivity described earlier in addition to representing the visual field outside of the central 10° and may be a candidate region for this function (Colby, Gattass, Olson, & Gross, 1988). In ST, the central region is treated differently from the periphery specifically to deal with the Boundary Problem; the two separate representations are clear in figure 4.2. The **Central Attentional Field** in the figure represents the central 10° of the visual field and all the responses of neurons of the top layer of the pyramid whose RFs are within this central area. The **Peripheral Attentional Field** in the figure represents the neural responses of early layers of the pyramid, say V1, V2, MT—areas early enough in the pyramid to have not been too strongly affected by the Boundary Problem—in the region outside the central 10° area.

The simple algorithm above hides a problem. Once the eyes move away from a fixation point, how does fixation not return to that point over and over (i.e., how does fixation not oscillate between strongest and second-strongest locations)? In the original Koch and Ullman (1985) formulation, location inhibition was included after an item was attended so that attention may shift to the next most salient item. In fact, the mathematics of the winner-take-all selection process demands this by definition—if one does not remove the current winner, the algorithm will blindly re-find this as the maximum in the set of its inputs. All models seem to have reached the same conclusion on this point. If however the covert system is linked with the overt system, a new dimension is added to the inhibition. Not only must locations within an image be inhibited but also locations outside the current image. When the eyes move to attend a peripheral item, previously attended items may not be present in the new image. Subsequent movement of fixation may bring those previously attended locations back into view; the result would be an oscillating system. This Inhibition of Return (IOR; Posner et al., 1985) plays an important computational role, but not with the breadth of that suggested experimentally (Klein, 2000). Here, we include a **Fixation History Map** (FHM), a representation of 2D visual space larger than the visual field containing the sequence of recent fixations, and it provides the source of location information for IOR used in a subsequent computation. Interestingly, Tark and Curtis (2009), using functional magnetic resonance imaging, found evidence for the frontal eye field (FEF) to be an important neural mechanism for visual working memory. Subjects performed an audio-spatial working-memory task using sounds recorded from microphones placed in each subject's ear canals. FEF activity persisted when maintaining auditory-cued space, even for locations behind the head to which it is impossible to make saccades. Therefore, they concluded that human FEF activity represents both retinal and extraretinal space, and as such, it is a good candidate for the FHM functionality that ST requires.

The FHM is centered at the current eye fixation and represents space in a gaze-centered system. The FHM is constructed as a 2D map that encodes position in the world; previously fixated locations are marked as 'on' and others 'off.' The 'on' locations decay to 'off' with a time constant that is either some default value or one that is set by task needs. These are all reset to 'off' at the end of the task. The FHM is updated on each fixation with an associated saccade history shift with direction and magnitude opposite to the trajectory of the eye movement so that correct relative positions of fixation points are maintained (Colby & Goldberg, 1999; Duhamel et al., 1992; see also Zaharescu et al., 2005). Further, a simple task influence plays a role here. If the task is sufficiently complex to require multiple fixations of the same item, then this task influence can reset the decay of fixation inhibition. It is doubtful that this will suffice in the general case; this does not address specific object-based IOR nor task-related issues that may override IOR (see Klein, 2000). Consider it as a first step.

The main fixation decision is made using the **History-Biased Priority Map** (HBPM), the closest representation in ST to the saliency map (Itti et al., 1998; Koch & Ullman, 1985). One difference is that the Saliency Map Model always has eye movement as output, whereas our model permits both covert and overt fixations. A second difference is that in the central area only one location is represented, the NCF, and in the periphery, priority is computed. Third, the particular computation differs as outlined earlier. A final difference is that this representation is always modulated by task demands that inhibit task-irrelevant locations and feature contributions (because the feed-forward computations on which both the NCF and the PPM is based are task-biased in advance). Like the Saliency Map Model, previous fixations are inhibited using the FHM representation. Our HBPM is more closely related to the Priority Map of Fecteau and Munoz (2006).

Algorithm 4.3 (and figure 4.2) describes the sequence of actions involved in one attentive cycle (the bold phrases refer to items in figure 4.2). The ordering of actions coarsely reflects their temporal sequence.

The level of resolution of the HBPM is an issue because it is the source of location information for saccade planning; it is necessarily coarse, perhaps at best, at the level of the number of columns in V1. As a result, the precision of each saccade is limited. If the fixation misses the target by a little so that the target falls within the suppressive surround of the resulting localization, then the target is not seen. It can only be seen when the suppression is released, and in the context of the algorithm this occurs after a commitment to make an eye movement has been made. Sheinberg and Logothetis (2001) describe such 'double take' saccades.

The elegant aspect of this framework is that it cleanly shows the extent of Neisser's (1967)—and then Wolfe, Klempen and Dahlen's (2000)—preattentive, attentive, and postattentive vision stages; Posner's (1980) orienting, alerting, and search functions of attention; and the saliency map/master map of locations of Koch and Ullman (1985) and Treisman and Gelade (1980). The preattentive stage begins with step 1 and ends with the completion of step 3. The attentive phase is between steps 4 and 9a (if required). The postattentive phase is composed of step 9b. Posner's alerting function is represented by the competition that selects the next target in step 6. His orienting process is the set of steps that realize the next fixation, namely steps 7 and 8a, and the search function is 9a. Finally, figure 4.2 shows ST's counterpart to the saliency map, the History-Biased Priority Map. But it is not quite a match; the Koch and Ullman saliency map does not include any task bias, and in ST all representations are biased by task. The closest may be that of Navalpakkam and Itti (2003) where task biases are included.

Algorithm 4.3

1. In advance of a new task, the **FHM** contains some sct of previously viewed locations.

2. Prime the processing network with **Task Information** using a top-down traversal of the processing network to **Suppress Task-Irrelevant Computations** (as step 2 of Algorithm 4.1).

3. Stimulus appears at input layer causing **Feed-Forward Activation** of neurons. During this feed-forward activation, representations in the **Peripheral Attentional Field** from the early layers of the pyramid are combined to derive the **Peripheral Priority Map**.

4. **Select** the **Next Central Focus** from the **Central Attentional Field**.

5. Combine **Next Central Focus, Peripheral Priority Map,** and FHM into **HBPM**. **FHM** negatively biases the **HBPM**.

6. **Select** the next fixation target, biased by **Task Information**.

7. **Update Fixation History Map** with the new fixation point shifting other remembered fixations appropriately in space. Task Information can reset decay time constants as needed.

8. Decide on an appropriate action for the winning fixation target:

  8a. If target is a peripheral one, then **Plan Overt Shift**

   8a-1. **Disengage Attention**, releasing suppressive surround if present;

   8a-2. Foveate target via **Saccade-Pursuit Controller** using location from **HBPM**;

   8a-3. Allow time for **Feed-Forward Activation** through pyramid;

   8a-4. **Select** neurons to attend in top layer.

  8b. If target is the central one, then **Plan Covert Shift** (if attention is to be maintained on same item, skip 8b-1)

   8b-1. **Disengage Attention**, releasing suppressive surround if present;

   8b-2. Attend **NCF** neurons in top layer.

9. If the task requires more than detection or categorization, then

  9a. Deploy the **localization/surround suppression** process;

  9b. **Reinterpret** the stimulus after surround suppression.

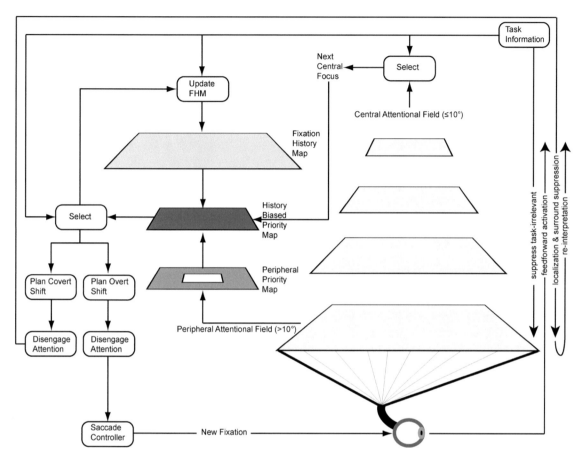

Figure 4.2
ST with fixation control. The diagram illustrates the algorithm in the text.

Differences with Other Models

First of all, ST does not rely on a single saliency map for all its attentional functionality. The view that attention is a *set* of mechanisms is the main distinguishing feature
between this model and others, particularly those that are direct descendants of the
original 1985 model of Koch and Ullman, which itself was an attempt to realize
Feature Integration Theory (Treisman & Gelade, 1980). The original Saliency Map
Model dealt only with the selection of a single spatial point of interest, of maximum
conspicuity. The first implementation and simulation of it was due to Sandon (1990).
Later, Itti and colleagues developed a new and expanded implementation (Itti et
al., 1998). He and his group have added task bias, motion, and other elements to it.

Throughout this development, the original form of the saliency model has remained intact and does not deal with attentive effects in any other representation of visual processing. The Selective Tuning view of attention includes [in fact predicted, in Tsotsos (1990a), figures 7 and 8, p. 440)] effects due to attentive processing throughout the visual processing network. The statement there is even stronger; attention *controls* the subnetwork that feeds neurons at the top of the visual processing hierarchy. To quote the description in that paper of the attentional beam idea (that also appeared in Tsotsos, 1988b):

> The output of a given unit at the top of the hierarchy is directly affected by the sub-hierarchy for which it is the root. Thus the beam must affect the branches and leaves of the selected sub-tree. The beam expands as it traverses the hierarchy, covering all portions of the processing mechanism that directly contribute to the output at its point of entry at the top. In other words, the effective receptive field of the output unit selected for attention is that entire sub-hierarchy, and the attentional beam must control that receptive field. The central portion of the beam allows the stimulus of interest to pass through unaffected, while the remainder of the beam selectively inhibits portions of the processing hierarchy that may give rise to interfering signals.

Recently, Gilbert and Sigman (2007) have suggested exactly the same.

ST uses recurrent tracing of connections to achieve localization. The idea of tracing back connections in a top-down fashion was present in the NeoCognitron model of Fukushima (1986) and suggested even earlier by Milner (1974). Within the Selective Tuning model, it was first described in Tsotsos (1991b, 1993), with accompanying details and proofs in Tsotsos et al. (1995). It also appeared later in the Reverse Hierarchy Model of Ahissar and Hochstein (1997). Only NeoCognitron and Selective Tuning provide realizations; otherwise, the two differ in all details. Fukushima's model included a maximum detector at the top layer to select the highest responding cell, and all other cells were set to their rest state. Only afferent paths to this cell are facilitated by action from efferent signals from this cell. In contrast, neural inhibition is the only action of ST, with no facilitation. The NeoCognitron competitive mechanism is lateral inhibition at the highest and intermediate levels. This lateral inhibition enhances the strongest single neurons thus assuming all spatial scales are represented explicitly, whereas ST finds regions of neurons, removing this unrealistic assumption. For ST, units losing the competition at the top are left alone and not affected at all—the nonattended visual world does not disappear as in NeoCognitron. ST's inhibition is only within afferent sets to winning units. This prediction of a space-limited suppressive surround firmly distinguishes the two approaches and, as the experiments described in chapter 8 will show, places ST ahead of NeoCognitron in terms of biological plausibility.

ST employs surround suppression in the spatial and feature domains to improve signal-to-noise ratio in neural response. Koch and Ullman's (1985) saliency map features a prediction that locations near the focus of attention are facilitated for next focus choice; the model includes a proximity effect that would favor shifts to neighboring locations (see p. 224 of their paper, the section titled "Proximity Preference"). In fact, Koch and Crick went on to show how an attentive suppressive surround was not biologically feasible, going through the options of attentive enhancement, suppression, and their combination in the development, explicitly rejecting the suppressive penumbra idea (Crick & Koch, 1990, p. 959). In Selective Tuning, this differs. Consider the following. Neurons have a preferred tuning, that is they are selective for certain kinds of stimuli. A preferred stimulus within its receptive field is the *signal* it seeks, whereas whatever else may lie within the receptive field is not of interest (the Context Problem); it can be considered *noise*. The overall response of the neuron is clearly a function of both the signal and the noise. The response to the signal would be maximized if the noise were suppressed (Reynolds et al., 1999). It was suggested that this might be realized using a Gaussian-shaped inhibition on the surround (Tsotsos, 1990a, pp. 439–440). This stood as a prediction for years but now enjoys a great deal of support. Also, this attentive suppression has an interesting side-effect: an apparent enhancement of neural response, because the 'noise' is removed (Tsotsos, 1990a, p. 441). This may be contrasted with the attention gain multiplier in the Biased Competition model. In ST the enhancement is a consequence of suppression, whereas in Biased Competition it is an explicit element. The points made in this paragraph are further detailed in chapter 8.

In general, ST differs greatly from Biased Competition. The Biased Competition (BC) model of visual attention has provided inspiration for many other studies and models (Desimone & Duncan, 1995; Reynolds et al., 1999). It is based on an equation that shows how an attentional bias may affect the response of a neuron that receives input from excitatory and inhibitory neuron pools. As a result, it shows how a receptive field might shrink-wrap a stimulus when it is attended. It also provides a good fit to the firing patterns of V4 neurons in macaque. In contrast, ST is not a single-neuron theory; BC is, as evidenced by the only formal description of it in Reynolds et al. (1999). BC does not provide a method for how a particular neuron may be selected nor for how attentional influence might arrive there. ST provides a network-based mechanism and shows how selection is accomplished and how the selection is communicated through the network. In BC, attention is just a multiplier, a constant integer value whose source and computation are left unspecified. They assume that attention has the effect of increasing the strength of signal coming from the population of cells activated by the attended stimulus. In ST, attention is a broad set of mechanisms, more closely connecting to the range of observations made by so many studies over the years. Finally, the effects of attentional modulation in biased competition are clearly manifested in a bottom-up order, from early to later visual areas, exactly the opposite from that in ST as well as exactly the opposite from experimental evidence (further detailed in chapter 8). A more detailed comparison of models will appear at the end of the next chapter once the mathematical formulation of ST is presented.

Summary

An overview of the ST theory shows its breadth and potential for its explanatory and predictive properties. This also shows the many ways in which ST is distinguished from others and, in most cases, has priority over many models for key ideas. By contrast with any other theory, ST integrates more of the functional elements of attention outlined in chapter 3. Within ST's algorithms and overall strategy, one can find commitments for the following elements: Alerting, Spatial Attentional Footprint, Covert Attention, Disengage Attention, Endogenous Influences, Engage Attention, Exogenous Influences, Inhibition of Return, Neural Modulation, Overt Attention, Postattention, Preattentive Features, Priming, Salience/Conspicuity Selection, Shift Attention, Search, Time Course, and Update Fixation History. Details on how these may be realized will be given in chapter 5. The Binding and Recognition elements will be presented in chapter 6. The weak element is the executive controller that is assumed outside the model at this time.

5 Selective Tuning: Formulation

The formulations of the elements included in the algorithms presented in the previous chapter are the subjects of this chapter. It is important to keep in mind—as was true in the early papers on the model—that there is no commitment to any particular decomposition of visual information (such as into edges or regions or surfaces, etc.) and that the model is applicable to any hierarchical decomposition as long as its basic assumptions are satisfied. These assumptions will be detailed as they arise throughout the chapter.

Objective

It was claimed in chapter 2 that attention is a set of mechanisms that tune the search processes inherent in vision. This tuning has the goal of optimizing but does not quite achieve optimality in the strict sense. Generally, optimization methods choose the best element from some set of available alternatives. This means finding values that best satisfy some objective function within a defined domain. As should be clear, the problem addressed here is multidimensional and has many variables, often conflicting, that must be simultaneously optimized. This necessarily involves trade-offs: to maximize one variable, another must be sacrificed. A typical multiobjective function could be considered that involves, say, functions Y_i, $1 \leq i \leq \eta$, which involve variables to be maximized, and functions Ω_j, $1 \leq j \leq v$, of variables to be minimized, each weighted by its relative importance. Although this is a normal procedure for such problems, things come to a grinding halt when one tries to characterize these functions and to know something about how to solve the overall objective for our domain. In other words, normally one needs to specify the variable ranges, any constraints among them that the solution must obey, whether this is a well-formed function, one that is differentiable, whether it is convex and has a unique global maximum or is a more complex landscape that needs different search methods, and so on (see, e.g., Papalambros & Wilde, 2000). Such a function for the structure and function of the brain—or of vision as a subtask—is very far from being available. The set of characteristics that the human (or animal) brain has optimized via its evolution is still an open problem.

Qualitatively, only a little can be said about what characteristics might be optimized. From a physical standpoint, minimizing the number and lengths of connections and minimizing the number of neurons required seem important. Minimizing time to make a decision is definitely ecologically important, and maximizing the probability of a correct decision is an obvious factor. Along with this, maximizing signal-to-noise ratio is a contributing element. Other factors such as packing—how to make a given number of neurons, connections, and their support mechanisms fit the volume and shape of the brain—or waste, heat, energy, and oxygen management all must ultimately also play a role. In what follows, a few small steps are made toward understanding elements that might contribute to the possible Y_i and Ω_j. The determination of a complete optimization framework must wait a bit longer.

Representations

The most central representational element of the model is the pyramid that has been a major part of the development in chapters 2 and 4. The pyramid concept is generalized here to reflect the fact that there are many different kinds of visual information that must be represented hierarchically. The need for this comes from two sources. The first is the separate maps idea of chapter 2, where it was argued that the ability to consider separate features as opposed to the ensemble of features helps with reducing computational complexity. To do so requires separable representations within the pyramid. The second motivation is clear in the wiring diagram of the visual areas of the macaque monkey by Felleman and Van Essen (1991) described in chapter 2. Using the laminar patterns of connections between areas (the cortex has six distinct layers defined by differences in neuron type and density and by connection types present), they proposed a hierarchy of visual areas. These laminar patterns are as follows:

· Ascending or feed-forward connections typically have origins in either of the deep cortical layers (laminae 5, 6) and terminate in lamina 4.

· Feedback connections terminate predominately outside of lamina 4 and originate from superficial laminae (laminae 1, 2, 3).

· Lateral connections terminate throughout the column and have origin in both deep and superficial laminae (but not lamina 4).

Felleman and Van Essen go on to give a set of criteria for determining hierarchical relationships among the visual areas in the cortex:

[E]ach area must be placed above all areas from which it receives ascending connections and/or sends descending connections. Likewise, it must be placed below all areas from which it receives descending connections and/or sends ascending connections. Finally, if an area has lateral connections, these must be with other areas at the same hierarchical level.

At first blush, this characterization of connectivity resembles that of a general lattice, as shown in figure 5.1. Formally, a lattice is based on a definition of a binary relation $\unlhd$ [to be read as 'is contained in' or 'is a part of'; $\leq$ is the usual symbol used (see Birkoff, 1967), but to avoid confusion with the arithmetic version of less-than-or-equal-to, we use this new symbol here]. The most basic properties of $\unlhd$ lead to the concept of a partially ordered set, or poset. Following Birkoff (1967), a **poset** is defined as a set in which the binary relation $x \unlhd y$ is defined, which satisfies for all $x, y,$ and z the following:

Reflexive Property   For all x, $x \unlhd x$.

Antisymmetry   If $x \unlhd y$ and $y \unlhd x$, then $x = y$.

Transitivity   If $x \unlhd y$ and $y \unlhd z$, then $x \unlhd z$.

If $x \unlhd y$ and $x \neq y$, then $x \lhd y$ and is read as x is properly contained in y. A poset D can contain at most one element a that satisfies $a \unlhd x$ for all $x \in D$. Similarly, there

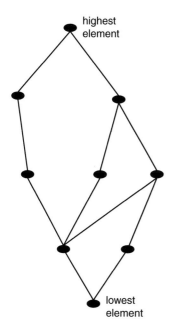

Figure 5.1
A hypothetical lattice structure.

can be only one element b that satisfies $x \trianglelefteq b$ for all $x \in D$. These, respectively, are known as the **least** (or infimum) and **greatest** (or supremum) elements of D. By extension, any two elements of D must have a unique least upper bound (called their **join**) and a greatest lower bound (called their **meet**). A **lattice** then is a poset where any two elements have a least element and a greatest element. A **chain** is a poset that is totally ordered; that is, given x and y, either $x \trianglelefteq y$ or $y \trianglelefteq x$ is true. Any single-neuron path through the visual system from retina to highest level is a neuron chain following this definition. Such a general lattice is illustrated in figure 5.1.

Thus far, the match with the general lattice structure and Felleman and Van Essen's ordering rules seems good. But there are some discrepancies. First of all, the question "What is an element of this lattice?" must be answered. If we consider a lattice organization for visual areas (not neurons), we must then ask "What area is the greatest element?" The least element can be safely considered to be the retina. In Felleman and Van Essen's hierarchy, the hippocampus is the top element. In the model to be described, the hippocampus and other high-layer areas are not addressed, and as a result the top two or three layers of Felleman and Van Essen's hierarchy are left out. A lattice where the greatest element is undefined is known as a **meet semilattice**. Any tree structure with its root as the least element is a meet semilattice. A lattice where the least element is undefined is known as a **join semilattice**. The next issue is that of the direction of connections; the partial order relation of a lattice provides for a single direction of connection and does not allow for bidirectional connections. Felleman and Van Essen report 121 reciprocal pairs of connections among the visual areas; the other 184 connections reported are unidirectional. Felleman and Van Essen describe 65 reciprocal linkages in which the pattern is explicitly identifiable as ascending in one direction and descending in the other. There are only five linkages that are identifiably lateral in both directions, and they question all in one way or another, as well as point out 10 possible exceptions to this pattern. We abstract from this a neater picture (admittedly requiring experimental confirmation) and define two lattices, one for the feed-forward connectivity and one for the feedback or recurrent connectivity. We name the former the **F-Lattice** and the latter the **R-Lattice**. It is an important part of the definition that these two lattices are composed of the same set of elements, the same set of visual areas. Only the relations among them differ. The F-Lattice is a meet semilattice with least element the retina. The R-Lattice is a join semilattice; however, this does not seem to suffice here because there is no source for the recurrent signals. We thus include as a single additional element the complex of brain areas that act as the executive controller and make this the least element of the R-Lattice. As the R-Lattice has a greatest element, the retina, it is no longer a join semilattice, but rather a lattice proper. The executive may or may not include the areas removed for the F-Lattice, and it does include prefrontal areas that are not in Felleman and Van Essen's hierarchy. This abstraction is appropriate for the theory we are developing even though it may be less of an ideal fit to the real neuroanatomy.

Next, we must address the lateral connections, again a relationship not part of a general lattice. However, given that we have the F- and R-Lattices, we may define a third lattice, the **L-Lattice**, using the operation of **direct product** (Birkoff, 1967). A direct product of two lattices D and Q is the set of all couples (x, y) with $x \in D$, $y \in Q$ and ordered by the rule that $(x_1, y_1) \trianglelefteq (x_2, y_2)$ if and only if $x_1 \trianglelefteq x_2$ in D and $y_1 \trianglelefteq y_2$ in Q. The direct product of any two lattices is also a lattice. This of course provides these couple relationships among any qualifying elements of the original lattices. Not all may be required, so as will be seen later when weights are associated with each relationship, those not needed will have a weight of zero. Overall, these three lattices provide us with a reasonable abstraction of the Felleman and Van Essen hierarchy, with a formal mathematical foundation, and of sufficient complexity and realism to enable a useful test of the concepts.

The final complication is our requirement for pyramid representations, also completely consistent with known characterizations of the sizes of the brain's visual areas. We thus define an element of each of the F- and R-Lattices to be an array, a retinotopic representation of the full visual field. These elements will be referred to as **sheets**—sheets of retinotopically organized neurons. Each sheet may be connected to more than one other sheet in a feed-forward, recurrent, or lateral manner, and these connections are represented by the F-Lattice, R-Lattice, and L-Lattice relationships, respectively. The definition of a pyramid requires that the number of elements in each sheet decreases moving higher in the pyramid. Let X and Y be sheets within the F-Lattice (and the R-Lattice as the elements are the same), and let $\|X\|$ and $\|Y\|$ be their cardinality, the number of locations in the array. In the F-Lattice, if $X \trianglelefteq Y$, then $\|X\| > \|Y\|$, and for these same elements of the R-Lattice, $Y \trianglelefteq X$, $\|Y\| < \|X\|$. In general, the determination of the content and exact form of these sheets is related to some combination of inputs from the layers below. In most of the usual pyramid formulations (for an overview, see Jolion & Rosenfeld, 1994), there are fixed rules for how the resolution changes layer to layer and how each value in the pyramid layers is computed. There are no such fixed rules in the visual system, and the transformation of information from layer to layer is unique. Due to the desire to not make the attention framework specific to any particular visual representation, the layer-to-layer transformations are left unspecified, and the presentation will apply to any definition.

Note that our sheets and Felleman and Van Essen's rules for laminar connections do not exactly match up. The laminae of the visual areas contain many neurons and of varying kinds and function. Connections may originate in one or more lamina and terminate in others. The only likely adjustment we can make is that each of our sheets represents a single kind of computation, and that a single visual area most probably is composed of many of these sheets. In this way, the match between our structure and real neuroanatomy is closer; it is not an exact match, but this level of detail is beyond the scope of our theory at this time.

This overall representation will be termed a **Pyramid Lattice**, or **P-Lattice** for short, and is considered as the loose union of the F-, R-, and L-Lattices defined above [it is possible to derive this formally, but it would require too many additional assumptions about the exact structure of the lattices—the interested reader can consult Birkoff (1967) for more]. Although these definitions might allow us to take advantage of the rich mathematics available within general lattice theory (Birkoff, 1967; Grätzer, 1978), the reformulation of what follows in those terms is a topic for future consideration. For now, this representational abstraction, although perhaps not reflecting the full diversity and variability of the real neuroanatomy of the visual cortex, certainly suffices for our purpose and provides a first formalization of that neuroanatomy.

It is assumed throughout that sheets and neural receptive fields are square in shape for convenience and with no loss of generality. In fact, in all subsequent diagrams, rectangular representations are always retinotopic presentations of the visual field. Assume there are L levels, so L—the executive controller—is the highest-level layer regardless of pathway. The input layer is layer 1. Any path (or chain) of sheets from level 1 to L represents a single pyramid. Specifically, the layer of sheets at level $L - 1$ represents the most abstract stages of visual processing. Figure 5.2 shows such a hypothetical P-Lattice; four distinct pyramids are easily seen within it.

Although the several pyramid problems in chapter 2 were described in the context of a single pyramid, they all apply to this lattice of pyramids. In fact, it should be clear that most are exacerbated by this expanded representation. Consider, for example, that lateral connections are not only within a sheet but can also be found among sheets in a layer. The issue of multiple foci of attention must also be reconsidered for the P-Lattice. In chapter 2, it was claimed that multiple foci would not be a reasonable strategy because it is difficult to determine if one attentive beam might cause interference with another.

The beams would have to be sufficiently far apart, and this seems difficult to determine in a dynamic, real-time fashion. In a P-Lattice, top-down beams might be separate at their origin—layer $L - 1$ of the structure—and then might traverse different pathways. In this way, perhaps it is possible to have multiple foci of attention as long as the kinds of neural tunings they address differ enough and as long as location in the visual field differs enough so the beams are kept separate throughout the P-Lattice. Scalf and Beck (2010) show experiments where those constraints are violated, and indeed, attention to multiple items is impaired. In contrast, Braun (1998b) summarizes many experiments with attention seemingly allocated to two tasks equally, others where attention favors one or another task, and still more

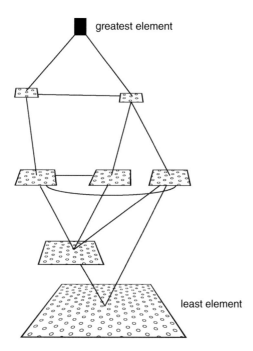

Figure 5.2
A hypothetical lattice of pyramids.

where attention is allocated outside the focus of attention. It is beyond most models to account for such results.

The consideration of representational issues such as the problem with information flow in a pyramid or P-Lattice representation is not common in the attention modeling literature, where the focus has been primarily on selection of point of fixation or on attentive neural response modulation. It is a major point of differentiation of the Selective Tuning approach from other models in that ST considers attention in a much broader manner. For the most part, the information flow problems require dynamic solutions that change from moment to moment depending on task and input; it is for this reason that it makes sense to include them in any discussion on attention [Anderson and Van Essen (1987) did the same when describing routing problems in the cortex]. Models that ignore these routing problems are not only incomplete but also lose out on incorporating the constraints that the problems provide.

A number of variables must now be introduced.

R_i represents the number of sheets in layer i, $1 \leq i \leq L$. $R_L = R_1 = 1$. Each sheet is a retinotopic, square array with no loss of generality. Each array element may be a

neural assembly that contains one or more neurons and connections (for convenience, such a neural assembly will be simply referred to as a neuron in what
follows). There is no constraint on the number of sheets in a layer.

ijxy is a 4-tuple that identifies the location of a particular neuron as being at location
(x,y) in sheet j of layer i, $1 \le j \le R_i$. Such a 4-tuple will be used as a subscript for
particular neuron types throughout.

u_{ij} gives the number of neurons in sheet j of layer i; $u_{11} = P$, the number of input
pixels (photoreceptors). It will be assumed that the sheet at the top of this lattice
has only a single element, $u_{L1} = 1$. This assumption has no obvious biological counterpart; it exists only to define the lattice and to provide connections to the $L - 1$
layer sheets. This single top node corresponds with the executive controller as mentioned earlier.

U_{ij} is the set of neurons in sheet j of layer i; the cardinality of the set is $\|U_{ij}\| = u_{ij}$.

g_{ab} is the strength of connection between two neurons, a and b, in the direction from
a to b. If $a = ijxy$ and $b = klvz$, then one neuron is at location (x,y) in sheet j of layer
i and the other at location (v,z) in sheet l of layer k. In effect, the set of all values
of g_{ab} define the full connectivity of the P-Lattice.

$r_{ijxy}(t)$ is the time-varying response of the neuron at location (x,y) in sheet j of layer
i at time t. $0 \le r_{ijxy}(t) \le Z$, and Z is its maximum.

There are several sets that represent connections between neurons:

$\overline{\wedge}_{ijxy}$ represents the set of feed-forward connections to neuron r_{ijxy}. In other words,
these are the partial order relationships for the F-Lattice defined earlier. This will
be specialized below by means of a superscript to distinguish the different kinds of
feed-forward connections in the model.

$\underline{\vee}_{ijxy}$ represents the set of recurrent connections to neuron r_{ijxy}. These are the partial
order relationships for the R-Lattice defined earlier. This will be specialized below
by means of a superscript to distinguish the different kinds of recurrent connections
in the model.

Ξ_{ijxy} represents the set of local connections of r_{ijxy}; that is, the neurons to which it is
connected within the same sheet. Again, this will be specialized below by means of
a superscript to distinguish the different kinds of local connections.

At this point in the development of the theory, there is no area lateral connectivity;
that is, the weights for all connections between sheets in the L-Lattice are zero. They
may be considered placeholders for roles yet to be determined for interarea computations. More variables will be introduced as they are needed; the above will
suffice to start the presentation.

It is not within the scope of this volume to delve deeply into the mathematics of dynamical systems in neuroscience. On the other hand, it is not possible to isolate or compartmentalize all the components of attentional processes so they can be formalized independently of how neurons and their responses are characterized. After all, the thesis here is that attention is a *set* of mechanisms. Attention is not an independent module or an add-on to any system—each of the mechanisms will affect different aspects of any neural formulation. As a result, making too strong a commitment to a particular formulation of neural processing would not be useful. The approach here is to show how, for a standard formulation of neurons and their networks, the various pieces might fit.

The Wilson volume on dynamical systems in neuroscience (Wilson, 1999) is an excellent source for the background of what is to follow. Koch's book (Koch, 1999) and Arbib's encyclopedic treatment (Arbib, 1995) are also wonderful sources. A thorough comparative paper by Izhikevich (2004) provides a very useful perspective on a broad span of models. Given that our goal is to understand attention and not all the complexities of neurons in detail, it is very tempting in the current context to use the simplest formulation of a neuron, namely, the McCulloch–Pitts version (McCullough & Pitts, 1943). The reasoning would be that much of what follows deals with how neural inputs are modulated and not with the details of single-neuron processing. Their neuron is a binary one, whose output $y(t + 1)$ at time $t + 1$ is '1' as defined by

$$y(t + 1) = 1$$

if and only if

$$\sum_{i \in I} g_{iy} x_i(t) \geq \kappa, \tag{5.1}$$

where the g_{iy} are weights $-1.0 \leq g_{iy} \leq 1.0$ specifying the strength of contribution from neuron i to y, the $x_i(t)$ are input values, the set I is the set of neurons that provide input for neuron y, and κ is a threshold. The McCullough–Pitts neuron provides a simple weighted-sum of inputs strategy and has been shown to suffice for models of various functions (logical NOT and AND for example). However, binary neurons will not suffice for Selective Tuning, and better realism is necessary. Although we cannot move along the realism dimension all the way to the Izhikevich neuron (Izhikevich, 2003, 2004), we will move a bit further toward neural realism by using the leaky integrator neuron (see any of the above-cited works for additional detail).

The formulation throughout is based on a rate model; that is, the neuron's response to its input is the number of spikes per second that it generates. Equation 5.2 defines stimulus intensity $P_y(t)$, the net postsynaptic potential reaching the site of spike generation for neuron y, as

$$P_y(t) = \sum_{i \in I} g_{iy} x_i(t), \tag{5.2}$$

where the weights and inputs are defined as for the McCullough–Pitts neuron. The response or spike rate S is given by

$$S[P(t)] = \begin{cases} \dfrac{ZP(t)^\xi}{\sigma^\xi + P(t)^\xi} & \text{for} \quad P(t) \geq 0 \\ 0 & \text{for} \quad P(t) < 0. \end{cases} \tag{5.3}$$

Z is the maximum response (spike rate), and σ, the semisaturation constant, determines the point at which S reaches half of its maximum. ξ determines the maximum slope of the function (i.e., how sharp the transition is between threshold and saturation). This is roughly a sigmoidal function with a lower asymptote of 0 and an upper asymptote of Z. It is important to note that equation 5.3 only represents the asymptotic or steady-state firing rate and that the response of a neuron varies exponentially over time as it approaches this value. The differential equation that describes this temporal variation of a single neuron's response or spike rate is

$$\frac{dr}{dt} = \frac{1}{\tau}[-r + S(P)], \tag{5.4}$$

where τ is a decay time constant. If $r(0) = 0$, the solution as a function of t is given by

$$r(t) = Ae^{-t/\tau} + \frac{1}{\tau}\int_0^t e^{-(t-\zeta)/\tau} S[P(\zeta)]d\zeta \tag{5.5}$$

where A is a constant dependent on the initial conditions. This equation describes the responses of cortical cells to a wide variety of time-varying stimuli (Wilson, 1999). Exact results are possible for constant input

$$r(t) = (1 - e^{-t/\tau})S(P). \tag{5.6}$$

Several additional elements will be introduced with the neural circuits that use them in the next section.

Neurons and Circuits for Selective Tuning

There have been many attempts to elucidate the cortical and subcortical circuitry of vision and of attention; our understanding is still evolving. The first ST circuit diagram appeared in Tsotsos et al. (1995) and was a coarse representation of types of computations and their connections with no attempt to identify any neural correlates. It simply provided a map for the interactions of the several types of units required for the computations made by the model. Since then, much has been learned that enables a new formulation, the topic of the following sections.

A number of authors have presented neural circuit diagrams for attentive processes at varying degrees of detail and specificity. Gilbert and Sigman (2007) show a schematic of the interactions of top-down, feedback, and local circuits. The simplest form of attentive influence for them is direct connection from neurons in higher cortical regions to pyramidal neurons in V1. They suggest that this might explain response selection or the attentional spotlight. They note that feedback between networks might gate subsets of neuronal inputs; for example, targeting inhibitory interneurons to eliminate the effect of horizontal connections. Their discussion focused only on attentional effects for V1 pyramidal neurons. Buia and Tiesinga (2008) show a model at a higher level of abstraction using three types of units: top-down, feed-forward, and excitatory (pyramidal) cells. Feed-forward input goes to both the excitatory pyramidal cells and to the feed-forward cells, whereas task or knowledge input goes to the top-down cells. There is local inhibition within the column for the feed-forward and excitatory cells, activated by cross-column projections that can be inhibited by the top-down cells. Top-down cells can directly inhibit the excitatory cells. Whereas Gilbert and Sigman do not formalize their model mathematically, Buia and Tiesinga do, and they show good single-neuron as well as local network properties.

There are several types of neurons required for ST to function. The connectivity among four classes of neurons—interpretive, bias, lateral, and gating—will be introduced in the following series of figures, designed as an incremental exposition of the overall network. The figures show a single assembly within any sheet. Each computes a single visual quantity (feature, object, etc.) at a single tuning profile. All elements of this single assembly are at the same (x, y) location. At the same location, however, there is also competition for representing the stimulus. As Hubel and Wiesel (1965) described, columns of neurons, each with a different tuning but the same spatial receptive field, are present in this model as well. Some are in competition whereas others may cooperate, and still others might be independent of one another.

Interpretive Neurons

These are the classical feature-detecting neurons and will be represented by r_{ijxy}. They receive feed-forward input from other areas that arrives in lamina 4 and provide an output to other areas from laminae 5 and 6. Their general behavior is governed by equation 5.7 (refined from equation 5.4):

$$\frac{dr_{ijxy}}{dt} = \frac{1}{\tau}\{-r_{ijxy} + S[P_{ijxy}(t)]\}, \tag{5.7}$$

where

$$P_{ijxy}(t) = \sum_{k \in \overline{\wedge}_{ijxy}} g_{k(ijxy)} r_k(t),$$ (5.8)

and $g_{k(ijxy)}$ are weights $-1.0 \leq g_{k(ijxy)} \leq 1.0$ specifying the strength of contribution from neuron k to r_{ijxy}. Figure 5.3 provides a simple circuit layout for the basic interpretive neuron. The figure makes explicit the presynaptic and postsynaptic parts of a synapse. The reason for this is a later circuit requires the postsynaptic signal (the weighted input) before it is integrated along the dendrite, as input. All other synapses in the figures will be distinguished as either excitatory or inhibitory only. In the figure, only T-junctions of lines are dendritic branches; any other lines or curves are continuous and cross over any they appear to intersect. The T-junction just at the apex of the pyramidal neuron in figure 5.3 is that point at which the value of P as defined by equation 5.8 can be found.

It is important to revisit the concept of receptive field in light of the P-Lattice representation used here. A receptive field is usually defined as the spatial region in the visual field where stimulation causes a neuron to fire. Here, we define the **Featural Receptive Field** (FRF) to be the set of all the direct, feed-forward inputs to a neuron, specifically, those in the set $\overline{\wedge}_{ijxy}$ and the full hierarchy that these connect to. These $\overline{\wedge}_{ijxy}$ inputs arise from the union of k arbitrarily shaped, contigu-

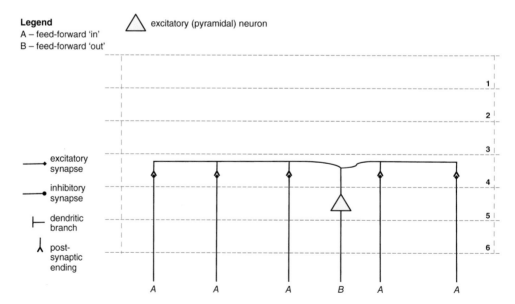

Figure 5.3
Illustration of the circuit involving a single interpretive neuron.

ous, possibly overlapping subfields from any feature map (sheet), and there may be more than one subfield from a feature map (within the definition of the F-Lattice). The overall contribution to a neuron is given in equation 5.8 for the neuron's FRF. Of course, this applies to each level of visual processing and to each neuron within each level. As a result, a hierarchical sequence of such computations defines the selectivity of each neuron. Each neuron has input from a set of neurons from different representations, and each of those neurons also has an FRF and their own computations to combine its input features. With such a hierarchy of computations, a stimulus-driven feed-forward pass would yield the strongest responding neurons within one representation if the stimulus matches the selectivity of existing neurons or the strongest responding component neurons in different representations if the stimulus does not match an existing pattern. At one level of description, this does not alter the classical definition. However, the region of the visual field in which stimulation causes the neuron to fire now has internal structure reflecting the locations of the stimulus features that are determined by the hierarchy of feature map subfields.

Bias Neurons

These provide top-down guidance for visual processing, whether the selection is for locations or regions in space, subranges of visual features, objects, events, or whole scenes to attend to. They are represented by B_{ijxy}. They act by suppressing the input to task-irrelevant interpretive neurons. The bias is realized as an axosomatic process; that is, it suppresses the net postsynaptic input to the interpretive neuron via a synapse on the cell body. For task-relevant neurons, the value is unity so there is no impact. The bias originates with the executive controller and is relayed to the next lower layer following the R-Lattice connectivity pattern. As the bias signal is a top-down one and is not necessarily spatially uniform across the lattice or any of its sheets, the Convergent Recurrence Problem arises. A simple rule can solve this; namely, that the bias signal is the minimum value of all the converging bias signals. Let $B_{ijxy}(t)$ be the bias value associated with neuron r_{ijxy} in layer i, representation j, location (x,y) at time t with real-value $0.0 \leq B_{ijxy}(t) \leq 1.0$ defined by

$$B_{ijxy}(t) = \min_{\beta \in \vee_{ijxy}^{b}} B_{\beta}(t), \tag{5.9}$$

where $\vee_{ijxy}^{b}$ is the set of bias units making feedback connections to r_{ijxy}. The default value of bias units is 1.0. Adding this bias to equation 5.7 in a straightforward manner yields

$$\frac{dr_{ijxy}}{dt} = \frac{1}{\tau}[-r_{ijxy} + B_{ijxy}S(P_{ijxy})] . \tag{5.10}$$

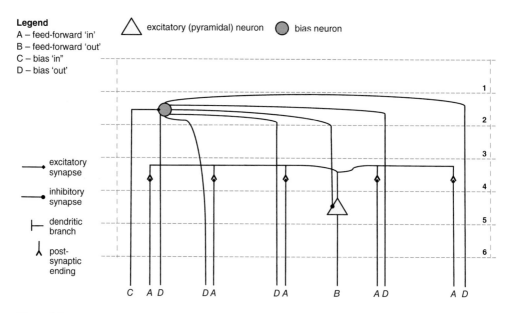

Figure 5.4
The bias circuit added to the interpretive one of figure 5.3.

The configuration of bias and interpretive neurons depicted in figure 5.4 performs the computation of equation 5.10. The nature of the bias computation is to inhibit any task-irrelevant units allowing the relevant ones to pass through the pyramid without interference. For example, if the task is to detect red items, the interpretive units that are selective for red stimuli would be unaffected while all other color-selective units would be biased against to some degree. If the neuron of equation 5.10 is one for which the input must be suppressed, the second term within the brackets on the right-hand side would be suppressed, perhaps to zero, by the bias multiplier. If there is no real input, then $S(P_{ijxy})$ would reflect only baseline firing of the input neurons, a small value but certainly not zero. A suppressive bias would drive this toward zero as well.

The bias signal determined for r_{ijxy} is relayed to lower-layer sheets, and the Spatial Spread and Interpolation Problems are relevant. ST assumes the trivial solution to both; that is, spatially uniform signals are relayed.

Lateral Cooperation Neurons

Perhaps the most studied and best understood of lateral neural computations, lateral inhibition is believed to provide an antagonist process that sharpens neural responsiveness spatially. The simplest formulation for lateral inhibition would be that specifying a neuron's response decay as a linear function of the weighted sum of

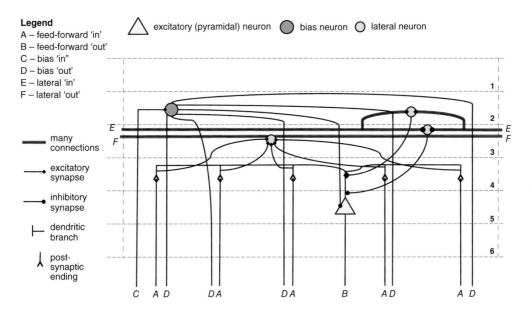

Figure 5.5
The lateral cooperation subnetwork added to the circuit of figure 5.4.

responses of its neighbors, where the weights are $0.0 \leq g_h \leq 1.0$. However, it is very useful to generalize lateral computation, as Rosenfeld, Hummel, and Zucker (1976) pioneered (see also Hummel & Zucker, 1983), later experimentally observed by Kapadia, Ito, Gilbert, and Westheimer (1995), in order to permit lateral influences to both inhibit and enhance neural response. To accomplish this, the range of the weights must include negative values. Incorporating this into equation 5.10 yields

$$\frac{dr_{ijxy}}{dt} = \frac{1}{\tau}\left[-r_{ijxy} + B_{ijxy}S\left(P_{ijxy} + \sum_{h \in \Xi^a_{ijxy}} g_h r_h\right)\right], \tag{5.11}$$

where $-1.0 \leq g_h \leq 1.0$, and Ξ^a_{ijxy} represents the connections horizontally across columns for neuron r_{ijxy}. g_h represents the weight, or degree of influence, from neuron r_{klvz} to r_{ijxy} where $h = (k,l,v,z) \in \Xi^a_{ijxy}$. Use of a simple linear cooperative process is sufficient to illustrate the point. The circuit realization of this is a different matter. Synapses do not have the breadth of function to dynamically permit both inhibition and enhancement. We require that one sum of contributions have a negative effect while a different sum has a positive one. As a result, this function appears in the circuit of figure 5.5 as a three-neuron subnetwork.

One neuron (the leftmost of the three in the figure) collects all the postsynaptic inputs to the interpretive unit and relays their sum to the neighboring neurons,

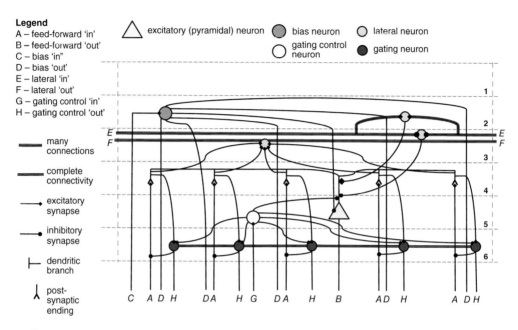

Figure 5.6
The complete network, with the addition of the selection circuit to that of figure 5.5.

represented by the connections in Ξ^a_{ijxy}. The other two neurons collect inputs from those same neighboring neurons and compute their weighted sums but with different weights. One set of weights is for the excitatory contributions (in the rightmost neuron), and the other is for the inhibitory ones (in the central neuron). The former sum provides enhancement and the latter inhibition. This is very much in the spirit of the compatibilities detailed in the relaxation processes of Rosenfeld et al. (1976), later adopted by many others in neural modeling. Those compatibilities differ not only depending on spatial neighbor relations but also by feature differences. The above will suffice to include both. Of interest is a recent finding: Adesnik and Scanziani (2010) find that horizontal projections in sensory cortex suppress layers of cortex devoted to processing inputs but facilitate layers devoted to outputs. It is clear that in order for this to operate, the full breadth of lateral cooperation described here is an important component.

Gating Network

This subnetwork is the most complex that ST requires. Figure 5.6 illustrates the full network adding in the gating network. This is the major mechanism by which selection of attended neurons is made and by which those neural activations are traced back down to their source, forming the path of the attentional beam.

This subnetwork is charged with the following tasks:

· Determine the winning subset of those inputs to the pyramidal neuron r_{ijxy} (the chains within the lattice representation).

· Suppress feed-forward connections to r_{ijxy} that correspond with the losers of the competition.

· Once the competition converges, transmit the values of the gating neuron γ_f down to the next layer, to become the gating control signals for the next layer neurons corresponding with $\overline{\wedge}_{ijxy}$.

The network in the figure differs for the special case of layer $L - 1$. In that case, the gating network applies to the direct responses of the excitatory neurons across the whole representation for each of the R_{L-1} representations, rather than the inputs to a particular neuron from an earlier layer. The formulation remains the same, but the participating neurons differ. One might think that connectivity might be a concern here; however, as this applies to the highest-level representations that are the smallest arrays of neurons, as long as $u_{(L-1)j}$ is less than some maximum number of connections, this is not a problem.

There are two kinds of neurons in this subnetwork. There is one gating control neuron for each r_{ijxy}. The gating control neuron acts as a switch; it either turns the competition 'on' or leaves it in its default 'off' state. Also, it suppresses any lateral influences on r_{ijxy}. If an 'on' gating control signal has reached this interpretive neuron, then the neuron is on the attentional beam's pass zone pathway. The goal then is to reduce signal interference due to the context of that neuron's input, and this includes any lateral contributions.

Let ς_{ijxy} be the gating control neuron for r_{ijxy}. Due to the Convergent Recurrence Problem, each r_{ijxy} may need to deal with a number of incoming gating control signals. The policy here is that if any gating control signal is 'on,' then the convergence of signals leads to an 'on' signal:

$$\varsigma_{ijxy} = \begin{cases} 1 & \text{if } \sum\limits_{a\in\underline{\vee}^c_{ijxy}} \zeta_a > 0 \\ 0 & \text{otherwise,} \end{cases} \tag{5.12}$$

where $\underline{\vee}^c_{ijxy}$ is the set of gating control signals converging onto r_{ijxy}. There is also one gating neuron, $\gamma_f, f \in \overline{\wedge}_{ijxy}$, for each of the feed-forward inputs to r_{ijxy}, $0 \le \gamma_f \le 1.0$.

The network of gating neurons is responsible for computing the subset of weighted inputs that form the strongest connected set. As a top-down traversal commences, ς_{Ljxy} is set to 1.0 for all j, x, y, and all the $\gamma_f = 1.0$. The value of γ_f falls as the competition proceeds to reflect the branch-and-bound pruning (see below) except for the winning neurons where it remains at 1.0. At the end of the top-down traversal, ς_{Ljxy}

is reset to 0.0. The inputs to each γ_f must be postsynaptic; that is, weighted inputs [as in the WTA scheme of Yuille and Geiger (1995)]. These neurons form a completely connected network, necessary for competition for strongest responses. More detail will be provided in the next section.

Selection

The method will be presented in several parts: general description of the strategy, formalization of the strategy for a single sheet, then for a single pyramid, and then for a P-lattice.

General Strategy

The major task the gating network must perform is to determine the winning subset of weighted inputs to the interpretive neuron. Most attention models use a Winner-Take-All process (e.g., see Koch & Ullman, 1985). However the process as formulated there has undesirable characteristics. It may not converge, particularly if there is more than one maximum value, and it requires computation time dependent on the number of competitors. Our process differs in these respects. One key distinguishing characteristic comes from the fact that it creates an implicit partial ordering of the set of neural responses. The ordering arises because inhibition between units is not based on the value of a single neuron but rather on the difference between pairs of neural responses, where the difference must be at least as great as a task-specific parameter θ, $\theta \geq 0.0$. Further, this process is not restricted to converging to single values as all other formulations; rather as will be apparent in the discussion, regions of neurons are found as winners. This will be termed the θ**-Winner-Take-All** (θ-WTA) process.

First, competition depends linearly on the difference between neuron response strengths in the following way. Neuron r_A will inhibit r_B in the competition if $r_A(t) - r_B(t) > \theta$. Otherwise, r_A will not inhibit r_B. The overall impact of the competition on r_B is the weighted sum of all inhibitory effects, each of whose magnitude is determined by $r_A(t) - r_B(t)$ for all the neurons with which it is competing.

Each input to the competition must be weighted by its role for the interpretive units that it feeds to reflect the importance of each input to the interpretive computation in the competition. It would not be necessary if all inputs to a given interpretive unit were equally weighted; this is not the case. If the largest valued input to the neuron is weighted negatively by its tuning profile, then it should not be considered as the most important input within the receptive field. Thus, the inputs to the gating network must be postsynaptic as shown in figure 5.6.

As a general statement of the goal of the gating network computation, we can say that the algorithm seeks subsets of locations, M_{ij}, in each sheet j in each layer i. Each element of M_{ij} is a set of locations (p,q) in sheet j, layer i. Beginning with the special case of layer $L - 1$ (recall how layer L contains only one element so the general process really begins in layer $L - 2$), the set of elements in M_{ij} is constrained by

$$\forall[(p,q) \in M_{(L-1)j}] \mid r_{(L-1)jpq}(t) - r_{(L-1)juv}(t) > \theta, \tag{5.13}$$

where

$$(u,v) \in (U_{(L-1)j} - M_{(L-1)j}) \text{ and } M_{(L-1)j} \subset U_{(L-1)j},$$

and the locations represented by the set elements are connected, as defined by

$$\forall[(p_1,q_1) \in M_{(L-1)j}], \exists[(p_2,q_2) \in M_{(L-1)j}] \mid |p_1 - p_2| \le 1 \text{ and } |q_1 - q_2| \le 1,$$
$$\text{for } p_1 \ne p_2, q_1 \ne q_2. \tag{5.14}$$

This is a special case because it must operate over all the responses at the highest layer of the network. Each of the gating neurons corresponding with the winning set $M_{(L-1)j}$ sends an 'on' gating control signal down to the next layer of the competition to all the columns from which its gating input originated. Again, the Spatial Spread and Interpolation Problems appear, and here, the trivial solution as for the bias neurons is adopted. In addition, those neurons not part of the winning set have their input connections suppressed. This action simultaneously solves the Context and Cross-talk Problems.

Then, and in the order $m = L - 1, L - 2, \dots, 2$, we seek the sets $G_{(m-1)nxy}$, where G is a set of locations as was M above, for each neuron for which the gating network competition has been turned on by the gating control neuron, where

$$\forall[(p,q) \in G_{(m-1)nxy}] \mid \rho(p,q) - \rho(u,v) > \theta,$$

$$(p,q) \text{ and } (u,v) \in \overline{\wedge}_{mnxy} \text{ and } n = 1,2,\dots R_m. \tag{5.15}$$

$\rho(\text{-},\text{-})$ is the postsynaptic input to r_{mnxy}. The set of locations $G_{(m-1)nxy}$ correspond with afferents of r_{mnxy}, and thus the layer is below that of r_{mnxy}. The region connectivity constraint applies equally here:

$$\forall[(p_1,q_1) \in G_{(m-1)nxy}], \exists[(p_2,q_2) \in G_{(m-1)nxy}] \mid |p_1 - p_2| \le 1 \text{ and } |q_1 - q_2| \le 1,$$
$$\text{for } p_1 \ne p_2, q_1 \ne q_2. \tag{5.16}$$

Each of the inputs to the selection process may be weighted by the strength of their involvement in the decision, and this will appear in the next section. How this characterization of the solution is converted to an algorithm follows.

Selection within a Single Sheet

The inputs to the selection process are the inputs to r_{ijxy}; that is, $r_f(t)$, $f \in \overline{\wedge}_{ijxy}$. The competition itself is formulated as:

$$\forall f \in \overline{\wedge}_{ijxy}, r_f'(t'+1) = R\left[r_f'(t') - \varsigma_{ijxy} \sum_{\lambda \in \Xi_{ijxy}^s, \lambda \neq f} \Delta(f,\lambda) \right]. \tag{5.17}$$

It is likely that such a process requires mediation by a set of interneurons, but these are not explicitly part of this discussion. At the time that the competition is started, that is, when ς_{ijxy} for r_{ijxy} has a value of 1.0, the clock, t', for the competition begins with $t' = 0$ for a real-world clock time of t; let $r_f'(0) = r_f(t)$ at this time. $\Delta(f,\lambda) = g_{\lambda(ijxy)}r_\lambda'(t') - g_{f(ijxy)}r_f'(t')$, if $0 < \theta < [g_{\lambda(ijxy)}r_\lambda'(t') - g_{f(ijxy)}r_f'(t')]$, and equals 0 otherwise. $g_{\alpha(ijxy)}$ is the weight on the input r_a for the computation of r_{ijxy}. The set Ξ_{ijxy}^s represents the set of gating neurons connected to r_{ijxy}. The gating control signal ς_{ijxy} (from equation 5.12) turns this competition on and off; when it has value 0, the response remains unchanged. R is a half-wave rectifier to ensure only positive values, $R(a) = (a + |a|)/2$. The weighting of each input, as seen in $\Delta(f,\lambda) = g_{\lambda(ijxy)}r_\lambda'(t') - g_{f(ijxy)}r_f'(t')$, is included to reflect the importance of each input to the computation. It would not be necessary if it were the case that all inputs to a given interpretive unit were equally weighted; this is not the case. If the largest-valued input to the computation is weighted negatively, then it should not be considered as a most important input within the receptive field. Using the weights in the manner above ensures that the largest input value is also positively weighted; it is the product of value and weight that is important to the computation of contributions in the selection.

Although this appropriately determines the set M_{ij} as described above, this is not sufficient because in the circuit diagram of figure 5.6, gating neurons modulate each input connection to r_{ijxy} multiplicatively to reflect the competition. We wish the competition first to converge and only then for the modulation of input connections to occur. We know that the competition has converged if for every $f \in \overline{\wedge}_{ijxy}$, $|r_f'(t' + 1) - r_f'(t')| \approx 0$ at some time on the competition clock (or at least less than some threshold value). Let the time of convergence be t_c. The real-world clock is now at $t + t_c$. Let the value of the gating neuron $\gamma_f(t)$, $f \in \overline{\wedge}_{ijxy}$, be the modulating multiplier for neuron f. Once each gating neuron achieves convergence, the modulating value of each gating neuron within the column of r_{ijxy} is

$$\gamma_f(t+t_c) = \frac{r_f'(t_c)}{r_f(t+t_c)}. \tag{5.18}$$

The winning set of inputs do not change during the competition and thus for those, $\gamma_f(t + t_c) = 1.0$. For the remainder $\gamma_f(t + t_c)$ approaches 0.0, effectively suppressing that input connection.

Once the competition converges, the competition at the next layer down must be initiated. The value of $\varsigma_{(i-1)---}$ is set to 1.0 (the notation means 'for any value of the last three subscripts') when each gating neuron detects that it has converged to its final value. Note that the process is not in lock-step; as the fate of each unit within the contribution is decided, its result is propagated downward asynchronously.

It was shown in Tsotsos et al. (1995) that this strategy is guaranteed to converge, that it has well-defined properties with respect to finding strongest items, and that is has well-defined convergence characteristics. The proofs are repeated here. Let the competitive contribution (second right-hand term within brackets) of equation 5.17 be represented by G.

Theorem 5.1 *The updating rule of equation 5.17 is guaranteed to converge for all inputs.*

Proof

1. As the contribution to unit i depends on a difference function, a partial ordering of units is imposed depending on response magnitude.

2. By definition, the largest response neurons (a unique maximum value is not needed) will receive a competitive contribution of 0 and will remain unaffected by the iterative process. The neurons with the smallest responses will be inhibited by all other neurons.

3. $G \geq 0$ by definition, and therefore all units that receive inhibition will have strictly negative contributions throughout and thus will decay in magnitude monotonically, iteration by iteration, or remain at zero.

4. The iterations are terminated when a stable state is reached (no units change in magnitude). The ones with the largest response do not change, and all other values decay to zero (the rectification ensures this).

It is thus trivially shown that the process is guaranteed to converge and locate the largest items in a competition.   ∎

The response of r_{ijxy} thus becomes

$$\frac{dr_{ijxy}}{dt} = \frac{1}{\tau}\left[-r_{ijxy} + B_{ijxy}S\left(\sum_{k \in \bar{\Lambda}_{ijxy}} \gamma_k g_{k(ijxy)}r_k + \hat{\varsigma}_{ijxy} \sum_{h \in \Xi_{ijxy}^a} g_h r_h \right) \right]. \tag{5.19}$$

The element $\hat{\varsigma}_{ijxy}$ requires a bit of explanation. One of the tasks for the gating network is to eliminate interference due to lateral contributions. If r_{ijxy} is on the pass path of attention, $\varsigma_{ijxy} = 1.0$. $\hat{\varsigma}_{ijxy} = 0.0$ if $\varsigma_{ijxy} = 1.0$, and is 1.0 otherwise. In other words, in the situation where r_{ijxy} is not an attended neuron, then the lateral contributions are allowed to affect it. If it is an attended neuron, then lateral contributions are suppressed.

The next step is to find the largest, strongest responding spatially contiguous region within the set of winners found by the above algorithm. The connectivity constraint needs to now be included and enforced. This can be accomplished by running a second competition but only among the neurons that survived the first competition. This second competition looks much the same as the first with two changes: the set Ξ^s_{abxy} is replaced by the set of winners, call this set W, found by the first step of the algorithm, and Δ is replaced by Φ, defined as

$$\Phi(a,b,x,y,w,z)=\mu(r_{abwz}(t)-r_{abxy}(t))\left(1-e^{\frac{\delta^2_{wzxy}}{\zeta^2}}\right), \tag{5.20}$$

and like the definition of Δ, Φ has the above value if that value is greater than θ, and 0 otherwise. μ controls the amount of influence of this processing stage (the effect increases as μ increases from a value of 1), δ_{wzxy} is the retinotopic distance between the two neurons, and ζ controls the spatial variance of the competition. The larger the spatial distance between units, the greater is the inhibition. A large region will inhibit a region of similar response strengths but of smaller spatial extent on a unit-by-unit basis. This strategy will find the largest, most spatially contiguous subset within the winning set. At the top layer, this is a global competition; at lower layers, this is competition only within receptive fields. It is important to note that this strategy will find one solution but not necessarily the optimal one; that is, the connectivity constraint is only approximately enforced.

We now turn to the convergence properties of this scheme. From the updating function, it is clear that the time to convergence depends only on three values: the magnitude of the largest unit, the magnitude of the second-largest unit, and the parameter θ. The largest unit(s) is not affected by the updating process at all. The largest unit(s), however, is the only unit to inhibit the second-largest unit(s). The contribution term for all other units would be larger than for the second largest because those units would be inhibited by all larger units. Along with the fact that they are smaller initially, this means that they would reach the lower threshold faster than the second-largest unit. Convergence is achieved when the units are partitioned into two sets: one set of units will have a value of zero, and the other set of units will have values greater than θ but those values will be within θ of each other. Therefore, the time to convergence is determined by the time it takes the second-largest element to reach zero. This makes the convergence time independent of the number of competing units. The amount of inhibition from the updating rule for the second-largest unit B where the largest unit is A is given by

$$B(t) = 2^t B(0) - (2^t - 1)A(0) \tag{5.21}$$

for t starting at 0, and both $B(0)$ and $A(0)$ are constant. Convergence is achieved when $B(t) = 0$. Convergence will thus require

$$\log_2\left(\frac{A(0)}{A(0) - B(0)}\right) \tag{5.22}$$

iterations. An even faster convergence could be obtained by setting a threshold for convergence that is greater than zero; that is, convergence would be achieved when $B(t) \leq \varepsilon$. In this case, the numerator of equation 5.22 becomes $A(0) - \varepsilon$. Equation 5.22 clearly shows that the more similar the values of the two items, the slower the convergence. There is no dependence on either topographic distance (as in Koch & Ullman, 1985) or numbers of competitors. A bound on this number of iterations is desirable. By definition of the updating rule, the differences between competitors must be at least θ, so the denominator of the logarithm can be no smaller than θ. Neither A nor B can be larger than Z. Thus, the upper bound on the number of iterations is given by

$$\log_2\left(\frac{Z}{\theta}\right). \tag{5.23}$$

A lower bound on number of iterations, in practice, is one.

Selection within a Pyramid

Now that the selection method has been detailed for a single sheet, it can be extended to a pyramid of sheets. The equations are the same as shown above; the only change is the participants in the competitions.

Theorem 5.2 *The θ-WTA algorithm is guaranteed to find a path (chain) through a pyramid of L layers such that it includes the largest-valued neuron in the output layer (m_L) and neurons m_k, $1 \leq k < L$, such that m_k is the largest-valued neuron within the support set (the set $\bar{\wedge}$ for that neuron) of m_{k+1} and where m_1 must be within the central region of the input layer.*

Proof   The proof is by induction on the number of layers of the pyramid. Theorem 5.1 proved that for a single layer, θ-WTA is guaranteed to converge and to find the maximum-valued elements in the competing set. This is true regardless of the type of computation that derived those values. The same single layer guarantees hold throughout the pyramid. Thus, the theorem is true for one layer.

There is an important reason for the restriction on the neuron that the method is guaranteed to find. Recall the Context and Boundary Problems. The absolute maximum value in the input layer is confounded by these two characteristics of pyramid processing and would not be preserved under all conditions. Thus, θ-WTA can only find the maximum values of those convolutions from layer to layer and not necessarily the maximum values that are inputs to those convolutions. This seems exactly what is required if those convolutions are measures of fit for features or events in the input.

Assume that for a pyramid of n layers, the theorem is true. By the induction principle, if it can be proved that the theorem holds for $n + 1$ layers (where the $n + 1$-th layer is added to the pyramid on the input layer side), the proof is complete for a pyramid with an arbitrary number of layers. Suppose that the beam path includes neuron m_n in the n-th layer. The θ-WTA process rooted at neuron m_n is guaranteed by theorem 5.1 to find the largest-valued neuron in the support set of node m_n in layer $n + 1$ and include it in the path.   ∎

The proof was specific for single winners of the θ-WTA algorithm but extends trivially to winning regions because all of the proof's components apply equally to each element within a winning region in an independent fashion. This provides strong evidence that the strategy of top-down tracing of connections works; the examples of the real system in operation given in chapter 7 will complete the proof of the efficacy of the method.

Selection within the P-Lattice

The final extension to the selection process is to show how it may operate on the lattice of pyramids defined early in this chapter. First, we must decide how the top layer, $L - 1$, of sheets is handled. If no additional machinery is added, the selection process outlined can proceed independently within each of the R_{L-1} sheets in that layer. A strongest responding region of neurons will be found for each, and each will then activate a top-down search within its pyramid. If, within the R_{L-1} sheets, only one sheet contains active neurons (e.g., if the others represent features or objects not present in the input), there is no problem and selection proceeds as if in a single pyramid. Moving to the more complex case where there are more active sheets than one, several cases can be identified. If the winning regions are completely spatially coincident—presumably, they arise due to the same stimulus—they are all selected, and the top-down tracing proceeds along each path independently. The proof of theorem 5.2 is sufficient to ensure the independent traversals will converge (and the examples of chapter 7 will demonstrate this). As the proof of theorem 5.2 was done by induction, it holds for any number of layers of a pyramid. Any level of a pyramid can thus play the role of the input layer; that is, the proof applies for a contiguous subset of layers of a pyramid. As a result, the theorem tells us that top-down tracings with multiple starting points will converge onto a shared common sheet within the P-Lattice if the cause of each traversal is the same stimulus. That shared common sheet is the greatest element of the R-Lattice.

Suppose the winning regions in the R_{L-1} sheets arise due to different stimuli; they may be only overlapping or completely disjoint spatially. A number of heuristics can apply, and some are explored in Tsotsos et al. (2008):

• Task-specific selection by the executive.

• Select the largest overall response either in terms of actual value or in spatial extent or in combination.

• Select the largest response in each sheet.

• If it were possible that sheets could be related by whether or not one encodes stimulus qualities that are complementary or mutually exclusive to one another, then this information might be useful. Regions within complementary sheets can be chosen together; among the mutually exclusive ones, the individual winning regions compete with each other, and the strongest is chosen.

The kind of visual entity that is represented is also important. If, for example, one sheet represents the outline of a face, another the eyes, and another the nose, then the regions will certainly not be spatially coincident even if they are in sheets at the same layer and arise due to a single face in the image. However, here the choice of visual decomposition would seem inappropriate. Each of these elements are part of a face, and the face should be represented at a higher-layer sheet. In other words, if there is an appropriate hierarchical decomposition of visual information, the likelihood of this problem diminishes. Many have described such part-based decompositions; for review see Tsotsos (1992b) and Dickinson (2009). There may be other heuristics that might be useful. In general, due to the heuristic nature of these approaches, the potential for error is real.

Competition to Represent a Stimulus

The above has been presented as if there were only one possible concept represented at each spatial location. That is, the lateral competition and cooperation across columns is represented explicitly in equation 5.19, but no similar concept is provided within a column. Certainly, the classical conception of a column includes many interpretive neurons, each representing different features or concepts, but all with the same receptive field (Hubel & Wiesel, 1965). Some are clearly in competition with one another (different orientations of lines, for example), whereas others are independent (color with oriented lines, for example). The ones that are independent are covered by equation 5.19. The ones that compete require some additions.

The type of competition would be exactly the same as in classic lateral inhibition (described earlier), namely, the strongest wins, although task bias may remove some possibilities from a given competitive set. ST provides no explicit mechanism of attention to affect this competition otherwise. However, the spatial or featural selection that has been described has the side-effect of modulating this competition. Suppose there is more than one separate stimulus within a receptive field. Also suppose there is at least one neuron that is selective for each stimulus. If, for any reason, attention is paid to one of the stimuli, ST's mechanism will spatially suppress the remainder of the receptive field for the neuron selective—call it neuron A—to that stimulus. In doing so, those neurons that are selective to the other stimuli—call them, B, C, and so on—but whose receptive fields have spatial overlap with the selected neuron will see their input suppressed and thus their response diminished. This in turn would lead to reduced inhibition directed to neuron A from B, C, and so on. The reduction in inhibition will lead to an increase in response of A. These are layer-by-layer effects. Motter (1993), and many since, showed that attention can lead to both increases and decreases in response. The above solution was first represented in Tsotsos, Culhane, and Cutzu (2001). The Biased Competition Model covers this issue as well but with a slightly different explanation (Reynolds et al., 1999); the Normalization Model of Attentional Modulation also demonstrates this nicely (Lee & Maunsell, 2009, 2010).

More on Top-Down Tracing

To this point, the only mechanism to guide the downward tracing is the computation of the gating networks. Is there ever a need to terminate a traversal because it is errant as was hinted at in the "Selection" section of this chapter? How would the system know if the traversal goes astray? The proof of theorem 5.2 is sufficient to guarantee that any top-down traversal in a single pyramid will converge on the strongest set of responses in the central region of the input layer. If the strongest responses are in the periphery, a second, independent mechanism deals with it. However, what happens for top-down traversals in the P-Lattice that do not have the same stimulus cause? To illustrate this issue, recall that layer $L-1$ of the P-Lattice represents R_{L-1} sheets; these sheets are the top layers of separate interacting pyramids within the P-Lattice. Now suppose that the selection process finds a different subset of winning neurons in each, different in that they do not have the same location and spatial extent. This is possible because they operate independently and only share bias or priming imposed by the executive. It is not difficult to imagine situations where there are many strong stimuli in a scene whose perception may conflict with one another. Fortunately, the key objective for this traversal provides what we need. Suppose one of the heuristics outlined in the previous section is applied. The point of the downward traversal is to identify the pathway of neurons that participate in the correct identification of an attended stimulus and to ameliorate or eliminate the effect of any surrounding context. The side-effect of these actions is that the responses of those neurons on the selected pathway will never decrease. They will remain the same or increase, necessarily so if conflicting context is reduced, and this was outlined in the previous section.

Reynolds and Desimone (1999) concluded:

[W]hen attention is directed to one of two receptive field stimuli, its effect depends on the underlying sensory interactions. In the absence of sensory interactions, attention to either individual stimulus typically is limited to a moderate increase in mean response. When sensory interactions do occur, the magnitude and direction of the observed attention effects depend on the magnitude and direction of the underlying sensory interactions. If the addition of the probe suppresses the neuronal response, then attention to the reference stimulus typically filters out some of this suppression. If adding the probe facilitates the response, attention to the reference typically filters out some of this facilitation. Attending to the probe magnifies the change that was induced by the addition of the probe. These linear relationships between selectivity, sensory interactions, and attention effects provide several constraints on the set of possible models of ventral stream visual processing.

They, and also Luck, Chelazzi, Hillyard, and Desimone (1997a), found increases due to attention, when sensory interactions are small, to be more than 60% in both V4 and V2 neurons in monkey. Reynolds and Desimone show that adding a second stimulus typically caused the neuron's response to move toward the response that was elicited by the second stimulus alone. Further, they found that if each of two different stimuli cause the neuron to respond equally, then if both are present in the receptive field, the response is the same as if only one were present; in other words, firing rate cannot distinguish them. The mechanism outlined in the previous section leads to exactly this behavior and is the counterpart of what Reynolds and Desimone call the sensory interaction. We will need to assume that this general pattern is true throughout the visual processing areas. We also need to assume that each neuron has only one preferred stimulus, and if that preferred stimulus is seen on any possible context, it will respond less than if it sees its preferred stimulus on a blank field. This does not preclude location or rotation invariance, for example, for the same stimulus. This means that a simple monitoring of the attended neurons at layer $L - 1$ to ensure response never decreases is sufficient to know that the top-down traversal is succeeding. If it is detected that the responses decrease, the traversal can be terminated, and a new one started. Alternatively, a back-tracking strategy can be used moving upward one level, finding an alternate set of winners, and retrying. The reasons for errors in the traversal might have their source in the heuristic nature of how the start of the traversals is determined as described in the previous section. This is one clear source of possible errors during complex scene perception whose correction may proceed on a hypothesize-and-test basis and, at the very least, requires more processing time.

Inhibition of Return

The algorithms presented in chapter 4 both include components that are related to the inhibition of return function, the first algorithm in step 8, and the second in step 6. The first of these specifically inhibits the pass zone of the attentional beam after a stimulus has been attended and thus those same connections are not available for use in determining the second fixation. The second of these inhibits previously fixated locations in the overall competition between overt and covert targets. It is assumed that these signals arise from an executive controller that is outside of the main algorithms presented here. Clearly, they must be tied to the task at hand. A detection task would require only the second kind of signal upon its completion, whereas a visual search task would require both kinds for each candidate target examined in a sequence.

Peripheral Priority Map Computation

As described in chapter 4, the determination of salience plays a very specific role in the overall model, and that role is intimately connected to eye movements (i.e., overt fixation). The computation of visual saliency is built on a first principles information theoretic formulation named Attention via Information Maximization (AIM; Bruce, 2008; Bruce & Tsotsos, 2005, 2009). In AIM, the definition of visual saliency includes an implicit definition of context. Visual salience is not based solely on the response of cells within a local region but on the relationship between the response of cells within a local region and cells in the surrounding region. Visual context may be equated to a measure of the information present locally within a scene as defined by its surround, or more specifically, how unexpected the content in a local patch is based on its surround and information seeking is the visual sampling strategy. Further, as mentioned earlier, task bias plays a role as well. It is not within the scope of this volume to provide all the details of AIM, and the reader should consult one of the above citations where all the detail is available.

The AIM algorithm would take as input the Peripheral Attentional Field, that is, the neural responses of early layers of the P-Lattice, say V1, V2, MT—areas early enough in the pyramid to have not been too strongly affected by the Boundary Problem—in the region outside the central 10° area. The expected annulus of visual field that would be affected by the Boundary Problem is small because of the small sizes of receptive fields involved and also the relatively few layers of additive effects. The computations of those visual areas would be already biased by task knowledge as shown in figure 4.2. Decisions regarding the selection of attentional fixations in the periphery are made on the basis of these early computations and in the central regions are made on the basis of fully abstracted visual processing. This is perhaps the key distinction between the Selective Tuning and Saliency Map Models. It also points to a very different way of testing fixation models.

Fixation History Map Maintenance

The combination of Peripheral Priority Map, Fixation History Map, and History-Biased Priority Map provide the inputs to the overt fixation control mechanism for ST. Within the algorithm presented in the section "Selective Tuning with Fixation Control" of chapter 4, all of the steps are straightforward except for step 7—update the Fixation History Map.

Each of the PPM, FHM, and HBPM is encoded in gaze-centered coordinates, that is, the point of gaze is always location (0,0). All other locations are relative to this origin. The dimensions of each (i.e., in terms of the visual angle of visual field they encompass) are left unspecified except for the following relationships:

• PPM has the same overall dimensions as visual area V1, but the central $10°$ of visual field are omitted.

• HBPM has the same dimensions as visual area V1, but the full extent of the visual field is represented.

• FHM represents a larger spatial extent than the HBPM.

The determination of the contents of each of these maps is accomplished as follows:

• The AIM method provides the computation of the PPM.

• HBPM is dynamically updated to represent the current central focus and the contents of the PPM. Also, the current contents of FHM inhibit the contents of HBPM on a location-by-location basis.

• Within the FHM, an (x,y) location that has previously been visited has an initial value of, say, 1.0, and this decays over time with some time constant, perhaps determined by task demands. If a fixation shift is covert, no changes to the map are needed save to update the new location within it. If the fixation is overt, then the coordinates of the whole map change. If the shift can be specified as a move from $(0,0)$ to location (x_{new}, y_{new}), then the contents of the entire map must be shifted by $(-x_{new}, -y_{new})$. Clearly, as the FHM must be of finite size, some previously viewed locations may fall off the map. Additional detail and discussion may be found in Zaharescu (2004) and Zaharescu et al. (2005).

Task Guidance

How exactly are the instructions given to a subject (e.g., when viewing a display during an experiment) used in ST? The fact that task guidance has been part of the model since its inception does not answer this question. Task instructions lead to the inhibition of all task-irrelevant computations in ST (see figure 4.2). For other models, for example that of Navalpakkam and Itti (2005, 2007), the task only biases the computation of the saliency map. The Navalpakkam and Itti model uses the task represented by keywords that are then matched to a world knowledge base to determine what features might be relevant. Those become the preferred features. They address complex instructions together with the full object recognition problem. The goal here is less grand.

For a great percentage of all visual attention experiments, especially those involving non-human primates, targets are shown to subjects visually. The target must be processed by the same system that will be used for test displays—this is obvious. But the analysis of the target by itself can be used to provide guidance. The following are available immediately after the target is interpreted:

• The image contrast might be used to determine a suitable value for θ.

• The size of the target can be used to determine δ and ζ.

• A location cue can be encoded by the position and configuration of the attentional beam; attend the cue but then do not disengage attention. The stimulus image will be processed initially with the cue location and extent intact yet its immediate surround suppressed.

• For unactivated sheets, that is, sheets that may represent features or stimulus qualities not present in the target, their bias signal, B, and control signal, ς, can be set to 0.

• For all locations within sheets that show some activity above a noise or resting firing rate threshold, the bias signal B passed downward is set to 1.0. Alternatively, the degree of activity could also play a role in the value of B. A sheet that is highly activated by the target could lead to a higher value of B.

This is already quite a lot of task-specific guidance. To be sure, more can be had from any instructions given via natural language, and the context of one's world knowledge also plays a role in how those may be interpreted. As a point of comparison, the gain parameter, which is effectively the only attentional control signal in the Biased Competition Model, does not appear in this list because there is no explicit mechanism of response enhancement in ST.

Comparisons with Other Models

Table 5.1 provides a snapshot of ST and five other models and how they mathematically represent neural responses under attentional influence. The models, in addition to Selective Tuning (ST), and the acronyms used are

Biased Competition (BC; Desimone & Duncan, 1995; Reynolds et al., 1999)

Feature-Similarity Gain Model (FSG; Boynton, 2005; Treue & Martinez-Trujillo, 1999)

Cortical Microcircuit for Attention (CMA; Buia & Tiesinga, 2008)

Normalization Model of Attention (NMA; Reynolds & Heeger, 2009)

Normalization Model of Attentional Modulation (NMAM; Lee & Maunsell, 2009)

A number of other models have been proposed as plausible implementations of biased competition or feature-similarity gain, pushing forward on the forerunner models above (e.g., Ardid, Wang, & Compte, 2007; Rolls & Deco 2002; Hamker & Zirnsak, 2006; Spratling & Johnson, 2004), but are not included here.

For each of the models, there is no evaluation of their actual results presented because each in its own way shows good matches to data and/or behavior. As a result, the point of this comparison is to clarify commonalities, differences, gaps, and strengths. The most immediate first impression of table 5.1 is how different all the formulations appear. But this seems to be more of a feature of the model scope and starting assumptions than of substance.

As a first point of comparison, all of the models except for ST are data-fitting models and not computational models using the definition of chapter 3. Each would take existing data and determine parameter values of a set of equations that provide the closest fit to the data. As such, equations with high degrees of freedom (most variables) and nonlinearities have the greatest potential to capture the data presented. They also are the least specific or have the least scientific value because a high-enough number of variables and nonlinearities may capture just about any data set. ST takes input images and determines responses to that input, a completely different approach because the data and/or behavior must be produced for specific input. Again, a computer program may behave in any manner its programmer sees fit; it too may have suspect scientific value unless it has been developed on a sound and principled theoretical foundation. The development of ST has been conducted on such a sound theoretical foundation, and all aspects of its realization have been guided by it.

Table 5.1
The mathematical formulation of the five models compared in this chapter. The reader should consult the original papers for further details.

Model	Single-Neuron Equation	Variables
Biased Competition (BC) (Desimone & Duncan, 1995; Reynolds et al., 1999)	$\dfrac{dy}{dt} = (B-y)E - yI - Ay$	$E = x_1 w_1^+ + x_2 w_2^+$, excitatory input for two stimuli within the same receptive field. $I = x_1 w_1^- + x_2 w_2^-$, inhibitory input for two stimuli within the same receptive field. The w's are positive and negative synaptic weights. $\lim\limits_{t\to\infty} y = \dfrac{BE}{E+I+A}$. B is the maximum response. A is a decay constant.
Feature-Similarity Gain (FSG) Model (Boynton, 2005; Treue & Martinez-Trujillo, 1999)	$R(x_i, c_i, y) = G(y)[H(x_i, c_i) + \delta]$	$H(x_i, c_i) = \dfrac{\sum_i [c_i F(x_i)]^2}{\sum_i c_i^2 + \sigma^2}$, where the x_i are features, the c_i their contrast. $F(x_i)$ is the linear response to each stimulus component. σ is a semisaturation term. δ is the inherent baseline-firing rate of the neuron. The gain factor $G(y) > 1$ for a preferred feature, $G(y) < 1$ otherwise.
Cortical Microcircuit for Attention (CMA) (Buia & Tiesinga, 2008)	$I_{E1} = I_{0,E1} + A_E[\beta_E c_1 + (1-\beta_E)c_2]$ $I_{FF1} = I_{0,FF1} + A_{FFI}[\beta_{FFI} c_1 + (1-\beta_{FFI})c_2]$ $I_{E2} = I_{0,E2} + A_E[\beta_E c_1 + (1-\beta_E)c_2]$ $I_{FF12} = I_{0,FF12} + A_{FFI}[\beta_{FFI} c_1 + (1-\beta_{FFI})c_2]$	Equations are those for each type of neuron in their network (see text). E, excitatory pyramidal neuron; FFI, feed-forward interneuron; A, an overall scaling factor; c, stimulus contrast; β, stimulus selectivity, $0.5 \leq \beta \leq 1$; I_0, constant offset current.
Normalization Model of Attention (NMA) (Reynolds & Heeger, 2009)	$R(x,\theta) = \left\lvert \dfrac{A(x,\theta)E(x,\theta)}{S(x,\theta)+\sigma} \right\rvert_T$	$E(x,\theta)$ is the stimulus drive at location x for orientation θ. $A(x,\theta)$ is the attentional field. $S(x,\theta)$ is the suppressive drive. σ is a constant that determines the neuron's contrast gain. $\lvert.\rvert_T$ specifies rectification with respect to threshold T. $S(x,\theta) = s(x,\theta) * E(x,\theta)$ ($*$, convolution). $s(x,\theta)$ gives the extent of pooling. Stimulus contrast is also included in the equations and is not shown here; see the paper for further details. $A(x,\theta) = 1$ everywhere except for the positions and features that are to be attended, where $A(x,\theta) > 1$.
Normalization Model of Attentional Modulation (NMAM) (Lee & Maunsell, 2009)	$R_{1,2} = \left[\dfrac{N_1 \cdot (I_1)^u + N_2 \cdot (I_2)^u}{N_1 + N_2} \right]^{1/u}$	Assumes two stimuli present in RF. $N_{attended} = (1-s)(1-e^{-\beta ac}) + s$, $\beta = 1$ for unattended items, $\beta > 1$ for attended items, α is the slope of normalization, c is stimulus contrast; s is the baseline of normalization. $I_j = \left[R_j^u + \dfrac{s}{N_j}(R_j^u - m^u) \right]^{1/u}$, direct input ($u$ is a free parameter to enable modeling of different summation regimens). $N = (1-s)(1-e^{-\alpha c}) + s$ is the normalization term.
Selective Tuning (ST) Model	$\dfrac{d r_{ijxy}}{dt} = \dfrac{1}{\tau} \left[-r_{ijxy} + B_{ijxy} S \left(\sum_{k \in \hat{c}_{ijxy}} \gamma_k g_{k(ijxy)} r_k + \hat{c}_{ijxy} \sum_{h \in \hat{c}_{ijxy}} g_h r_h \right) \right]$	See equations earlier in this chapter.

ST and BC are based on the time-varying version of the popular leaky integrate-and-fire neuron formulation; NMAM is based on the constant input version (see equation 5.6). CMA is based on the classic Hodgkins–Huxley model, and the remainder of the models seem to be more custom designed. Note that Izhikevich (2004) points out that the integrate-and-fire model has quite poor realism in comparison with real neurons, whereas the Hodgkins–Huxley model is perhaps the best. The tables are turned, however, when it comes to practicality; Hodgkins–Huxley is very expensive computationally and suited only for few neuron simulations, whereas integrate-and-fire is easy to implement and is suitable for large networks especially if analytic properties are of interest. The Izhikevich neuron model seems to exhibit the best of both realism and efficiency, but seems less intuitive as to how to include the effects being explored here. It may be that the various basic neuron models were not designed with the goals needed for this sort of computational exploration.

BC, FSG, NMA, and NMAM are single-neuron models. NMA goes beyond a single neuron in that it takes larger visual fields into account. Specifically, it takes as input the attentional field, the stimulus drive, and the suppressive drive and produces a population response. As the authors describe it, the attentional field is the strength of the attentional modulation as a function of receptive field center and orientation preference. The attention field is multiplied point-by-point with the stimulus drive. The suppressive drive is computed from the product of the stimulus drive and the attention field and then pooled over space and orientation. The response is computed by dividing the stimulus drive by the suppressive drive. Such a divisive normalization is also present in NMAM and FSG as well, although it takes different forms. CMA employs a network of several neurons; there are top-down interneurons (TDI), feed-forward interneurons (FFI), and excitatory pyramidal neurons (E) arranged in two columns of one neuron of each type. Stimulus inputs come to the FFI and E cells. E cells provide excitatory input to the FFI cells in the opposite column while receiving inhibition from the FFI and TDI cells in the same column. FFI cells also receive inhibition from the TDI cell in the same column. TDI cells receive input from outside the system (top-down inputs). In addition, the TDI cells are connected among themselves via mutual inhibition. In contrast, ST operates over the complex, anatomically realistic, P-Lattice architecture. This, coupled with ST's set of basic equations, permits network-wide attentional effects.

ST and BC do not take stimulus contrast into account, whereas the remaining models do. It seems difficult to know what value the contrast parameter might take in a feed-forward system. One would need to know which stimulus is to be attended, to segment it in the scene, and then compute its contrast with the background. By this time, however, it has already been attended and analyzed. Although contrast may be a good variable to include in a data-fitting model strategy, it seems less so in a computational model.

The next dimension along which these models may be compared is the manner in which attention is incorporatcd. CMA encodes attention by modifying a linear contrast parameter in the equations for the E and FFI neurons. Similarly, BC, FSG, NMA, and NMAM all provide a single parameter that controls attention; this is a bias or gain whose value changes from 'attended' to 'unattended' values. For example, in BC, attention is implemented by increasing by a factor of 5 both excitatory and inhibitory synaptic weights projecting from the input neuron population responding to the attended stimulus. In NMAM there is a parameter that takes values equal to 1 for unattended stimuli and larger for attended ones. Its effect is multiplicative; it multiplies the product of slope of normalization and contrast in the exponent of the response function. These models are all silent on how this value is set or how selections may occur. CMA is also silent in this regard. ST, on the other hand, has the selection mechanism completely integrated within the basic equations. Further, it is consistent with the conclusions of Khayat et al. (2010) who observed that attention can be best considered as modulating inputs to neurons, both spatial and feature: ST's equations do exactly this, manipulating neural inputs to achieve the required attentive effect.

ST provides for several mechanisms due to attention: task-specific bias, selection of strongest responses, modulation of lateral computations, and surround suppression. Going back to the taxonomy of attentional mechanisms presented in chapter 3, we see that much is covered by ST (◆):

• Selection mechanisms include selection of
    · spatiotemporal region of interest ◆
    · features of interest ◆
    · world, task, object, or event model
    · gaze and viewpoint
    · best interpretation or response ◆
• Restriction mechanisms are those dealing with
    · task relevant search space pruning ◆
    · location cues ◆
    · fixation points
    · search depth control during task satisfaction
    · modulating neural tuning profiles ◆
• Suppression applies in a number of ways, among them
    · spatial and feature surround inhibition ◆
    · inhibition of return ◆
    · suppression of task-irrelevant computations. ◆

It is difficult to see how the other five models deal with most of these. Note how enhancement or inhibition of response is not in this list; these are manifestations that result from various combinations of these mechanisms. It may be that these other models focus on modeling the actual data too strongly rather than on modeling the underlying causes for the changes in the data. Things look worse for all the models except for ST if the full list of attentional elements from chapter 3 is considered; chapter 8 will detail how ST fares in that comparison. It seems that most models were not developed with the breadth of attention as a goal.

Summary

This chapter has laid out the important details regarding how Selective Tuning may be realized. To be sure, insufficient information is given here for enabling one to develop a computer implementation. But this was not the goal. The primary goal is to develop the underlying theory in such a way so that it transcends implementation with a major focus on its predictive power for human visual attention. In comparison with several other models, the only reasonable conclusion is that it is perhaps a bit premature to make decisions on which formulation is best. Each seems to have desirable elements, and none seem to include a full picture of attentive neural processes. But it is clear that the richness required for progress on this issue is already in place.

Chapter 6 will continue the theoretical development, and chapter 7 will present many examples of the current implementation that will serve to illustrate the breadth and depth of the model. Chapter 8 will detail the many predictions for human visual attention.

6 Attention, Recognition, and Binding

This chapter begins with its punch line: Attention, recognition, and binding are intimately related. This is not a common position, particularly for computational vision research, and it is difficult to overcome the momentum of the fields involved. Part of the problem is that there is virtually no agreement on what these terms really mean. The literature over the past 50 years and more has caused the terms *attention*, *recognition*, and *binding* to become so loaded with different and conflicting meanings that their true nature is masked. The previous chapters were dedicated to a particular theory of attention, and hopefully what is meant by *attention* in this book is clear by now. Figure 6.1 provides a diagrammatic summary of the major attentional mechanisms described earlier. It should be as clear that this decomposition is not claimed to be complete and that other components may be discovered as our understanding develops. However, at this point, the three major mechanisms and their subclasses cover a large majority of the observed phenomena that an attention—indeed, a vision—theory must include.

Next, the same must be done for the terms *recognition* and *binding*, although it will not be to the same level of detail. Once all three terms are better explained, the relationships among them will be explored.

It should be pointed out that this exercise—trying to define what vision may be, what recognition is, what binding means—has occupied many in the past. The list of previous authors dealing with attention has been given; those who have dealt with the other issues include Pylyshyn (1973), Milner (1974), Grossberg (1975), Gibson (1979), Zucker (1981), Barrow and Tenenbaum (1981), von der Malsburg (1981), Marr (1982), Poggio, (1984), Biederman (1987), Aloimonos (1992), Wandell and Silverstein (1995), Treisman (1996, 1999), Palmer (1999), Roskies (1999), Singer (1999, 2007), Ullman (2000), Perona (2009), and Dickinson (2009), among many others. It is not clear that we have much agreement although elements seem to repeatedly appear. It is a testament to the intrinsic difficulty of providing definitions for these topics.

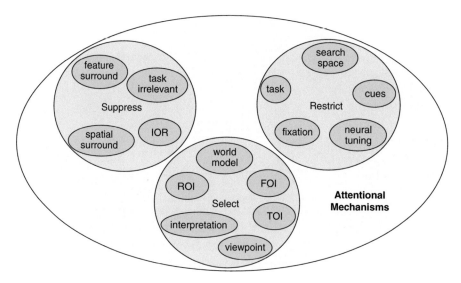

Figure 6.1
A Venn diagram of the key attentional mechanisms. IOR, inhibition of return; ROI, region of interest; TOI, time of interest; FOI, feature of interest.

What Is Recognition?

In computer vision, the definition of recognition has varied over the past 50 years. It seems that it is always intertwined with the recognition technique used (see Hanson & Riseman, 1978; Tsotsos, 1992b; also, the series of proceedings of the International Conference on Computer Vision from 1987 onwards). It is not possible to detail this evolution here; it has already been done well by Dickinson (2009). A list of currently studied recognition tasks is provided by Perona (2009):

Verification   Given an image patch, is a particular target present, yes or no?

Detection and Localization   Given a complex image, is an exemplar of a given category present and where?

Classification   Given an image patch or full image, can it be classified into one of a number of categories?

Naming   Given a complex image, name and locate all objects from a large set of categories.

Description   Given an image, describe it (environment, what objects, actions, relationships, etc.).

These are very interesting because of their relationship to previous discussions in this book. The first problem seems to be identical to the Visual Match problem proved to be NP-Complete if a pure feed-forward strategy is used. The Description task includes the tasks Yarbus presented to subjects that seemed to require task-directed scanning of the image; but certainly no eye movements are suggested by the current computer vision approaches. Classification can be considered as a set of Visual Match problems if the category is represented by enumerating all instances (a brute-force solution). So its worst-case complexity is also bad. Naming and Description can likely be decomposed into sequences of Verification, Detection, Localization, and Classification problems with computations for determining relationships and the like.

Dickinson uses the terms *categorization* and *abstraction* (Dickinson, 2009) where Perona uses *detection* and *classification*. This highlights the need for a standard terminology. Dickinson also points out that much of what recognition, broadly speaking, needs was already laid out by researchers in the 1970s and is only being rediscovered in recent years. However, that rediscovery is also accompanied by powerful new algorithmic tools. Dickinson stresses:

1. the importance of shape (e.g., contours) in defining object categories;

2. the importance of viewpoint-invariant, 3D shape representations;

3. the importance of symmetry and other nonaccidental relations in feature grouping;

4. the need for distributed representations composed of sharable parts and their relations to help manage modeling complexity, to support effective indexing (the process of selecting candidate object models that might account for the query), to support object articulation, and to facilitate the recognition of occluded objects;

5. the need for hierarchical representations, including both part/whole hierarchies as well as abstraction hierarchies;

6. the need for scalability to large databases; that is, the "detection" or target recognition problem (as it was then known) is but a special case of the more general recognition (from a large database) problem, and a linear search (one detector per object) of a large database is unacceptable;

7. the need for variable structure; that is, the number of parts, their identities, and their attachments may vary across the exemplars belonging to a category.

Certainly points 4, 5, and 6 resonate strongly with what has been said in previous chapters here. The remainder deal with aspects of visual representation, a topic a bit beyond the current scope. Nevertheless, these may be considered as a solid foundation for future recognition research.

Categorization to Dickinson means the same as it does to most human vision experimentalists. A further perspective from the biological sciences is useful.

Macmillan and Creelman (2005) provide good definitions for many aspects of recognition as they are related to experimental paradigms. **One-interval experimental design** involves a single stimulus presented on each trial. Between trials visual masks are used to clear any previous signal traces. Macmillan and Creelman wrote their specifications to have broader meaning than just for vision, and in fact their task descriptions apply for any sensory signal. Let there be K possible stimuli and M possible responses from a subject. A **Classification** task sorts those stimuli using the responses. Classification has many subtypes. If $K = 2$ (i.e., there are two possible stimuli), the task is **Discrimination**, the ability to tell the two stimuli apart. The simplest example is a **Correspondence** experiment in which the stimulus is drawn from one of two stimulus classes and the observer has to say from which class it is drawn. This is perhaps the closest to the way much of modern computer vision currently operates. A **Detection** task is where one of the two stimulus classes is null (noise), and the subject needs to choose between noise and noise plus signal. In a **Recognition** task, neither stimulus is noise. This seems to be what Perona meant by Verification. More complex versions have more responses and stimuli. If the requirement is to assign a different response to each stimulus, the task is **Identification**. The **Categorization** task requires the subject to connect each stimulus to a prototype, or class of similar stimuli (cars with cars, houses with houses). Perona's Classification task is exactly this as is Dickinson's Categorization. The **Within-Category Identification** task has the requirement that a stimulus be associated with a particular subcategory from a class (bungalows, split-level, and other such house types, for example). Responses for any of these tasks can be of a variety of kinds: verbal, eye movement to target, the press of a particular button, pointing to the target, and more. The choice of response method can change the processing needs and overall response time.

In **N-interval designs**, there are N stimuli (out of the possible K) per trial. In the **Same-Different** task, a two-interval task, a pair of stimuli is presented on each trial, and the observer must decide if its two elements are the same or different. For the **Match-to-Sample** task, N stimuli are shown in sequence, and the observer must decide which of the sequence matches the first one. **Odd-man-out** is a task where the subject must determine the presence of an odd stimulus from a set where all stimuli are somehow similar while one is not. The tasks just described are summarized in figure 6.2.

This forms a better starting point for us. This choice of starting point is not arbitrary. If our goal is to develop a theory of human visual processing, then the definitions used by experimentalists are the only ones to use because otherwise we would be comparing apples with oranges—comparing results arising from particular experimental methods with theories and their realizations that may have different testing methodologies and different underlying assumptions would not lead to any progress

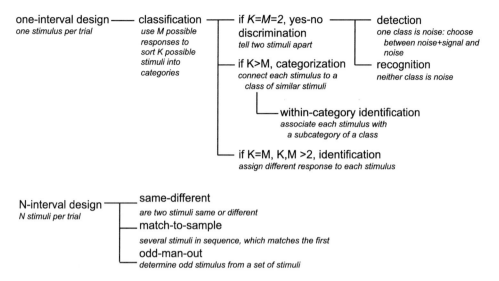

Figure 6.2
A partial taxonomy of experimental tasks involving different kinds of recognition.

and would only further confuse this difficult area of inquiry. Here, the definitions of Macmillan and Creelman are used.

More complex designs are also used by experimentalists, and Macmillan and Creelman detail many; the point here is not to summarize their entire book. Rather, the point is to present the definitions that we need and to stress that if computational theories wish to have relevance to human vision, they need to consider and explicitly match the experimental context and procedure for each task when comparing their performance with experimental observations.

It is possible to summarize experimental methods and provide a very generic template of what a typical experiment might have as its elements, keeping in mind that this is not intended to represent all possible experiments. Figure 6.3 shows this template. The template includes many options: there may be one or more cues provided visually or otherwise, there may be task specific instructions, there may be a fixation point, there may be one or more stimuli presented in one or more images in a sequence; the timing of presentation may be varied; there may be a need for subjects to select one stimulus over another, and so on. Variations in timings or inclusion of cues, repetitions, masks, display contents, response methods, subject feedback (and more) lead to an enormous breadth of possible experiments. Basically, recalling the decomposition of attentional mechanisms, these different components of an experiment seem to overlap quite well. It seems that attentional mechanisms—whether they were ever regarded as such by the

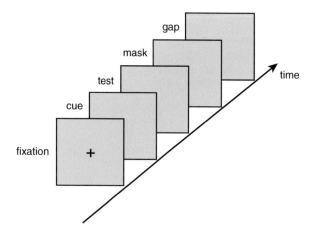

Figure 6.3
A hypothetical template for experimental design showing some of the typical elements that are part of an experimental setup.

experimenters—are inextricably intertwined with the experimental methods for recognition themselves.

All experiments require a response from the subject, a response that in some cases requires location knowledge—to varying degree—of the stimulus perceived. This leads us to define a new task that is not explicitly mentioned in Macmillan and Creelman, the **Localization** task. In this task, the subject is required to extract some level of stimulus location information to produce the response dictated by the experimenter. That level of location information may vary in its precision. Sometimes it may be sufficient to know only in which quadrant of the visual field a stimulus is found; other times a subject may need to know location relationships among stimuli, and so on. In fact, this may be considered as an implicit subtask for any of the standard tasks if they also require location information to formulate a response. Throughout the following, adding a superscript "L" to the task name will denote a task that also includes localization. The reason for this departure from the taxonomy of Macmillan and Creelman is that localization is a key component that distinguishes tasks. In contrast with many other proposals, it is not assumed that location is 'free' (i.e., without computation cost).

For a task where there is more than one stimulus in a sequence but where response is required for each stimulus for the same task, an additional notational change is needed. In fact, 'waves' or 'cascades' of stimuli continually flow through the system. We denote this kind of task with the prefix "R-." Thus, a task such as Rapid Serial Visual Presentation (RSVP) is an example of **R-Classification**. Finally, let us package all two-or-more interval designs, visual search, odd-man-out, resolv-

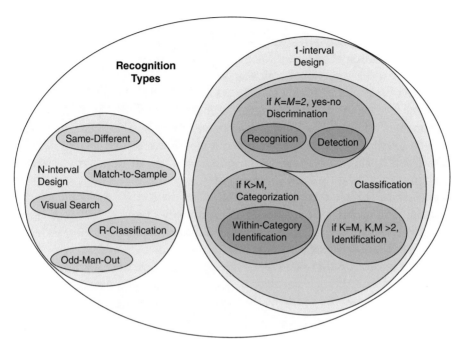

Figure 6.4
A Venn diagram of the revised recognition tasks, based on figure 6.2 but including the new tasks described in the text. Each of the types may include the Localization component as described in the text.

ing illusory conjunctions, determining transparency, any task requiring sequences of saccades or pursuit eye movements, and more as the **Extended Classification Task** for ease of reference. The recognition types are summarized in figure 6.4.

We now have a much better description of what recognition—or rather, the various kinds of such tasks—means. It is based on standard definitions in experimental perception, has many contact points with some uses of the terms in computer vision, and extends those standards to reflect 'hidden' tasks that are implied by subject response. We now turn to the binding issues.

What Is Visual Feature Binding?

A great deal of effort has gone into the discovery and elaboration of neural mechanisms that extract meaningful components from the images our retinae see in the belief that these components form the building blocks of perception and recognition. The problem is that corresponding mechanisms to put the pieces together again have been elusive even though the need is well accepted and many have studied the problem. This Humpty-Dumpty-like task has been called the **Binding Problem**

(Rosenblatt, 1961). Binding is usually thought of as taking one kind of visual feature, such as a shape, and associating it with another feature, such as location, to provide a unified representation of an object. Such explicit association, or binding, is particularly important when more than one visual object is present to avoid incorrect combinations of features belonging to different objects, otherwise known as **illusory conjunctions** (Treisman & Schmidt, 1982). Binding is a broad problem: visual binding, auditory binding, binding across time, cross-modal binding, cognitive binding of a percept to a concept, cross-modal identification, and memory reconstruction. The literature on binding and proposed solutions is large, and no attempt is made here to review it (but see Roskies, 1999).

As discussed in chapter 2, location is *partially* abstracted away within a hierarchical representation as part of the solution to complexity (Tsotsos, 1990a). A single neuron receives converging inputs from many receptors, and each receptor provides input for many neurons. Precise location is lost in such a network of diverging feed-forward paths yet increasingly larger convergence onto single neurons. It cannot be fully represented, and this is a key reason why binding is a real problem. Imagine how difficult the task becomes with the P-Lattice representation proposed in chapter 5. Any stimulus will necessarily activate a feed-forward diverging cone of neurons through all pathways, and in each case, neural convergence causes location information to be partially lost. Furthermore, there is no *a priori* reason to think that coordinate systems or magnifications or resolutions are constant throughout the system, so there may be large differences in all of these at each level. How can location be recovered and connected to the right features and objects as binding seems to require? How is the right set of pathways through this complex system identified and bound together to represent an object?

Three classes of solutions to the binding problem have been proposed in the literature. Proponents of the **Convergence** solution suggest that highly selective, specialized neurons that explicitly code each percept [introduced as **cardinal cells** by Barlow (1972), also known as **grandmother cells**] form the basis of binding. The main problem with this solution is the combinatorial explosion in the number of units needed to represent all the different possible stimuli. Also, whereas this solution might be able to detect conjunctions of features in a biologically plausible network (i.e., a multilayer hierarchy with pyramidal abstraction), it is unable to localize them in space on its own (Rothenstein & Tsotsos, 2008), and additional mechanisms are required to recover location information. **Synchrony**, the correlated firing of neurons, has also been proposed as a solution for the binding problem (Milner, 1974; Singer, 1999; von der Malsburg, 1981, 1999). Synchrony might be used to signal binding but is not sufficient by itself, as it is clear that this can at most tag bound representations, but not perform the binding process. The **Co-location** solution proposed in the Feature Integration Theory (Treisman

& Gelade, 1980) simply states that features occupying the same spatial location belong together. Because detailed spatial information is only available in the early areas of the visual system, simple location-based binding is blind to high-level structure. At best, then, this may be a useful idea for the early stages of visual processing only.

It is important, given the debate over binding and vagueness of its definition, to provide something more concrete for our purposes. It is as important to point out that the remaining discussion will focus on feature binding only. Here, a visual task—any of those defined earlier—will require a **Visual Feature Binding** process if:

the input image contains more than one object each in different locations (may be overlapping),

the objects are composed of multiple features,

the objects share at least one feature type,

the objects that satisfy these conditions are located centrally in the visual field.

Given the clear bias of processing for the central $10°$ of the visual field in human vision, described in chapter 2, binding problems might only arise if these conditions are true within those $10°$, not in the periphery (in the periphery, one cannot determine if these conditions are satisfied). If these conditions are not met, then a binding process is likely not required. This definition not only differs from previous ones but also has the property that it shows the dependence on image content for the determination of binding actions. Its justification arises from considerations of the circumstances of feed-forward stimulus activation of the P-Lattice that would lead to ambiguity in terms of category, components that define the category, and location of those components. As laid out so well by Reynolds et al. (1999), there are many scenarios where decision-making by neural response without attention will lead to incorrect results.

Four Binding Processes

The previous three sections outlined novel perspectives on the meaning of the terms *attention*, *recognition*, and *binding*. Recognition specifies the kind of visual task to be performed and sets up the decision-making process for that task; feature-binding needs are determined by the content of the stimuli on which the task is to be performed; and attention supplies the mechanisms that support both. The three must coexist.

Regardless of visual task, it is the same pair of eyes, the same retinal cells, the same, LGN, V1, V2, and so forth, that process all incoming stimuli. Each step in the processing pathway requires processing time; no step is instantaneous or can be assumed so. In experiments such as those defined above, the timings for each of the input arrays are manipulated presumably to investigate different phenomena. There are many variations on these themes, and this is where the ingenuity of the best experimentalists can shine. The argument made here is to use time as an organizational dimension; that is, the most effective way of carving up the problem is to cut along the dimension of time. The process of binding visual features to objects in each of the recognition tasks differs, and different sorts of binding actions take different amounts of processing time.

Consider the one-interval Discrimination Task (as long as no location information is required for a response) and its several subcategories: Correspondence, Detection, Recognition, and Categorization. Detecting whether or not a particular object is present in an image seems to take about 150 milliseconds (Thorpe, Fize, & Marlot, 1996). Marr, in his definition of full primal sketch, required about this time to suffice for segregation, as mentioned earlier, and thus his entire theory falls within this task, too. This kind of 'yes–no' response can also be called 'pop-out' in visual search with the added condition that the speed of response is the same regardless of number of distractors (Treisman & Gelade, 1980). The categorization task also seems to take the same amount of time (Evans & Treisman, 2005; Grill-Spector & Kanwisher, 2005). Notably, the median time required for a single feed-forward pass through the visual system is also about 150 milliseconds (Bullier, 2001). Thus, we conclude that a single feed-forward pass suffices for this visual task, and this is completely in harmony with many authors. These tasks do not include location or location judgments, the need to manipulate, point, or other motor commands specific to the object, and usually all objects can be easily segmented, as Marr required and reflected in the criteria presented earlier. That is, the background may provide clutter, but the clutter does not add ambiguity.

Convergence Binding achieves the Discrimination Task via hierarchical neural convergence, layer by layer, to determine the strongest responding neural representations in the processing hierarchy. This feed-forward traversal follows the task-modulated neural pathways through the 'tuned' visual processing hierarchy. This is consistent with previous views on this problem (Reynolds & Desimone, 1999; Treisman, 1999). This type of binding will suffice only when stimulus elements that fall within the larger receptive fields are not too similar or otherwise interfere with the response of the neuron to its ideal tuning properties. Such interference may be thought of as 'noise' with the target stimulus being 'signal.' Convergence Binding provides neither a method for reducing this noise nor a method for recovering precise location. The accompanying attentional process is the selection over the task-relevant representation of the strongest-responding neurons.

For an R-Classification Task (or one of its specialized instances), the feed-forward pass can be repeated. As each stimulus wave flows through the system, if inspection of the results at the top of the hierarchy suffices, Convergence Binding suffices here, too.

To provide more detail about a stimulus, such as for a within-category identification task, additional processing time is required, 65 milliseconds or so (Evans & Treisman, 2005; Grill-Spector & Kanwisher, 2005). If the highest levels of the hierarchy can provide the basic category of the stimulus, such as 'bird,' where are the details that allow one to determine the type of bird? The sort of detail required would be size, color, shape, and so forth. These are clearly less abstract entities, and thus they can only be found in earlier levels of the visual hierarchy. They can be accessed by looking at which feature neurons feed into those neurons that provided the category information. One way to achieve this is to traverse the hierarchy downward, beginning with the category neuron and moving downward through the needed feature maps. This downward traversal is what requires the additional time observed. The extent of downward traversal is determined by the task; that is, the aspects of identification that are required. **Partial Recurrence Binding** can find the additional information needed to solve the Identification Task if the required information is represented in intermediate layers of the processing hierarchy. Some aspects of coarse location information may also be recovered with a partial downward search (such as in which quadrant the stimulus lies). Partial Recurrence Binding can be directed by task requirements.

If detailed or precise localization is required for description or a motor task (pointing, grasping, etc.), then the top-down traversal process must be allowed to complete, and thus additional time is required. These are the **Discrimination**[L] *Tasks*, or simply, **Localization Tasks**. Recall that Perona's list of recognition tasks also included this. How much time? A lever press response seems to need 250–450 milliseconds in monkey (Mehta et al., 2000). During this task, the temporal pattern of attentional modulation shows a distinct top-down pattern over a period of 35–350 milliseconds poststimulus. The 'attentional dwell time' needed for relevant objects to become available to influence behavior seems to be about 250 milliseconds (Duncan, Ward, & Shapiro, 1994). Pointing to a target in humans seems to need anywhere from 230 to 360 milliseconds (Gueye, Legalett, Viallet, Trouche, & Farnarier, 2002; Lünnenburger & Hoffman, 2003). Still, none of these experiments cleanly separate visual processing time from motor processing time; as a result, these results can only provide an encouraging guide for the basic claim of our model and further experimental work is needed.

Behavior (i.e., an action relevant to the stimulus) requires localization. The precise location details are available only in the earliest layers of the visual processing hierarchy because that is where the finest spatial resolution of neural representation can be found. As a result, the top-down traversal must complete so that it reaches these earliest layers for location details. Note that intermediate points in the top-down traversal can provide intermediate levels of location details; full traversal is needed only for the most precise location needs.

A downward traversal may be partial not only because of the task definition but also because a full traversal is interrupted and not allowed to complete either because new stimuli enter the system before there is enough time for completion or because not enough time is permitted due to other tasks. The result is that there is the potential for errors in localization, and these may lead to the well-known illusory conjunction phenomenon (Treisman & Schmidt, 1982). A variety of different effects may be observed depending on when during the top-down traversal the process is interrupted with respect to the input.

Full Recurrence Binding achieves the Localization Task. If Convergence Binding is followed by a complete top-down traversal, attended stimuli in each feature map of the P-Lattice can be fully localized. Recurrent traversals through the P-Lattice "trace" the pathways of neural activity that lead to the strongest-responding neurons at the top of the hierarchy.

Full Recurrence Binding can determine the location and spatial extent of a stimulus discrimination object/event for images such as those defined for Convergence Binding, where there is no ambiguity and proper can occur without a special binding process. It can also do so for images that contain ambiguity. This means explicitly that segmentation for such images is not immediate in the Marr sense, that there are multiple objects in an image that share features and thus a simple convergence binding faces ambiguity and fails to find a clear winner.

Iterative Recurrence Binding is needed for the Extended Classification Task and for the R-Classification^L Task, and perhaps for others as well. Iterative Recurrence Binding is defined as one or more Convergence Binding–Full Recurrence Binding cycles. The processing hierarchy may be tuned for the task before each traversal as appropriate. The iteration terminates when the task is satisfied.

There are at least two types of Iterative Recurrence Binding. **Type I Iterative Recurrence Binding** is the more obvious one; namely, multiple attentional fixations are required for some task (e.g., visual search). **Type II Iterative Recurrence Binding** permits different pathways to be active for the same stimulus and fixation. Consider a stimulus depicting motion-defined form where a square of random elements rotates on a background of similar random elements. A rotating square is perceived even though there is no edge information present in the stimulus. After one cycle of Full Recurrence Binding, the motion can be localized and the surround suppressed. The suppression changes the intermediate representation of the stimulus so that any edge-detecting neurons in the system now see edges, edges that were not apparent because they were hidden in the noise. As a result, the motion is recognized, and with an additional processing cycle the edges can be detected and bound with the motion. This is clearly an instance of a concept that has been present

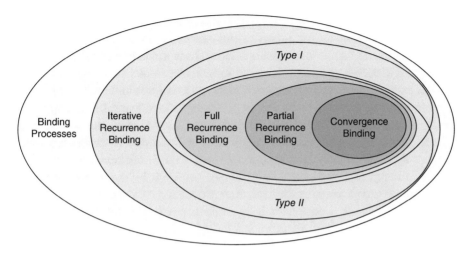

Figure 6.5
A Venn diagram of binding processes described in the text.

in computational vision for a long time (for a historical perspective, see Tsotsos, 1992b). An appropriate quote comes from Barrow and Tenenbaum (1981):

A major problem with the sequential program segmentation (segmentation followed by interpretation) used by both Roberts (1965) and Barrow and Popplestone (1971) is the inherent unreliability of segmentation. Some surface boundaries may be missed because the contrast across them is low, while shadows, reflections, and markings may introduce extra lines and regions.

Barrow and Tenenbaum advocated an Interpretation-Guided Segmentation process, where initial segmentations trigger possible interpretations that then guide improvements in segmentation, and the cycle continues until the task is completed. Type II Iterative Recurrence Binding may be considered an instance of exactly the same idea.

These several kinds of binding processes are shown in a Venn diagram in figure 6.5 to make clear their interrelationships. It is unlikely that this diagram is complete, and other forms of binding processes may be discovered in the future. However, this schematic does provide a unique foundation for organizing the concepts around binding issues.

Binding Decision Process

Most of what is required to implement the binding processes within ST has already been presented in chapter 5. One key remaining aspect is how the decision to use one or the other type of binding is made. Figure 6.6 gives the algorithm in its simplest form. For this algorithm—clearly a part of the executive controller—it is assumed that the kind of visual task is known in advance. Three kinds of tasks are included. Classification is the class where no location judgment or object manipulations are needed (i.e., no visually activated or guided behavior), and no conflicts in the images are expected. In the second task, Within Category Classification, a bit more is needed. Here, there is some visually guided behavior, but not much detail is needed for it. Tasks requiring Localization or in the class of Extended Classification tasks class require detailed observations to support visually guided behavior. For the first two tasks of the figure, if the processing thought sufficient by the task description is found to not be satisfactory for the task, then processing moves to the next-higher task. For example, if for a particular image one expects convergence binding to suffice but it does not, partial recurrence binding is tried. As in Posner's cueing paradigm, when the cue is misleading, processing takes longer. Similarly here, if the expectation does not match the stimulus, processing is revised until it does. In the case of free viewing, with no particular task, one may assume a Classification task; that is, one where no specific judgments of the perceived world are needed. If something is seen where this does not suffice, the system automatically moves to a perhaps more appropriate strategy.

Putting It All Together

All of the elements have now been laid out so that we may complete the puzzle of how attention, binding, and recognition may be connected. The mechanisms of attention, the types of recognition tasks and their observed response times, a set of four novel binding processes, and a control algorithm for choosing among them have been detailed. The algorithmic and mathematical details for each of the attentional mechanisms appeared in chapters 4 and 5. The details on how the various recognition processes actually occur and the specific visual representations that support them are beyond the scope of this book. The intent of the attention theory is to be applicable to any visual representation that satisfies the representational structure constraints of chapters 4 and 5. Evidence of its performance for a particular visual representation is shown in the next chapter. A second example of the kind of visual representation and recognition method that easily fit to Selective Tuning is the Learned Hierarchy of Object Parts (LHOP) theory of Leonardis and colleagues (Fidler & Leonardis, 2007; Fidler, Boben, & Leonardis, 2009). This is a generic framework for learning object parts and creating a hierarchy for categorization that satisfies the constraints for Selective Tuning as laid out in chapter 5.

The connections among attention, recognition, and binding are laid out in figure 6.7 and table 6.1. Figure 6.7 redraws and expands on figure 4.1. The new elements

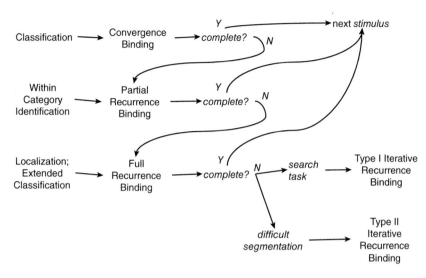

Figure 6.6
A flowchart of the algorithm for the binding decision process.

Table 6.1
A summary of the relationships among attention, binding, and recognition

Recognition task	Attention	Binding
Priming	Suppression of task-irrelevant features, stimuli, or locations; restriction to location cues, fixation point; selection of task success criteria	N/A
(R-)Classification (R-)Discrimination (R-)Detection (R-)Categorization (R-)Recognition (R-)Identification	Response selection	*Convergence Binding:* feed-forward convergence
Within-Category Identification	Response selection Top-down feature selection	*Partial Recurrence Binding:* top-down branch-and-bound until task completed
Localization Discrimination^L Classification^L	Top-down feature and location selection	*Full Recurrence Binding:* top-down branch-and-bound until localization completed
Extended Classification R-Classification^L	Sequences of convergence and recurrence binding, perhaps with task priming specific to each pass	*Iterative Recurrence Binding:* more than one task-relevant attentional cycle

*The asterisk beside Convergence Binding is a reminder that, as described in the text, those tasks are satisfied by Convergence Binding alone only if the constraint on the stimulus that there is an easy figure-ground segregation (within one feed-forward pass) is also satisfied. Otherwise, as shown in figure 6.6, a more complex binding procedure is needed. The notation '(R-)' means that the task is optionally repeated; recall earlier in the chapter where the prefix 'R-' was defined as signifying a repetitive task.

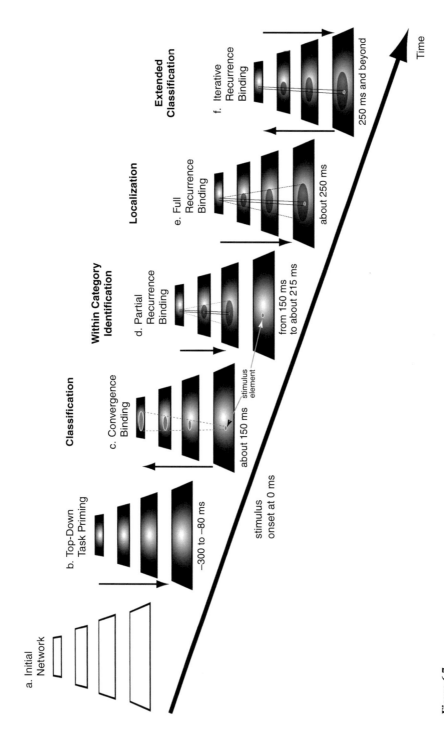

Figure 6.7
Tasks, attentional mechanisms, and binding processes organized along the dimension of processing time.

of figure 6.7 are the timings of processes, described earlier in this chapter, and the associated tasks. At best this is an approximation; the range of possible experimental variations does not lend itself to such a simple characterization, and the observed task timings show broad intervals that overlap with other tasks. Still, this can be considered a first-order organization of task type, attentional mechanisms and binding processes, and shows that the various views appearing in past literature all have a place even including the claims that binding is not a real issue (those that assume Convergence Binding with Marr-like segmentation quality suffices for all stimuli). For the Classification task, and if the image content is sufficiently simple (i.e., does not satisfy the constraints of the earlier section "What Is Visual Feature Binding" of this chapter), no obvious binding process is needed. Neural convergence suffices; here, this is the simplest binding process, Convergence Binding.

In addition to emphasizing that figure 6.7 is at best a first-order approximation, it is important to mention that the final stage—Extended Classification—is only a 'catch-all' stage. That is, experimental designs more complex than localization have not been at this time fully analyzed to see what subclasses they may represent and how the attentional and binding mechanisms may contribute to them. The challenge is to use this starting point as a means for organizing existing and defining new experimental and computational theories that might add flesh to the skeleton.

Table 6.1 provides a snapshot of the connections between the types of binding processes and attentional mechanisms proposed by Selective Tuning for each of the kinds of recognition tasks. It basically provides some of the labels and detail that would have overly cluttered figure 6.7. Figures 6.6 and 6.7 and this table give the full picture of the ST strategy for how attention, binding, and recognition are interdependent.

Summary

The connections between attention, binding, and recognition have been discussed with the goal of showing how these are tightly coupled and depend on each other. None are monolithic processes, and each has many subelements. The decompositions of attentional mechanisms and of binding processes are novel to the Selective Tuning approach. The recognition decomposition was borrowed in large part from Macmillan and Creelman (2005) but was enhanced and modified to include other tasks, such as Localization, and linked to views in computer vision such as those of Dickinson (2009) and Perona (2009).

The binding solution has some interesting characteristics that may be considered as predictions requiring investigation in humans or non-human primates:

1. Given a group of identical items in a display, say in a visual search task, subsets of identical items can be chosen as a group if they fit within a receptive field. Thus, the slope of observed response time versus set size may be lower than expected (not a strictly serial search). This is partially supported by the observations by Reynolds et al. (1999) concerning identical stimuli within a receptive field for V2 and V4 neurons.

2. There is no proof that selections made at the top of several pyramids will converge to the same item in the stimulus array. Errors are possible if items are very similar, if items are spatially close, or if the strongest responses do not arise from the same stimulus item.

3. Binding errors may be detected either at the top by matching the selections against a target, or if there is no target, during the binding attempt by checking the changes in neural responses as described toward the end of the previous chapter. The system then tries again; the prediction is that correct binding requires time that increases with stimulus density and similarity. In terms of mechanism, the ST model allows for multiple passes, and these multiple passes reflect additional processing time.

4. The mechanism of ST suggests that detection occurs before localization and that correct binding occurs after localization. Any interruption of any stage may result in binding errors.

ST has a number of important characteristics:

• a particular time course of events during the recognition process covering the simplest to complex stimuli that can be directly compared with qualitative experimental time courses;

• an iterative use of the same visual processing hierarchy in order to deal with the most complex stimuli;

• iterative tuning of the same visual processing hierarchy specific to task requirements;

• suppressive surrounds due to attention that assist with difficult segmentations;

• a particular time course of events for recognition ranging from simple to complex recognition tasks;

• a top-down localization process for attended stimuli based on tracing feed-forward activations guided by localized saliency computations.

Each of these may be considered a prediction for human or non-human primate vision. It would be very interesting to explore each.

7 Selective Tuning: Examples and Performance

The preceding chapters presented the theorems, strategies, data structures, logic, algorithms, and mathematics that define the Selective Tuning model. They have been extensively tested in many published papers and used by many other labs. However, the entire structure of figure 5.2 has not been tested as an integrated whole; many, but not all, of the pieces have been examined. This chapter will give many examples of these tests and provide discussion for a variety of features of the model.

To test the model effectively, some commitment to a representation of visual information must be made. The model was derived, formulated, and presented in a manner as independent from such commitments as possible expressly so that it would apply equally to any representational choices within the constraints presented. Here, most of the examples rely on a representation of visual motion processing. Others require shape or color processing. Some examples are rather old, others new, and thus visualizations differ across the examples; this is the nature of development over the long period of time during which Selective Tuning has been actively pursued. Color and animation are used extensively, and the color plates or the supplementary website (<http://mitpress.mit.edu/Visual_Attention>) should be viewed for those examples. The examples where a color version of a figure or an animation is provided on the Web have figure or movie numbers with the suffix "W."

The next section begins with a description of the main representation that is used in this chapter. Other representations will also be used, and these are described as they occur.

P-Lattice Representation of Visual Motion Information

The P-Lattice structure will be used to represent the visual information on which many of the following ST demonstrations are based. The choice of visual motion as the demonstration domain was made due to long-standing interest in motion perception. Note that this is a pure motion representation—there is no concept of edge or texture or depth or luminance and so on. Four distinct areas of the visual cortex are simulated in the model: V1, MT, MST (medial superior temporal), and 7a. These four areas are known to participate in the processing of visual motion (for a review, see Orban, 2008). There is no claim that the resulting model is a complete or fully biologically faithful replication of these visual areas. The model consists of 684 feature maps each of which encodes the entire visual field. These are the sheets of the P-Lattice, depicted in figure 7.1. The V1 layer contains 72 sheets, MT contains 468 sheets, MST has 72 sheets, and 7a has 72 sheets. Each of these groupings of sheets forms a hypercolumn structure although the diagram separates the maps for visualization purposes. V1 encodes translation at 12 directions and in three speed bands. V1 includes two main groupings of 36 sheets each:

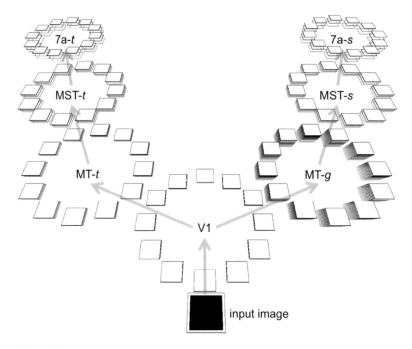

Figure 7.1
Full P-Lattice of the motion model. This shows the P-Lattice sheets that comprise visual areas V1, MT, MST, and 7a. Each rectangle (sheet) represents a single type of selectivity applied over the full image at that level of the pyramid. Position of a sheet around the ring of sheets represents direction of selectivity. The three sheets at each direction represent the three speed selectivity ranges in the model. In area V1, the neurons are selective to 12 different directions and 3 different speeds (low, medium, and high). Each area following area V1 has two parts: one where neurons are tuned to direction and speed, much like in V1 (the translational pyramid on the left), and the second part where neurons have more complex characteristics and are able to encode complex motion patterns, such as rotation, expansion, and contraction (the spiral pyramid on the right). The stack of sheets in area MT represents particular angles between motion and speed gradients.

one set performs spatiotemporal filtering on the input and feeds the filter results to the next set that integrates those results over the receptive field. Each area following area V1 has two compartments operating in parallel, one for translational motion (MT-t, MST-t, 7a-t) and one for spiral motion (MT-g, MST-s, 7a-s). Each of the sheets in the figure is drawn as having a thickness due to the fact that there are three speed tunings for each motion direction (three separate sheets). The translational compartments MT-t, MST-t, and 7a-t all have 36 sheets each, 3 speed tunings for each of 12 directions of translation. A translation motion sheet connects to the sheet of similar direction and speed in the next-higher translation motion area everywhere in the P-Lattice. MT-g includes three speeds but also 12 gradient directions for each local motion direction, so a total of 36 sheets for each of the 12 directions, and these appear in the figure as a stack of 36 rings for the 12 directions. An MT-g neuron receives input from three V1 sheets that encode the same direction of motion but are tuned to different speed bands. MST-s and 7a-s each have 36 sheets, 3 speed tunings for each of 12 complex motion patterns: rotations, contraction, expansion, and their combinations. MST-s neurons get input from a ring of MT-g sheets (i.e., one of the 36 rings of sheets that compose MT-g as shown in the figure), specifically, all sheets with the same gradient angles and speed tuning but all local translation directions. Finally, 7a-s neurons represent a coarser resolution version of the MST-s computation. All of these connections are reciprocal, however in the recurrent passes, only those that survive competition are active. More description for each area with mathematical formulations is relegated to appendix C. There, equations for the computation of P used in equation 5.4 of chapter 5 are given. The Selective Tuning functionality is integrated within this P-Lattice.

Priming

How is the representation of figure 7.1 affected if task information for priming is available? The next three figures provide examples. Figure 7.2 shows how priming for a rightwards motion affects the full P-Lattice. The effect on the translation side is easy to see. Recall that priming is realized in ST as an inhibition of the nonrelevant features or objects. Bias against non-rightwards motion (dark areas in the figure) is applied in a Gaussian-weighted fashion. That is, the strongest suppression is for leftwards motion, and suppression decreases in a Gaussian manner between the left and right directions. However, on the spiral side there is no impact. The reason is that the connectivity patterns here are different than those on the translation side as described earlier, and priming for a given direction has only a small effect on the sum of all the directions that form the input to an MST-s neuron. Figure 7.3 shows how priming for a location affects the network.

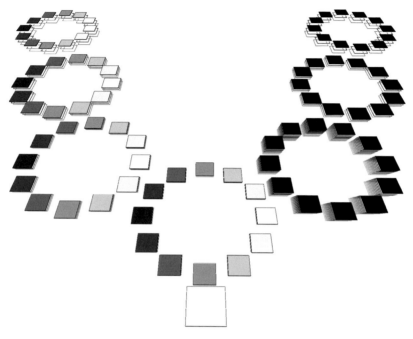

Figure 7.2
The P-Lattice of figure 7.1 but primed for rightwards motion. Darker shading represents greater inhibition.

Here, the result is more intuitive, and the inhibited regions are clear in all layers. Suppose there is both a rightwards motion direction and location component to the priming. The result is in figure 7.4. The combination of the previous two examples is easy to see. Nevertheless, depending on the particular representation of visual information used, these results are not obvious, and one can imagine that progressively complex kinds of priming instructions may in fact lead to counterintuitive bias patterns.

An early example of the impact of priming in the model simulation appeared some time ago in Dolson (1997). Dolson enhanced ST to allow position-invariant object recognition and introduced cooperation between features into the Selective Tuning Winner-Take-All framework to consider the spatial relationship between features when selecting winners. He demonstrated this with example recognition networks in which objects are represented as hierarchical conjunctions of parts and features culminating in the activity of one unit. He showed that the attentional beam that follows from the selection of such an object unit tightly encompasses the object in the image. Also, he showed that top-down inhibitory bias signals allow the selection of objects having particular low-level features.

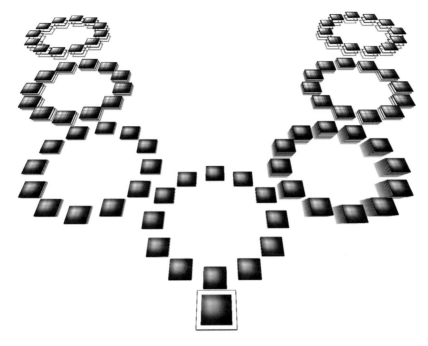

Figure 7.3
The P-Lattice of figure 7.1 but primed for location, specifically a position somewhat to the left of and above the center of the image. Darker shading represents greater inhibition.

The examples shown here are for an image containing two hollow rectangles, each a different color, and overlapping spatially (figure 7.5; color figure 7.5W).

The network is shown in figure 7.6. The network is designed to know about open rectangles of different colors. Details on how this network was constructed can be found in Dolson (1997). His network computed the following features, by layer in a feed-forward manner as a first pass, in order of processing:

Layer 1

Red-center minus green-surround

Green-center minus red-surround

Blue-center minus yellow-surround

Layer 2

Fine

Coarse

Blurred red and green colors

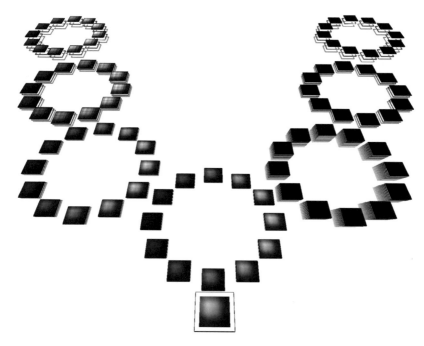

Figure 7.4
The P-Lattice of figure 7.1 but primed for rightwards motion at a particular location. Darker shading represents greater inhibition.

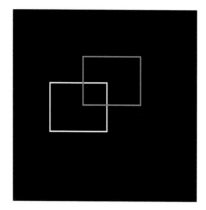

Figure 7.5 (color figure 7.5W)
Stimulus consisting of a red open rectangle (top item) and green open rectangle, the red overlapping the green [from Dolson (1997) with permission of the author].

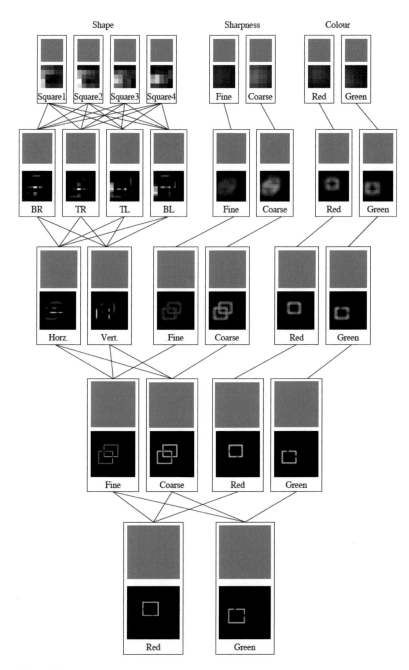

Figure 7.6
The result of a single feed-forward pass through the network of Dolson, defined to recognize different kinds of open rectangles. Each panel in this diagram contains a map of interpretive units below a map of (neutral) bias units. Note the confusing responses in many of the feature maps [from Dolson (1997) with permission of the author].

Layer 3

Horizontal edge

Vertical edge

Blurred Fine and Coarse sharpness

Blurred red and green colors

Layer 4

Bottom right corner

Bottom left corner

Top right corner

Top left corner

Blurred Fine and Coarse sharpness

Blurred red and green colors

Layer 5

Small square

Medium square

Large square

Very large square

Blurred Fine and Coarse sharpness

Blurred red and green colors

Each feature is shown in the lower part of each vertical panel in the figure; the upper part represents the bias weight map for that feature. The connecting lines between panels show the network feature map connectivity pattern. Figure 7.6 shows the result of the first processing pass for the input of figure 7.5W. It is clear that in many of the feature maps, there are many false and conflicting responses. If a top-down bias is applied in advance for, say, the red figure, the network would favor red features (the actual biases in this examples were red 0.25, green 0.75; fine 0.2, coarse 0.65; remaining shape biases were left at 0.5). The effect is shown in figure 7.7. The bias weight maps are shown in the upper parts of the network panels of figure 7.7, and their impact can be seen in the lower half of the panels. The top layer clearly has its greatest responses in the Red, Coarse, and Square 4 representations. Also clear is how the top-down bias permits one of the stimuli to be processed preferentially.

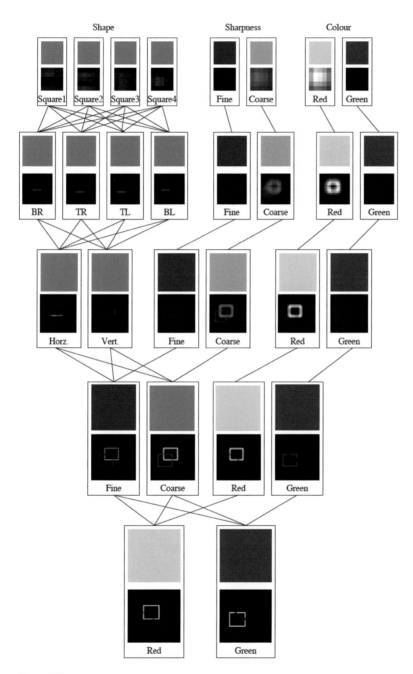

Figure 7.7
Task biases have been applied before the feed-forward pass in this example of Dolson's network and are shown in the various levels of intensity in the bias maps. The resulting set of responses is very different than in figure 7.6 and allows an easy segmentation of the red open rectangle [from Dolson (1997) with permission of the author].

Results After a Single Feed-Forward Pass (Convergence Binding)

A number of examples will now be shown to illustrate the performance of a single feed-forward pass through the motion representation. The simplest example is that of a single graphical object in motion on a blank background. Imagine the synthetic graphical object of figure 7.8 (movie 7.8W) rotating in a clockwise direction at some medium speed. Before continuing, a notational aside must be inserted. In figure 7.9 (plate 1; color figure 7.9W), a color wheel is shown that is used to label responses in the examples to follow. Color thus plays an important role in these examples (see the color plates or the Web page). As seen in these color wheels, a different color is used for each of the spiral motions; the same colors have different meaning when appearing in the translation part of the P-Lattice. There they refer to direction of

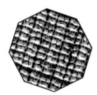

Figure 7.8 (movie 7.8W)
A single image from a video sequence of a synthetic, textured hexagon, rotating clockwise.

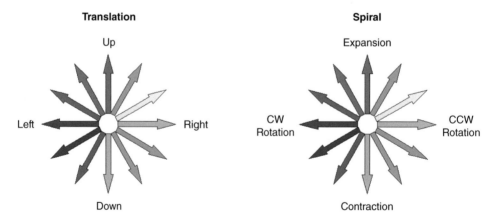

Figure 7.9 (plate 1; color figure 7.9W)
The color wheels used to code for motion direction and spiral motion class. The translation coding is on the left, and the spiral coding is on the right. The directions in between vertical and horizontal give combinations of the nearest orthogonal directions. The same color coding is used for the velocity gradient representations where it represents the direction of increasing gradient with respect to the local vector of translation, which by convention is set to be vertical. For example, if the gradient is coded green (as in counterclockwise rotation), it means that the direction of increasing value of velocity is perpendicular to the local direction of translation. CW, clockwise; CCW, counterclockwise.

translation, whereas in the spiral side of the P-Lattice they refer to kinds of spiral motion—clockwise, counterclockwise, approach or recede, and combinations of these. There is no additional coding for motion speed.

The image sequence of figure 7.8 (movie 7.8W) would activate the feed-forward network as shown in figure 7.10 (plate 4; color figure 7.10W). No cleaning up of the responses was performed (bounding box, outlier elimination, morphology, etc.) in this or any of the examples in this chapter. The output shown is always the direct result of ST's processing with no enhancements. This figure is a complex one, and reading it requires some guidance. Not all of the sheets present in figure 7.1 can be shown, obviously, so a reduced format appears in the subsequent figures. Areas 7a-t and 7a-s are not shown at all (nor for most of the following examples) because they would add no new component to this illustration other than a reduced resolution of area MST. Nine rings of 12 rectangles (sheets) each are shown, with 12 radial lines connecting groups of 9 rectangles. The radial lines are colored following the color wheel coding and have different meaning for different groups of rings. Each rectangle represents the response of one kind of neural selectivity; for example, the topmost rectangle in the figure represents upward translation at a fast speed. The inner three rings represent the spiral selectivities of area MST-s, the middle three rings are those of the gradient neurons of MT-g, and the outer three are the translation neurons of area V1. Within each group of three rings, the outer one is for fast motion, the middle for medium speed, and the inner for slow speed. Translation is shown only for V1 even though each of the areas has representations of translation. The MT-g responses shown are summary ones, because for each direction of local motion there are 12 gradient tunings. A sample of 12 different responses appears in figure 7.11. As a result, each rectangle shows only the maximum value on a point-by-point basis of all the gradient neurons at that position; for example, the maximum across the 12 responses shown in figure 7.11. This is only for this illustration; the algorithm does not use such a local maximum. The color-coding matters, so the reader is encouraged to see the color version (plate 4; color figure 7.10W).

There are a number of points to be emphasized regarding figure 7.10. The most obvious point is that even with this most simple motion stimulus, response is seen in almost all of the sheets. As such, a nontrivial problem of recombining responses into a single percept is present even here where it is clear that there are no responses due to other stimuli. A second point is that the single largest and strongest responding set of features is in the sheet to the left of the center, on the horizontal line, second closest to the center. This is an MST-s spiral sheet, for a medium-speed clockwise rotation, the correct percept for this stimulus. As a result, a simple inspection of the maximum response across MST-s sheets suffices to detect this. This corresponds, of course, with the Selection attention mechanism operating for Convergence Binding. A detection task such as this may be completed after a single

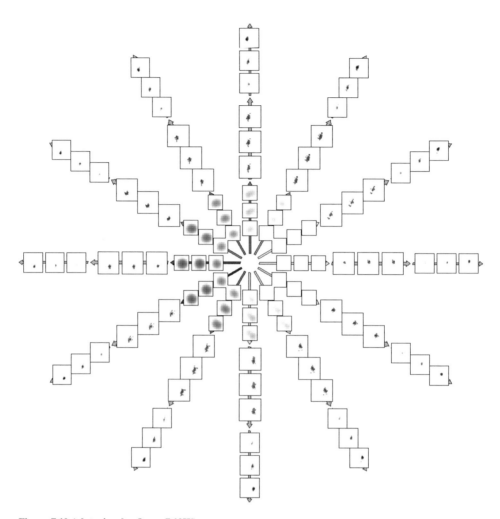

Figure 7.10 (plate 4; color figure 7.10W)
The representation of neural responses after the first feed-forward pass for the stimulus in figure 7.9. Areas V1 (outer three rings of sheets), MT-g (middle three rings of sheets), and MST-s (inner three rings of sheets) only are shown. The spokes give the colors of the coding color wheel with all the sheets along a spoke selective to appropriate, related feature qualities (outer sheets for direction, middle sheets for velocity gradient, inner sheets for spiral motion). MT-g depicts only the maximum response by location of all the gradient responses for ease of illustration only. The color coding in these sheets follows the color wheel. See text for more detail.

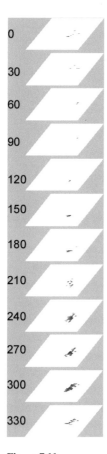

Figure 7.11
The 12 velocity gradient representations for a single local direction. The maximum at each point across the 12 representations is used for display purposes in the figures. Such a feed-forward maximum is not part of ST's computations.

feed-forward pass using a simple algorithm on the highest-level representations. A third point arises from a careful inspection of the spatial locations of responses. Moving around a particular ring of sheets, it is clear that responses basically cover the spatial extent of the stimulus. It is as if the stimulus is cut into 12 pie pieces by the neural selectivities of V1, then passed on to MT-g, and then reassembled for the response in area MST. This is only possible because of the choice of representation. Use of the gradient neurons is key because although the optic flow vectors for a rotating object as a whole cover all directions, the gradients of local motion all point in the same direction across the whole object. The representation of spatial derivatives of velocity in the brain was suggested by Koenderink and Van Doorn (1976)

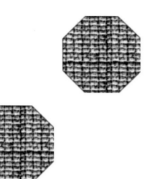

Figure 7.12 (movie 7.12W)
A single image from a video sequence of two synthetic, textured hexagons, the top one rotating clockwise and the lower one counterclockwise, both with the same speed.

and by Longuet-Higgins and Prazdny (1980) and shown to have human neural correlates by Martinez-Trujillo et al. (2005). More details are provided in appendix C.

Suppose now that two of these hexagons are presented to the same processing hierarchy as shown in figure 7.12 (movie 7.12W), both hexagons rotating in opposite directions but with the same speed. Figure 7.13 (plate 5; color figure 7.13W) shows the feed-forward response. The responses of each sheet are now more complex, with all sheets showing response. It is no longer such a simple matter to do a detection task: there are now two major peaks of the same value but for differing motion categories. Even if one peak is chosen arbitrarily, it is not possible to do a simple localization of the stimulus because there are now multiple groups of responses that contribute to each at the MST-s level—these neurons receive input from a ring of MT-g neurons—and the ambiguity only worsens further down in the hierarchy. Recall that the figure only gives the maximum response in the MT-g rings and that this maximum representation is for illustration only. All the MT-g rings contribute to the MST-s neurons. The point here is that Selection after Convergence Binding on its own will not suffice to unambiguously classify and localize the two stimuli.

Results from a Single Feed-Forward Pass Followed by a Single Recurrent Pass (Full Recurrence Binding)

The ambiguity presented in the previous example can be resolved by the recurrent binding process described in chapter 6. An example of this follows. The input for this demonstration is an image sequence showing a rotating square of noise embedded in noise (figure 7.14; movie 7.14W). In other words, this is an example of pure motion-defined form. There is no form information at all in the input, and as should be clear, there are no form neurons in the visual processing network of figure 7.1

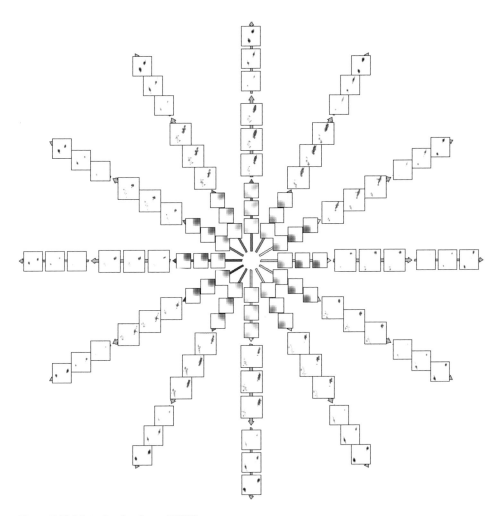

Figure 7.13 (plate 5; color figure 7.13W)
The neural responses to the stimulus of movie 7.12W using the same representation scheme as for figure 7.10.

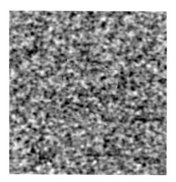

Figure 7.14 (movie 7.14W)
A single frame from an image sequence with a square rotating clockwise and receding into the image plane. Both background and square are composed of the same noise elements. This is an example of pure motion-defined form. The border of the rectangle is slightly enhanced for visibility in this figure.

of any kind. Figure 7.15 (plate 6) shows the final step of the recurrent traversal. The movie shows the entire recurrent progression (movie 7.15W). The color of the top-down beam that connects the selected neurons in each representation gives the motion category (from the color wheel)—a mix of clockwise rotation and receding motions at medium speed. This demonstrates some very important characteristics of ST. First, the motion representation used is significantly more powerful than many others that deal only with translational motion and would be blind to the motion shown. Second, ST's output is consistent with the many observations that show how humans can detect and categorize isolated visual stimuli with a single feed-forward pass. The color of the beam is the motion category; it can be detected by simple inspection at the top before localization in this example as in the first example of the previous section. But the stimulus shape or extent or precise location is not available through such a simple inspection. Finally, and perhaps more interestingly, one can see how the different spatial elements of the motion are selected from within each layer by following the progression of the recurrent pass over time. All of the components of motion eventually converge in the input layer, and the result segments the moving square neatly from the noise. This demonstrates the top-down localization process, but the example does not end here. It will be continued later.

Attending to Multiple Stimuli (Type I Iterative Recurrence Binding)

Returning to the synthetic hexagons, suppose there are two hexagonal textured objects in an image sequence (figure 7.16; movie 7.16W). The upper item is rotating counterclockwise while the lower one is rotating clockwise, occluding the other and at a slower speed. The first fixation finds the upper hexagon, and the second fixation

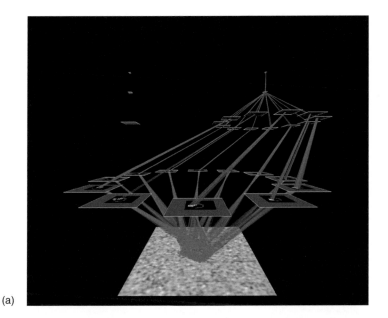

(a)

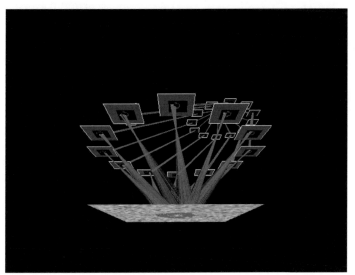

(b)

Figure 7.15 (plate 6; color figure 7.15W; movie 7.15W)
The completed, localized attentional beam for the stimulus of movie 7.14W. The lowest level of representation is the input image. The large ring of rectangles in the middle of the figure represents the V1 sheets. On the upper right side is the spiral pyramid and on the upper left side is the translation pyramid. Even though the translation portions of the hierarchy are active (as in figure 7.13), the overall response for the spiral motion was strongest and drove the recurrent localization process. Movie 7.15W gives the full time-varying progression. (a) The selected localized pathways are shown, colored following the color wheel to denote motion type, and converge on the stimulus square in the input. (b) A different viewpoint of the same structure, showing the detected stimulus. As well, the individual parts of each representation that are selected (in color) and inhibited (black) are shown allowing a clear view of the parts-based reunification of features into a whole shape. The dark rectangle within the V1 sheets shows the extent of the suppressive surround.

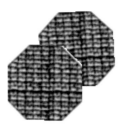

Figure 7.16 (movie 7.16W)
A single frame from a synthetic image sequence depicting two identical textured hexagons where the top one is rotation counterclockwise, the bottom one clockwise, but at a slower speed.

finds the lower one (figure 7.17, plate 7, and color figure 7.17W; figure 7.18, plate 8, and color figure 7.18W). This is a simple instance of Type I Iterative Recurrence Binding, the kind of processing that a visual search task would require, for example, if the task included not only detection but also some degree of localization. If both hexagons were similarly positioned but now rotating in place with the same speed and direction, the system could not tell them apart on the basis of motion alone, as is seen in figure 7.19 (plate 9; color figure 7.19W). The reason is that within a single receptive field there is ambiguity—the neuron simply sees motion of the same kind everywhere and thus cannot tell the two stimuli apart. This is exactly as has been found experimentally in monkey (see Lee & Maunsell, 2010). Without a location-specific or form-specific cue, ST cannot tell these two objects apart.

Suppose now there are three hexagonal textured objects. The large one in the lower right of the image is translating toward the upper left while rotating, the top one is rotating, and the small one on the left is translating to the right (figure 7.20; movie 7.20W). There is no representation in the system for the combined motions of the large item. Figures 7.21, 7.22, and 7.23 (plates 10, 11, and 12; color figures 7.21W, 7.22W, and 7.23W) make it clear that the model correctly finds each object, localizes it properly, and identifies the motion category (by color). Of interest is the first fixation; the object that has a compound motion and causes no difficulty. The spiral and translation portions of the motion hierarchy analyze the input independently, and selection can proceed along each dimension separately yet still converge on the same object. The convergence of the independent recurrent tracings onto the common source stimulus is a consequence of theorem 5.2 in chapter 5 as was alluded to in that chapter.

Empirical Performance of Recurrence Binding (Localization)

An additional example of pure motion-defined classification and localization follows. This is a real image sequence, not synthetic, created by imaging an 'e-puck' robot

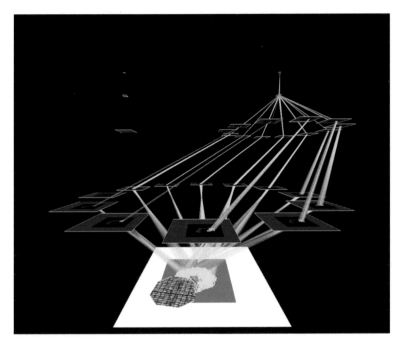

Figure 7.17 (plate 7; color figure 7.17W)
ST localizes the first stimulus and categorizes the motion type correctly. The localization is accurate except for the very center of the stimulus where insufficient motion texture does not permit categorization.

from above. The robot is camouflaged using circular cutouts of a background of leaves as shown in figure 7.24 (movie 7.24aW) and moving on that same background. Figure 7.24a shows one of the frames of movie 7.24aW that shows a single translating e-puck. The tracking and localization shown in figure 7.24b (movie 7.24bW) is quite good and has not been 'cleaned' in any way, reflecting the complete result of downward tracing of connections through the network (the color denotes the direction of classified motion). We evaluated the quality of the top-down localization algorithm by counting the number of pixels on the object in the original movie and by counting the localized pixels in the processed one. The image sequence contained 40 frames. In these, there were a total of 123,720 pixels on the moving object. As the localization is accomplished by top-down tracing of connections in the network, counting pixels that are correctly found by the tracing process is a valid performance measure. It would reveal how many of those connections found their correct target on the journey from area 7a downward. The algorithm correctly found 115,561 pixels (93.4%), missed 8,159 pixels (6.6%), and identified 19,502 pixels (15.8%) as false positives. Quantization errors are surely to blame for some of these errors as is the lack of lateral cooperation computation through most of the representation in this

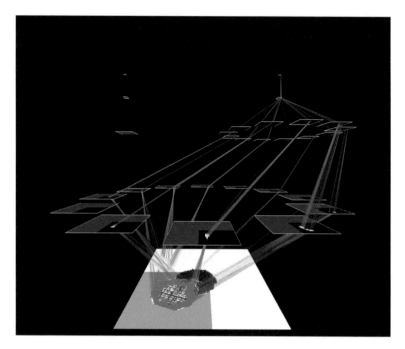

Figure 7.18 (plate 8; color figure 7.18W)
Once the first stimulus is attended, it is inhibited (Inhibition of Return), and the second is attended and localized and its motion is characterized. Here, due to the slower speed of rotation, more of the center region cannot be categorized.

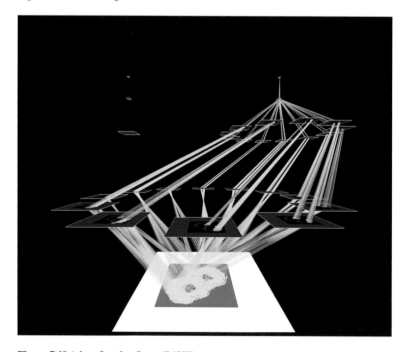

Figure 7.19 (plate 9; color figure 7.19W)
The same stimuli as in figure 7.16 but here both are rotating in the same direction and at the same speed. There is now ambiguity as there is insufficient information to permit the two objects to be segregated.

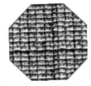

Figure 7.20 (movie 7.20W)
A single frame from an image sequence that shows three synthetic textured hexagons of different sizes and each undergoing a different motion. The largest is rotating and translating upward to the left. The top one is rotating, and the smallest one is simply translating to the right.

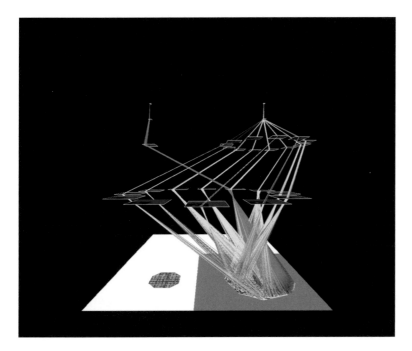

Figure 7.21 (plate 10; color figure 7.21W)
The first stimulus is attended, the largest one that is both rotating and translating. Its size is sufficient in this scenario to guarantee its first selection. Of greater interest is the fact there is no single neuron that represents this category of motion; it is a combination of both translation and spiral, yet ST is still able to detect, categorize, and localize the stimulus. The large gray rectangle on the input representation is the attentive suppressive surround.

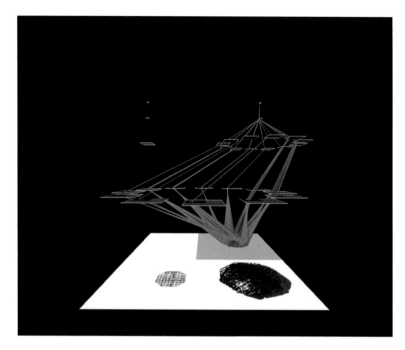

Figure 7.22 (plate 11; color figure 7.22W)
Once the first attended stimulus in inhibited (black), the second strongest stimulus is attended. This is pure spiral motion.

implementation. Nevertheless, any simple bounding box or outlier removal algorithm applied to the raw results would yield near-perfect results, so this experiment was quite successful. A second quantitative measure was also computed, namely, the image distance of the centroid of the localized pixels to the true centroid of the moving object, calculated in the standard way. The moving disk has a diameter of 63 pixels. The median separation of centroids was found to be 3.3 pixels with standard deviation 1.38. This measure is important because if the localization is to be used to guide behavior, there must be sufficient accuracy for it to be useful. Whereas other more common measures use bounding boxes and point to regions, here, an explicit segmentation is given with good accuracy for its centroid.

We repeated this with a different image sequence again of pure motion and found at http://i21www.ira.uka.de/image_sequences/. This is shown in movie 7.25aW (figure 7.25a shows one of the frames). Here, we were interested to see how the shadows would affect the selection and recurrence process. The tracking can be seen in movie 7.25bW (figure 7.25b shows one of the frames). The block had an image extent of 57 × 86 pixels. For this example, the same data was computed. In the 45 frames of the sequence, there were 182,585 pixels on the moving object, and the algorithm

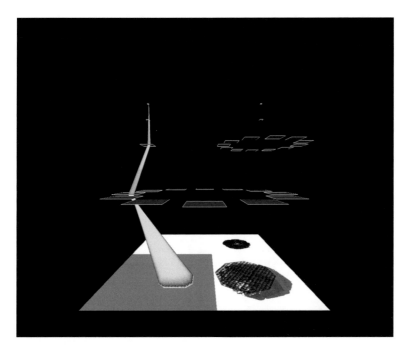

Figure 7.23 (plate 12; color figure 7.23W)
The third stimulus is next attended, a pure translation motion. Note how by the time the third fixation is made, the previously attended objects have moved.

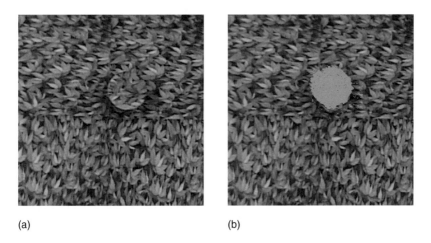

(a)   (b)

Figure 7.24 (movie 7.24a,bW)
(a) A single frame from an image sequence made by laying leaf-textured wallpaper on the floor, mounting a cutout of the same wallpaper on top of an e-puck robot, and directing the robot to translate across the surface. (b) The robot is tracked almost perfectly and segmented from the background.

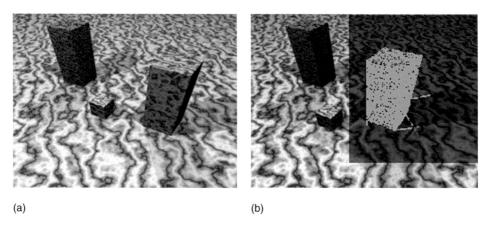

(a)   (b)

Figure 7.25 (movie 7.25a,bW)
(a) A single frame from a time-varying image sequence, obtained from the Web, of textured objects moving on a textured background. (b) The moving block is tracked with high accuracy except for some shadow edges.

found 162,936 pixels (89.2%) correctly, missed 19,649 pixels (10.8%), and identified 20,909 pixels (11.4%) as false positives. The distance between true and computed centroid has a median value of 3.5 pixels with standard deviation of 0.26 pixels. The shadows in this case cause a small degradation compared with the previous example; however, considering there are no other mechanisms except for motion processing, these are excellent results.

Visual Search

Having observed examples of how ST's Type I Iterative Recurrence Binding process operates, we are in a position to see how this extends to visual search tasks and whether or not ST's performance is the same as that observed in experiments.

Culhane (1992) and Culhane and Tsotsos (1992) described the first detailed implementation of ST and showed several nice examples of the performance of the localization mechanism for a variety of visual inputs. Culhane created the example in figure 7.26 (color figure 7.26W) that was presented in Tsotsos et al. (2001). In this example, an image of several colored blocks is attended. The P-Lattice here is composed of multiple pyramids for luminance and color opponent cells only. The algorithm is instructed to search for blue regions, and it attempts to do this by searching for the largest, bluest region first. This test image is shown on the right half of each figure part with the regions selected outlined in yellow, with blue lines between them showing the derived scan path. The left side of each image shows a four-level visual processing pyramid. The task bias is applied to the pyramid to tune its feature com-

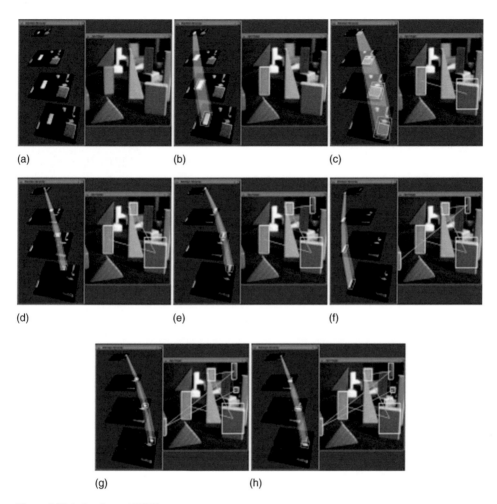

(a)   (b)   (c)

(d)   (e)   (f)

(g)   (h)

Figure 7.26 (color figure 7.26W)
Sequence of fixations to largest, bluest stimuli. The first panel at the top left (panel a) shows the initial representation after the primed first feed-forward pass. The remaining seven panels show the sequence of fixations for large blue objects. The left side of each panel shows a four-level visual processing pyramid, biased for the color blue. Then the θ-WTA algorithm selects the largest, bluest one first in (b), inhibits that region, and then repeats the process six more times (panels c through h) [from Tsotsos et al. (2001), with permission of The MIT Press].

putations, and the result is that the regions within each layer of the pyramid that remain are those that are blue. The left side of figure 7.26a shows the set of blue objects represented. Then the θ-WTA algorithm selects the largest, bluest one first, selected in figure 7.26b, inhibits that region, and then repeats the process six more times. Note that the system does not know about objects, only rectangular regions. Thus, although it appears to select whole blocks sometimes, this is only due to fortuitous selections. Nevertheless, even in this simple example, the performance of ST is exactly as expected.

More complex examples follow. Rodríguez-Sánchez et al. (2007), Simine (2006), Lai (1992), Liu (2002), and Zhou (2004) have shown a number of visual search tasks for which ST performs quite well, some compared in a qualitative manner with specific behavioral experiments. These experiments are now briefly presented, and the reader may wish to consult the original papers for more detail.

The motion processing representation given earlier was not used for the first two of the following experiments; it was used for the last one in this section. The object representation used for the first example is described in detail in Rodríguez-Sánchez et al. (2007). It consisted of a V1 representation of oriented lines, a V4 representation of curvature, and an inferotemporal (IT) representation of simple shapes.

In this first example, the stimulus patterns are the same as used in Nagy and Sanchez (1990), examining a color similarity search. They showed that feature search can be inefficient if the differences in color are small. Rodríguez-Sánchez et al. used the CIE values from their experiments converted to RGB (red, green, blue) with a fixed luminance (Y) of 0.25. The task is to find the redder circle among 5, 10, 15, 20, and 25 distractors for two conditions: small and large color differences. The target and distractors were randomly positioned on a black background.

Figure 7.27a (movie 7.27aW) shows ST's result for a typical visual search trial within this experiment. In figure 7.27a, the target and distractors have small color differences, and several shifts of attention were needed to find the redder item (white outline). In figure 7.27b, the number of fixations as a function of set size is shown for ST's performance. The gray line represents results for large color differences, and the black line represents results for small color differences. As in Nagy and Sanchez (1990), ST's results show that color search is inefficient if the color difference is small between target and distractors (slope = 0.39) and efficient if the difference is large (slope = 0.01).

In a second visual search example, the experiment of Bichot and Schall (1999) was followed. Bichot and Schall showed that monkey visual search reaction times are comparable with those of humans; namely, they show that the conjunction of two different features (shape and color) is steeper than feature search, but shallower than what was obtained by Treisman and Gelade (1980). They report slopes of 3.9 ms/item. Searching for a rotated *T* among rotated *L*s, Egeth and Dagenbach (1991)

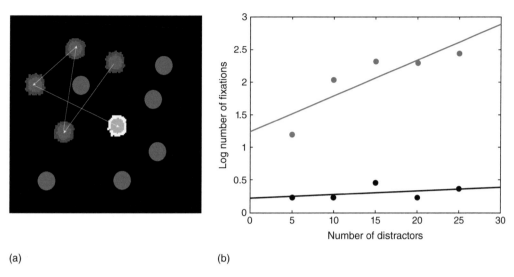

(a)   (b)

Figure 7.27 (movie 7.27aW)
Visual search results. (a) Example where the target and distractors have small color differences, five shifts
of attention were needed to find the redder item (white outline). (b) The number of fixations as a function of set size. Gray line: large color difference. Black line: small color difference [adapted from
Rodríguez-Sánchez et al. (2007) with permission of the author].

reported that this search was quite inefficient (20 ms/item), less efficient than conjunction searches. To find a *T* among *L*s is more inefficient than a conjunction search,
which is less efficient than a simple feature search. Rodríguez-Sánchez et al. (2007)
examined ST's performance for visual search involving feature search (find a circle
among arrows), conjunction search (find a red circle among red arrows and green
circles), and inefficient search (find a rotated *T* among *L*s). Figure 7.28a (movie
7.28aW) gives a typical scan trace for ST's fixations for a trial in this experiment.
Figure 7.28b shows the number of shifts of attention as a function of set size for
feature search (light gray), conjunction search (gray), and inefficient search (black).
The qualitative result is exactly the separation of tasks found for human subjects
by the above experimenters; namely, the steepest line corresponds with looking for
a *T* among *L*s (inefficient search, slope of 0.49), followed by conjunction search
(slope of 0.36), and feature search is practically flat (slope of 0.00).

The following experiment uses the motion representation described earlier in
this chapter. Simine (2006) (also appears in Rodríguez-Sánchez et al., 2007) compared the performance of the model with human data by reproducing the experiment described in Thornton and Gilden (2001). The stimulus images consisted of
a random noise background, where every pixel was randomly assigned a value
between 0 and 255, on which motion patterns were superimposed, also composed
of random intensity dots. The dot motion was confined to a square aperture, and

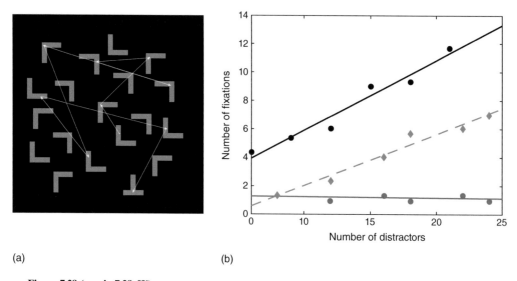

(a)   (b)

Figure 7.28 (movie 7.28aW)
Inefficient search: Find the rotated T among Ls. (a) Ten fixations were needed to find the T. (b) The number of shifts of attention as a function of set size for feature search (light gray), conjunction search (gray), and inefficient search (black) [adapted from Rodríguez-Sánchez et al. (2007) with permission of the author].

these apertures could be placed in four possible positions in the visual field (see figure 7.29a; movie 7.29aW). Six motion types were examined and are illustrated in figure 7.29b: upward and downward translation, clockwise and counterclockwise rotation, and expansion and contraction. For each type of motion there were six trial blocks with 10 trials in each block. The number of targets and distractors was varied between blocks. The blocks contained either 1 target and 0 distractors, 1 target and 1 distractor, 1 target and 3 distractors, 2 targets and 0 distractors, 2 targets and 2 distractors, or 4 targets and 0 distractors. The only difference between targets and distractors was the direction of motion. For example, for clockwise-rotating targets, the distractors were rotating counterclockwise, and for expanding targets distractors were contracting, and so on. The reaction time is expressed in terms of the number of frames needed to find the target. Figure 7.30a–d shows the results of the experiment. The left half of each panel shows the output of the model, and the right half of each panel is the data reported by Thornton and Gilden. The complex motion patterns produce nearly linear dependence with set size. There is no decline in the response time (RT) as the number of targets increases, and there is a nearly linear rise of response times as the number of distractors increases. The rotating motion shows the steepest slope among the complex motions, in agreement with the human data. Although no direct quantitative comparison can be done, we

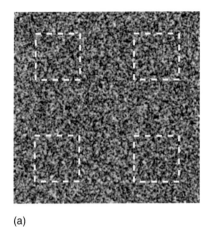

(a)

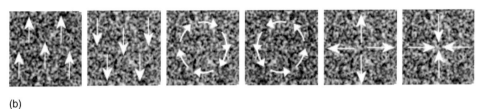

(b)

Figure 7.29 (movie 7.29aW)
(a) Possible positions of the motion patterns in the input images. (b) The six motion patterns used in the experiment, from left to right: translation up and down, clockwise and counterclockwise rotation, and expansion and contraction.

can see that qualitative similarity is definitely present. There is the exception of the translation data, however. It seems that the response time of the model increases sharply with the number of distractors, and this is inconsistent with the psychophysical findings that show that the response time to the translational patterns increases only slightly as the number of distractors increases. Perhaps some larger-scale grouping process, or Gestalt-like mechanism, is at play here; ST does not include this explicitly. However, if two stimuli that are identical fall within the same receptive field, ST cannot tell them apart in its current design (as shown in figure 7.19). If the spacing of the stimuli in the Thornton and Gilden experiment was matched to the sizes of receptive fields modeled in the ST implementation, the anomalous result found may be ameliorated. For each of the four sets of curves, the quantization of time into frames for our version of these experiments would also have an effect on the comparison.

The next example of visual search is for an overt search task, described in detail in Zaharescu et al. (2005) and Zaharescu (2004). The stimuli and tasks used by

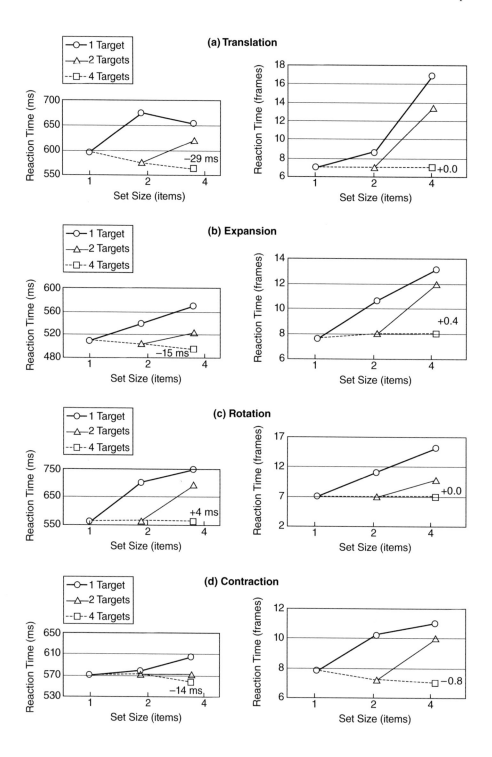

Motter and Belky (1998a,b) were used to test the parts of the overall ST model of figure 4.2 dealing with eye movements. To conduct the test, the model was used to generate gaze changes for a robotic binocular camera system, the TRISH (Toronto Iris Stereo Head) head (Milios, Jenkin, & Tsotsos, 1993). Rather than graphical stimuli on a computer screen, the stimuli were set up on a black panel. The black vertical wooden panel is a square 75.1 cm per side placed 67 cm away from the base of the TRISH head (figure 7.31; color figure 7.31W). Up to 24 red bars and 24 green bars were arranged on the blackboard. Each of the bars is cut out of cardboard and is of size 5.5 × 1.5 cm. The size of the distractors and the distance of the blackboard from the TRISH head were chosen such that the distractors would appear to have the size in the image plane similar to that of distractors in the Motter and Belky experiments. The camera provides 640 × 480 pixel images, with 24-bit color depth. Performance was very good for both feature and conjunction searches; however, due to the accumulating calibration errors from the robot head, this was less suitable for a quantitative assessment than hoped. The entire setup was then simulated on a computer and trials run to determine overall performance. Figure 7.32 (color figure 7.32W) shows a typical trial in the experiment. Zaharescu (2004) compared the number of fixations to recognize a target versus set size that ST required with those values in the experiments of Motter and Belky (1998b) as shown in figure 7.33.

The curves are both monotonically increasing at approximately the same overall slopes. They apparently differ by a constant factor, and this is understandable as there would be many parameters involved to bring results closer to monkey results that are not part of ST. Figure 7.34 shows a second comparison, the distribution of saccades between the Zaharescu implementation of ST and the results reported by Motter and Belky (1998a). Although the overall shape of the two curves is quite similar, differences may be due to the fact that microsaccades in the eye controller that serve to accomplish fine alignment after initial eye movement are not implemented. Further, there is no grouping mechanism in ST (as explained earlier), and a grouping mechanism would lead to fewer fixations. The shift of the ST curve to higher number of saccades is likely due to these differences.

One more example illustrates overt fixations for the motion representation of figure 7.1. Suppose again that the stimulus image sequence depicts motion-defined form, but this time there is one object translating and one rotating (movie 7.35W; figure 7.35 shows one frame from the movie with the stimuli outlined so they can be seen). ST can detect one of the targets, localize it, then do the same for the other.

◀ **Figure 7.30**
(a–d) Search results for the model on the stimuli used by Thornton and Gilden (2001). The right half of each panel shows the data from Thornton and Gilden, and left half shows the output of ST [adapted from Simine (2006) with permission of the author].

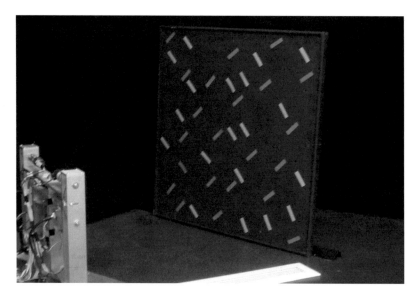

Figure 7.31 (color figure 7.31W)
The physical setup for the active search experiments using the TRISH binocular robot head and physical stimuli as in Motter and Belky (1998a,b) [adapted from Zaharescu (2004) with permission of the author].

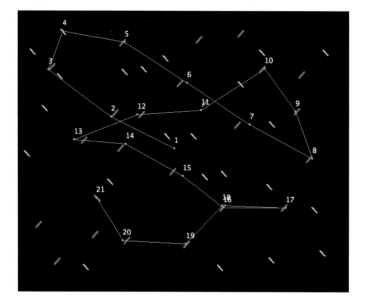

Figure 7.32 (color figure 7.32W)
The scan path of ST in a typical visual search trial: a search for a red bar oriented to the left, beginning with fixation in the center [adapted from Zaharescu (2004) with permission of the author].

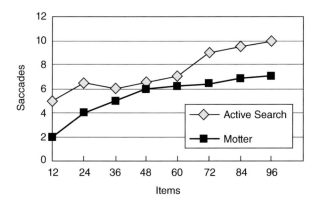

Figure 7.33
Comparison between conjunction search times exhibited by ST's active search algorithm and those reported by Motter and Belky (1998b) [adapted from Zaharescu (2004) with permission of the author].

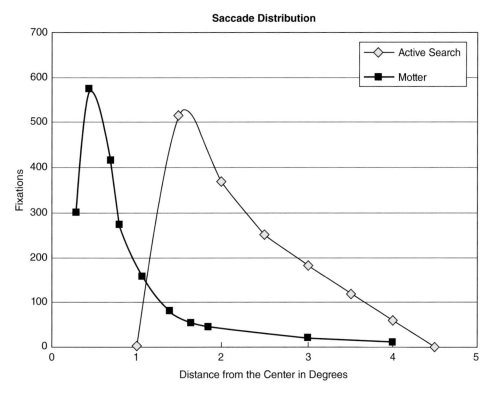

Figure 7.34
Saccade distribution comparison between ST's active search algorithm and the results in Motter and Belky (1998a). The main difference is due to the lack of corrective micro-saccades in ST used to accomplish alignment after initial eye movement (adapted from Zaharescu 2004 with permission of the author).

The placement of the stimuli in this example, however, puts one in a central location and one in a peripheral position. The peripheral computation components of figure 4.2 are included here. Figure 7.36a (movie 7.36W) is one frame of the animation showing the first fixation, and figure 7.36b shows the second. Note that the contents of the visual field itself change after the first overt fixation in order to bring the second target into the central region of the visual field (i.e., there is an overt gaze shift). This cannot be seen in the input representation of the figure, of course, but can be seen in the processing stages themselves.

By way of summary, this section showed ST's performance for visual search experiments involving object shape, color, and motion and included covert as well as overt fixation changes. Stimulus configurations examined were direction of translational motion, direction of rotation, contraction versus expansion, Ts among Ls, small versus large color differences for colored circles, circle among arrow shapes, and red bars versus green bars. Although this is only a small set of the large number

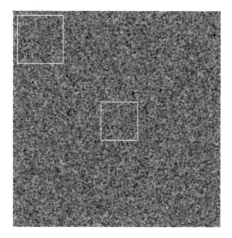

Figure 7.35 (movie 7.35W)
This is the first frame of movie 7.35W. The two moving squares are defined only by their motion as explained in the text, but for this figure are highlighted with white rectangles. The movie shows their motions.

Figure 7.36 (movie 7.36Wa; movie 7.36bW)   ▶
(a) A single frame from the movie that shows two stimuli, both motion-defined forms, one located centrally and the other peripherally. At this time instant, the central item is attended—it is a translating square shape. The peripheral stimulus can clearly be seen in the upper left corner of the representation of layer V1. Note that even though it is pure translation, some activation on the spiral side of the representation also is evident. (b) A single frame from the movie that shows two stimuli, both motion-defined forms, one located centrally and the other peripherally. At this time instant, the item that was peripheral in (a), but as a result of an overt fixation is now central, is attended—it is a rotating square shape. The previously central item that is now in the periphery can be seen in the lower right corner of the translation representations.

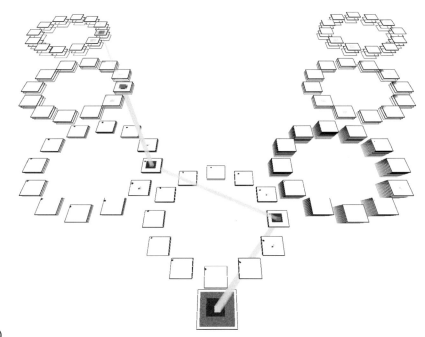

(a)

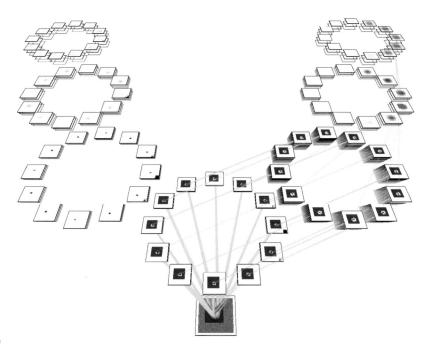

(b)

of stimuli that have been examined in human experiments, it is representative of a significant number, and the strong qualitative agreement between human and ST results is good evidence for ST's ability to deal with the visual search elements of attention.

Type II Iterative Recurrence Binding

As described in chapter 6, Type II Iterative Recurrence Binding involves going over the same input stimulus more than once and without a change of fixation. The point is to use an initial analysis as a seed that then can anchor subsequent analyses until a task is completed. Rothenstein et al. (2008) show several examples and provide details on the mechanism.

The recovery of shape from motion is a particularly good illustration of Type II Iterative Recurrence Binding, especially in cases where the shape information is not even present in the input image, and motion detection is a clear prerequisite to shape detection. As such, this example is the continuation of the example of figure 7.14 (movie 7.14W). Following the format of figure 6.7 that showed how the different binding processes are related along a timeline, figure 7.37 (plate 13; color figure 7.37W) consists of the motion processing system described earlier and a shape-processing network. Only the translation portion of the motion process is shown because this demonstration involves only translation. There was no priming in advance. The stimulus consists of a translating diamond shape in the left upper half of the image and a translating square shape in the right lower half of the image (see the figure). The shape network can detect basic geometric shapes and consists of a layer of first-order edge detectors (four directions, one scale), a second layer for pairs of parallel lines, and a third layer for spatially related pairs of pairs of parallel lines. Each layer has lower spatial resolution than the previous. With stimulus onset, all elements of the processing network are activated in a feed-forward manner, in parallel, with the result as shown in the first panel along the timeline of the figure. Note how the shape pathway is effectively blind to the motion of the two shapes. Figure 7.38 (plate 14; color figure 7.38W) shows an enlarged representation of areas 7a-t, MST-t, MT-t, and V1 to emphasize the ambiguity these stimuli give rise to. The Recurrence Binding process of ST then selects a peak within 7a-t and localizes the corresponding pixels in the input image. The parts of these four sheets that represent the selected spatial regions layer by layer are shown in green with the suppressive surround in red in the middle panel of figure 7.37 and in figure 7.38. What becomes apparent by the end of the recurrent pass (middle panel of figure 7.37) is that the selected shape—the diamond—is now isolated from its surround. As it becomes isolated, the shape network—which is continually activated

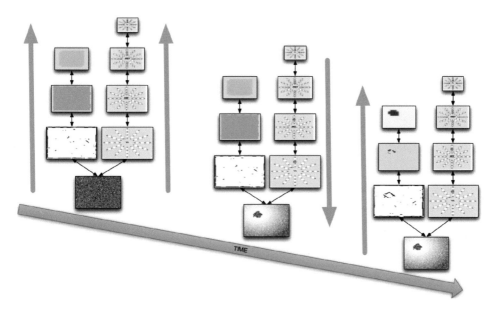

Figure 7.37 (plate 13; color figure 7.37W)
The sequence of Convergence Binding, Recurrence Binding, and Type II Iterative Recurrence Binding for motion-defined form stimuli. The text provides details.

by the input throughout this process—now sees input that fires its edge-detecting neurons and then the line and shape neurons. The ending configuration of the subsequent full feed-forward pass is in the final panel of figure 7.38. In this case, the purpose is to detect not only the kind of motion but also the shape of the moving object. It further implies that the detection of motion takes time that depends on the time for a first feed-forward pass and that the time required for determination of shape is longer, perhaps twice as long again. It is clear that combinations of task priming, selection-based tuning, and multiple passes of this kind each with their own tunings can lead to very complex behavior that dynamically adjusts the network to current input and task.

Saliency and AIM

As described in chapter 5, the saliency portion of ST's Peripheral Priority Map is determined using the AIM algorithm (Bruce, 2008; Bruce & Tsotsos, 2005, 2008, 2009). Other saliency models define saliency in terms of local feature contrast loosely based on observations concerning interaction among cells locally within primate visual cortex. Although this succeeds at simulating some salience-related behaviors, there is little to explain why the operations involved in the model have

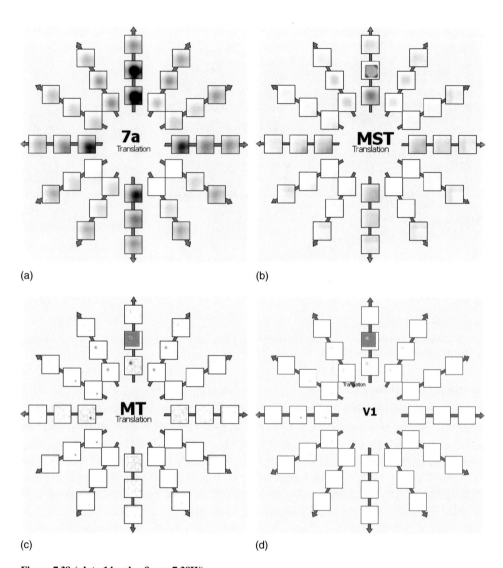

Figure 7.38 (plate 14; color figure 7.38W)
(a–d) Enlarged versions of the four motion sheets in the middle panel of figure 7.37. See text for details.

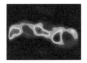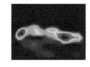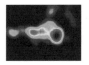

Figure 7.39 (plate 2; color figure 7.39W)
A qualitative comparison of AIM output with the experimental fixation data. From left to right: The image processed by AIM. AIM output with a 31 × 31 spatiochromatic basis. Output of the Itti et al. (1998) algorithm. Experimental fixation density representing the extent to which each pixel location was sampled on average across 20 observers. Original image modulated by the output of AIM. Hotter (redder) areas correspond with more salient regions.

the structure that is observed and, specifically, what the overall architecture translates into with respect to its relationship to the incoming stimulus in a principled quantitative manner. AIM considers the role that the properties of visual stimuli play in sampling from the stimulus-driven perspective and provides the following:

1. A computational framework for visual saliency built on first principles of Information Theory.

2. A definition of visual saliency in which there is an implicit definition of context. The definition of visual salience is not based solely on the response of cells within a local region but also on the relationship between the response of cells within a local region and cells in the surrounding region. This includes a discussion of the role that context plays.

3. Consideration of the impact of principles underlying neural coding on the determination of visual saliency and visual search behavior. A variety of visual search behaviors are seen as emergent properties of principles underlying neural coding combined with information seeking as a visual sampling strategy.

Although AIM is built entirely on computational constraints, the resulting model structure exhibits considerable agreement with the organization of the human visual system. For details on the formulation of saliency, its theoretical underpinnings, justifications, and comparisons with human fixation patterns, please see the papers cited in the previous paragraph.

Several examples and performance evaluations have appeared previously in the papers cited earlier, and two additional examples appear here. Figure 7.39 (plate 2; figure 7.39W) shows a qualitative comparison of AIM output with experimental fixation data. From left to right, the figure gives the image to be processed; AIM output with a 31 × 31 spatiochromatic basis; output of the Itti et al. (1998) algorithm; experimental fixation density representing the extent to which each pixel location was sampled on average across 20 observers; and the original image modulated by the output of AIM. Brighter areas (hotter areas in the color version) correspond with more salient regions, for this example as well as the next. Figure

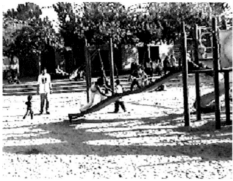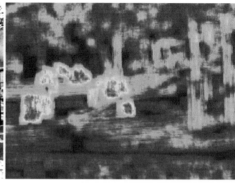

Figure 7.40 (plate 3; movie 7.40W)
A single frame from the park playground video sequence and a single frame of corresponding AIM algorithm output. Output is based on an $11 \times 11 \times 6$ (x,y,t) basis of spatiotemporal filters. Redder areas correspond with more salient regions.

7.40 (plate 3; movie 7.40W) shows a single frame from a video sequence depicting the output of AIM when applied to a video sequence or a park playground scene. Output is based on an $11 \times 11 \times 6$ (x,y,t) basis of spatiotemporal filters. The left side of the video shows the original sequence, and the right side shows the AIM output. Further quantitative comparisons can be seen in Bruce and Tsotsos (2009).

Summary

This chapter has focused on showing how Selective Tuning can be used for a very wide variety of input stimuli. It shows the quality of ST's performance and also how its performance compares with relevant experimental observations. It is not difficult to conclude that Selective Tuning exhibits strong and broad relevance to biological attention, to attention for computer vision, and for the list of attentional elements of chapter 3. Some readers may wonder about the relative lack of real images as test stimuli. Whereas several current models of visual classification use a handful of oriented line detectors as the only feature and then develop complex multidimensional feature descriptors based on these for a learned classifier, the work here makes no such assumption that a few simple features suffice. If in fact a few simple features sufficed for human vision, then we would not see the enormous number of different kinds of neural tunings that have been observed. The human visual system seems far more complex, and it is not so easy to see how the single final stage learned classifier is consistent with the neurobiology of human vision. It is clear that those other models can obtain good classification performance for tightly constrained and limited domains. But this is not the same as a theory for general human vision; that is the goal here.

There are of course many directions for improvement, but the approach shown in this chapter and in the next of insisting on tests for a broad spectrum of attentional elements is the only one that will lead to a full theory of attention. A focus on one element alone may lead to a better single-task model, but it would not be the case that it also fits into the broader context of attention. In this vein, the next chapter examines the set of predictions that ST has made for biological attention as well as the manner in which ST provides explanations for the attentional elements of chapter 3.

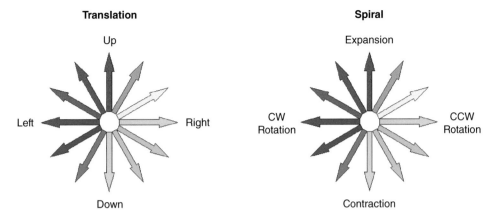

Plate 1 (figure 7.9; color figure 7.9W)
The color wheels used to code for motion direction and spiral motion class. The translation coding is on the left, and the spiral coding is on the right. The directions in between vertical and horizontal give combinations of the nearest orthogonal directions. The same color coding is used for the velocity gradient representations where it represents the direction of increasing gradient with respect to the local vector of translation, which by convention is set to be vertical. For example, if the gradient is coded green (as in counterclockwise rotation), it means that the direction of increasing value of velocity is perpendicular to the local direction of translation. CW, clockwise; CCW, counterclockwise.

 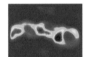 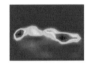 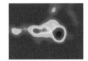

Plate 2 (figure 7.39; color figure 7.39W)
A qualitative comparison of AIM output with the experimental fixation data. From left to right: The image processed by AIM. AIM output with a 31 × 31 spatiochromatic basis. Output of the Itti et al. (1998) algorithm. Experimental fixation density representing the extent to which each pixel location was sampled on average across 20 observers. Original image modulated by the output of AIM. Hotter (redder) areas correspond with more salient regions.

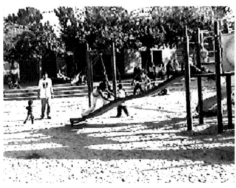 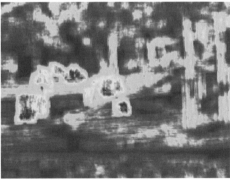

Plate 3 (figure 7.40; movie 7.40W)
A single frame from the park playground video sequence and a single frame of corresponding AIM algorithm output. Output is based on an 11 × 11 × 6 (x,y,t) basis of spatiotemporal filters. Redder areas correspond with more salient regions.

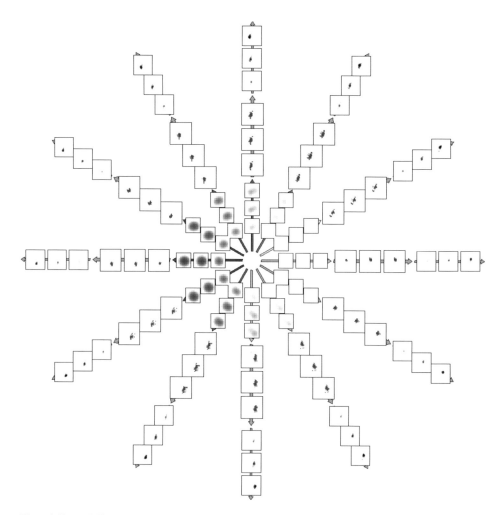

Plate 4 (figure 7.10; color figure 7.10W)
The representation of neural responses after the first feed-forward pass for the stimulus in Figure 7.8. Areas V1 (outer three rings of sheets), MT-g (middle three rings of sheets), and MST-s (inner three rings of sheets) only are shown. The spokes give the colors of the coding color wheel with all the sheets along a spoke selective to appropriate, related feature qualities (outer sheets for direction, middle sheets for velocity gradient, inner sheets for spiral motion). MT-g depicts only the maximum response by location of all the gradient responses for ease of illustration only. The color coding in these sheets follows the color wheel. See text for more detail.

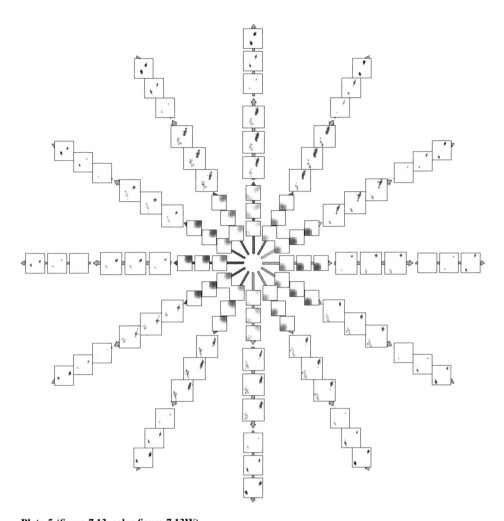

Plate 5 (figure 7.13; color figure 7.13W)
The neural responses to the stimulus of movie 7.12W using the same representation scheme as for plate 4.

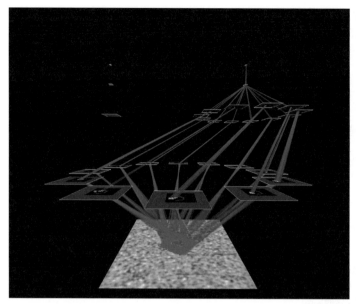

(a)

(b)

Plate 6 (figure 7.15; color figure 7.15W; movie 7.15W)
The completed, localized attentional beam for the stimulus of movie 7.14W. The lowest level of representation is the input image. The large ring of rectangles in the middle of the figure represents the V1 sheets. On the upper right side is the spiral pyramid and on the upper left side is the translation pyramid. Even though the translation portions of the hierarchy are active (as in plate 5), the overall response for the spiral motion was strongest and drove the recurrent localization process. Movie 7.15W gives the full time-varying progression. (a) The selected localized pathways are shown, colored following the color wheel to denote motion type, and converge on the stimulus square in the input. (b) A different viewpoint of the same structure, showing the detected stimulus. As well, the individual parts of each representation that are selected (in color) and inhibited (black) are shown allowing a clear view of the parts-based reunification of features into a whole shape. The dark rectangle within the V1 sheets shows the extent of the suppressive surround.

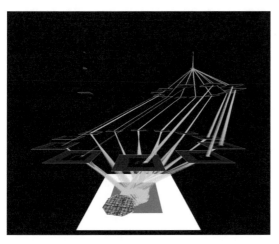

Plate 7 (figure 7.17; color figure 7.17W)
ST localizes the first stimulus and categorizes the motion type correctly. The localization is accurate except for the very center of the stimulus where insufficient motion texture does not permit categorization.

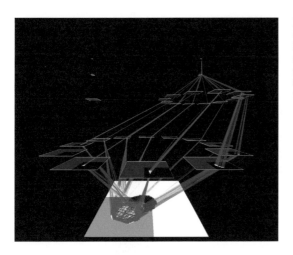

Plate 8 (figure 7.18; color figure 7.18W)
Once the first stimulus is attended, it is inhibited (Inhibition of Return), and the second is attended and localized and its motion is characterized. Here, due to the slower speed of rotation, more of the center region cannot be categorized.

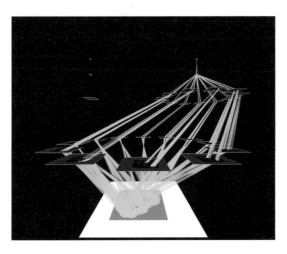

Plate 9 (figure 7.19; color figure 7.19W)
The same stimuli as in figure 7.16 but here both are rotating in the same direction and at the same speed. There is now ambiguity as there is insufficient information to permit the two objects to be segregated.

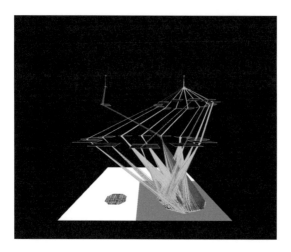

Plate 10 (figure 7.21; color figure 7.21W)
The first stimulus is attended, the largest one that is both rotating and translating. Its size is sufficient in this scenario to guarantee its first selection. Of greater interest is the fact there is no single neuron that represents this category of motion; it is a combination of both translation and spiral, yet ST is still able to detect, categorize, and localize the stimulus. The large gray rectangle on the input representation is the attentive suppressive surround.

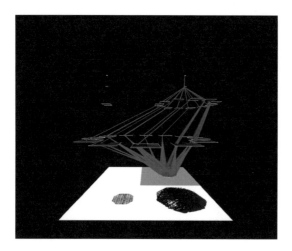

Plate 11 (figure 7.22; color figure 7.22W)
Once the first attended stimulus in inhibited (black), the second strongest stimulus is attended. This is pure spiral motion.

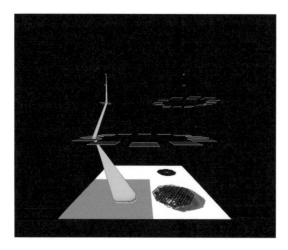

Plate 12 (figure 7.23; color figure 7.23W)
The third stimulus is next attended, a pure translation motion. Note how by the time the third fixation is made, the previously attended objects have moved.

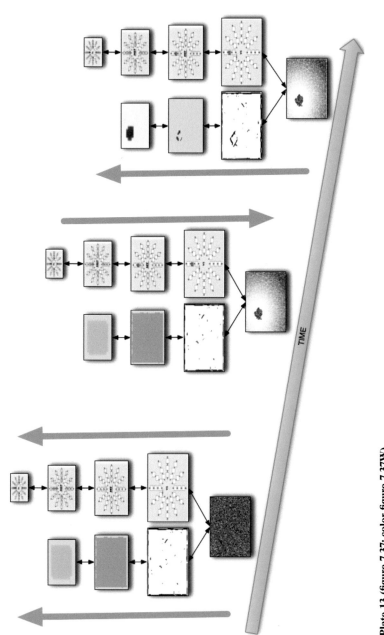

Plate 13 (figure 7.37; color figure 7.37W)
The sequence of Convergence Binding, Recurrence Binding, and Type II Iterative Recurrence Binding for motion-defined form stimuli. The text provides details.

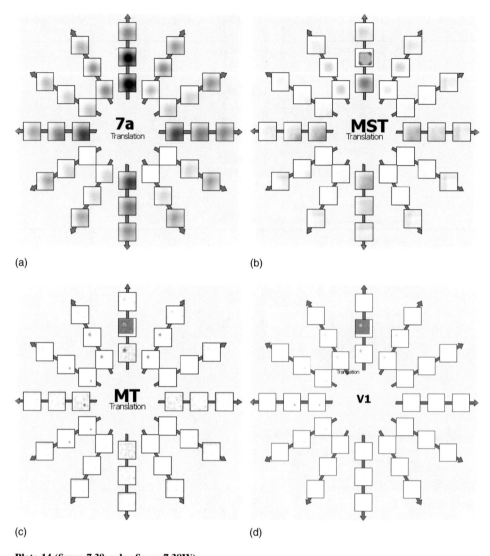

(a)

(b)

(c)

(d)

Plate 14 (figure 7.38; color figure 7.38W)
(a–d) Enlarged versions of the four motion sheets in the middle panel of plate 13. See text for details.

8 Explanations and Predictions

By now it should be clear that the driving motivation behind the development of the Selective Tuning theory and model is to understand visual attention in the brain. To see how well the theory and model satisfies this motivation, we must look at how well the body of existing experimental evidence is explained by ST and also at what predictions were made and how they have fared over the course of time. Here, we follow the scientific method completely, and just so there is no question, this is summarized in figure 8.1.

Observations of nature lead to the creation of a theory. Usually, the reason is to attempt to understand nature in a formal manner. Good theories not only explain existing observations but also provide predictions about what has not yet been observed. Those predictions foster new experiments and, often, novel experimental tools and designs. Closing the loop, new experiments lead to new observations that can be used to support, refine, or refute the theory. The work on the Selective Tuning theory began with the desire to discover a formal understanding of why attention is an important component of perception.

The success of any approach is judged in the expected manner: does it further our understanding of the problem domain? How much of our current understanding is explained by the theory? Does the theory make predictions that drive new research? To this end, it will be important to include a bit of historical context because many of ST's predictions were made in various early papers. One of those predictions was that single-neuron attentional effects can be observed in all visual areas in the cortex where there is convergence (many-to-one mapping) of neural signals. Its earliest instance was in Tsotsos (1990a, p. 439), where it was written that there is a top-down attentive tuning process for the whole processing hierarchy; that is, for all elements that contribute to a neuron's response. This may seem obvious now because so much experimental work has appeared to support it. However, at the time it was made, the only good support for single-neuron attentional modulation was in area V4 in macaque monkey (Moran & Desimone, 1985; they did see small effects in IT but none in V1). In fact, models were

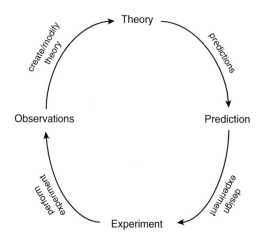

Figure 8.1
The classical scientific method.

developed that included only V4 attention (e.g., Niebur et al., 1993). Another early prediction in the same paper was that the attentional effects are observed first in the higher-order areas and move downward to the early areas of visual cortex (e.g., from IT down to V1 and LGN). Again, this was not viewed as a real possibility (see Desimone, 1990). Only very recently, as will be described below, has evidence appeared to support this. In what follows, the time that the predictions were made matters and shows that the predictions indeed foreshadowed results to come.

Another important consideration is the level of abstraction and scope of models. Usually, models do not cover the entire scope of a problem, and Selective Tuning is no exception. The gaps of coverage will become apparent during the following paragraphs. Models that address neural-level processes have great difficulty in providing explanations for behavioral observations. Similarly, behavior-based models have difficulty with neural-level explanations. ST covers a middle ground and can provide some explanations at behavioral as well as neural levels.

This chapter is structured into three main sections. The first, "Explanations," presents how well Selective Tuning includes and explains the attentional elements of chapter 3—an important test for any model or theory that purports to model human visual attention. The second section, "Predictions with Experimental Support," presents many of the predictions of the theory, details the reasoning behind them, and lists supporting experimental evidence. The third section, "Some Supporting Evidence," summarizes several of the experiments performed by us with the goal of discovering evidence supporting Selective Tuning.

Explanations

The previous chapter included many examples of how ST performs, and because some of the examples were derived directly from experimental observations, they may also be considered as explanations for those phenomena. We will begin with the functional elements of attention as presented in chapter 3 to structure this section. This not only provides connections to the elements of attention described earlier, but also it makes clear where the theory fits well, where it might not, and how other models may also be evaluated in the same manner. It also permits some structure to the unmanageably large body of experimental observations, where it sometimes seems as if some experiments tap into an unspecified subset of these functional elements (perhaps this is the reason for some of the difficulties of this field). For each of the elements, the corresponding paragraph will begin with a repetition of the short statement that characterized it in chapter 3 (without a repetition of references this time). Then, this will be followed by an elaboration of the functional element plus a short description of how it can be seen within the ST theory. This organization also presents a challenge to other models. To what degree do other conceptualizations of attentive processing in vision satisfy each of the main elements of attention listed here? Some comments regarding this will be included in what follows, but only where they help differentiate Selective Tuning from other proposals.

Alerting   The ability to process, identify, and move attention to priority signals.

First, one must clarify what a 'priority signal' is. Excellent discussions on this appear in Serences and Yantis (2007) and Fecteau and Munoz (2006). Priority, in those works, is the combined representation of salience and relevance. They summarize evidence that the oculomotor network shares features with the Saliency Map concept. They show that to be consistent with neurophysiology, the concept of the Saliency Map must be broadened to include top-down influences; that is, the relevance of the signal. Interestingly, Fecteau and Munoz argue that the neural expression of salience changes across tasks, which indicates that different tasks are not tapping into the same processes but different processes with similar manifestations in behavior. They conclude that the priority map appears to be a property of a network and not of a single area.

   It is clear that the ST theory and algorithms satisfy exactly the structures and function described by Fecteau and Munoz as well as Posner's characterization of Alerting. ST's History-Biased Priority Map includes conventional saliency as well as task bias and is the main representation used to determine if attention should be reoriented in a covert or overt manner. The fact that task can affect the whole network (figure 4.2) is consistent with the network concept of Fecteau and Munoz.

Attentional Footprint   Optical metaphors describe the 'footprint' of attentional fixation in image space and the main ones are spotlight, zoom lens, gradient, and suppressive surround.

There are many descriptive terms regarding the attentional footprint, or signature, in retinotopic representations. The spotlight metaphor due to Shulman et al. (1979) has dominated the literature with several other ideas playing smaller roles in the thinking of the attention community. In ST, the spatial footprint is the attended stimulus plus its suppressed surround. This is an abstraction at best; the true nature of this footprint is with respect to the neuron being attended and it exists in spatial as well as feature domains. An attended stimulus is surrounded by suppression up to the extent of the receptive field within which it lies. It is due to local disambiguation within a receptive field and is the solution of the Context Problem from chapter 2. The size of the surround is determined by the attended neuron. The attended neuron is the one that represents the information that satisfies the current task of the vision system. The size of that RF—somewhat determined by the position in the P-Lattice of the visual area it belongs to—is what sets the extent of the surround. It is easy to compare this with other metaphors. Consider the caricature of these in figure 8.2.

In the cases of the spotlight, zoom lens, and gradient, two characteristics are apparent. There is no manipulation of the contents of a receptive field and thus no solution to the Context Problem; and second, they are early selection schemes and imply the visual system as a whole sees only the attended area while the remainder of the visual world disappears. The ST footprint, however, makes is clear that both of these are properly handled. The remainder of the visual world does not disappear, and the Context Problem is solved.

A secondary point is that the Selective Tuning footprint does not necessarily have the idealized shape shown in the figure. The extent and shape of the footprint is determined by the shape and extent of the receptive field of the attended neurons. In other words, if a square item is being attended within an oval receptive field, then the suppressive surround has the complex shape shown in figure 8.3. This will have implications for experimental methods that are designed to detect it.

Binding   The process by which visual features are correctly combined to provide a unified representation of an object.

Chapter 6 provided detailed discussion of binding within ST. Not only was a novel position proposed, namely the tight connections between binding, recognition, and attention, but also a set of four novel binding processes—convergence, partial recurrence, full recurrence, and iterative recurrence—was incorporated into ST. These clearly distinguish ST from other models. Saliency Map Models are silent with

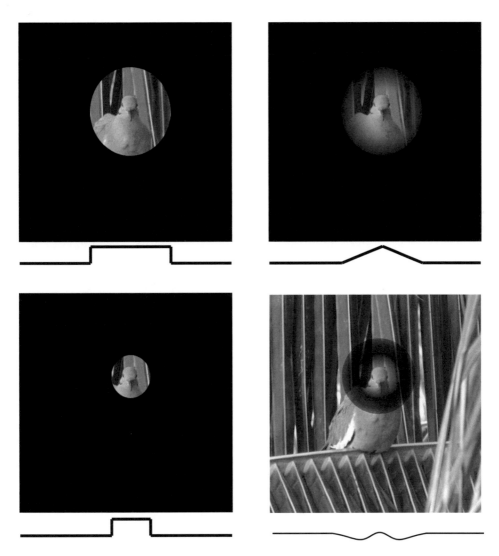

Figure 8.2
Four of the metaphors that characterize the spatial footprint of attention ("black" signifies attentional suppression of signal). Top left, spotlight; top right, gradient; bottom left, zoom lens; bottom right, suppressive surround.

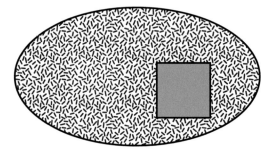

Figure 8.3
The shape of the suppressive surround (textured area) for a hypothetical oval receptive field and square stimulus.

respect to binding. Emergent Attention models have no methods to address binding but believe it will simply occur as needed. In an important sense, these models are not testable because they make no commitments. Temporal Tagging models do explicitly discuss binding and rely on the detection of groups of similarly oscillating neurons to determine binding yet provide little detail on how this might occur.

Covert Attention Attention to a stimulus in the visual field without eye movements.

The attention literature abounds with observations where subjects' eye movements are monitored and trials discarded if eye movements are detected. Because covert fixations can only be inferred, many have tried to detail their existence using response time characteristics, but this has inherent difficulties (Chelazzi, 1999; Townsend, 1990; Wolfe, 1998b). Perhaps an alternate route is via the predictions of a theory of covert fixation. Predictions of a Saliency Map Model cannot be used because they are inherently overt attention models; all are tested on eye movement patterns. Selective Tuning certainly allows for covert fixations; the first algorithm in chapter 4 deals entirely with covert shifts, and the second algorithm integrates them with the overt fixation system. Predictions that arise from this algorithm may be useful in supporting the existence of covert fixations. These predictions are

A. In step 8 of algorithm 4.1, ST inhibits the pass zone connections to permit the next strongest item to be processed. If it were possible to observe such a suppression of the neural pathways that a previously attended stimulus traverses, then this would be evidence of a cortical—and not oculomotor—process preparing for a covert shift.

B. In step 5 of algorithm 4.1, ST implements a layer-by-layer top-down search through the hierarchical WTA based on the winners in the top layer. If a sequence of such top-layer winners could be observed and no eye movements accompany them, this would be direct evidence of a change of attentional fixations.

Disengage Attention   The generation of the signals that release attention from one focus and prepare for a shift in attention.

Posner and colleagues hypothesized that such signals must be present, and this seems reasonable. Certainly, the decision to change fixation must be accompanied by the appropriate control signals that would act on that decision. This may be done in a fixed manner such as a cycle with fixed timing that always changes fixations every so many milliseconds, or perhaps dependent on task demands. The fact that there can be more than one reason for change of fixation necessitates a decision algorithm and accompanying control signals. Selective Tuning includes such explicit signals within its overall algorithm (see figure 4.2).

Endogenous Influences   An endogenous influence is an internally generated signal used for directing attention. This includes domain knowledge or task instructions.

Task influences permeate every aspect of processing within ST. How exactly they are coded from knowledge or task instructions is mostly outside ST (although see the section "Fixation History Map Maintenance" in chapter 5).

Engage Attention   The actions needed to fixate a stimulus whether covertly or overtly.

ST includes this functionality as can be seen from algorithm 4.3 and from the examples of chapter 7.

Executive Control   The system that coordinates the functional elements into a coherent unit that responds correctly to task and environmental demands.

Egeth and Yantis (1997), Yantis (1998), and Yantis and Serences (2003) provide excellent overviews of the topic and describe a large number of relevant behavioral observations that help illuminate the different aspects of the control problem. Corbetta and Shulman (2002) go further and, using brain-imaging studies, provide a neuroanatomic map of how the brain's nonvisual areas combine to provide attentional control. Much of their motivation and thus logic behind the map is to relate neurologic damage to functional anomalies. These papers point the way nicely to future research that might clarify issues related to attentional control.

ST has a rather weak functionality regarding executive control at least with respect to the just-cited works. Algorithm 4.3 presented in chapter 4 is the executive controller for ST. The decision algorithm for selection of binding process in chapter 6 is also a component of the executive. What brain area is responsible for this remains unanswered. How exactly task instructions are interpreted, represented, and used, how long-term and short-term memory are represented and used, how tasks are directed and completion detected, or other factors, are not addressed.

Exogenous Influences   Exogenous influence is due to an external stimulus and contributes to control of gaze direction in a reflexive manner. Most common is perhaps abrupt onsets.

In ST, algorithm 4.3, the ability to control gaze based on data-driven processes is evident through the Peripheral Priority Map. The processing path that a strong peripheral (outside of about the central $10°$ of visual field) stimulus takes may be considered reflexive if the alternate path is considered deliberate (nonreflexive). Certainly an abrupt onset or offset can be detected by the simple mechanism described in Wai and Tsotsos (1992) and Tsotsos et al. (1995) for change detection. There, 'on' and 'off' center-surround operators were used, defined in a standard manner, as well as their time derivatives. If the time derivative of one of these 'on' operators at a given location exceeded a threshold while the center region response alone also exceeded a threshold, then an onset event was detected. For offset events, the same strategy is used. This computation can be part of the overall input to the Peripheral Priority Map. The competition of step 6 in algorithm 4.3 could have a default state, where—unless task information provides a different priority—onsets or offsets win the competition and thus immediately lead to an appropriate change of gaze.

   Exogenous cues can also lead to object-based attention as shown by Reynolds, Alborzian, and Stoner (2003) and Fallah et al. (2007). Object-based cueing certainly is within the ST framework. If a representation of objects is part of the overall P-Lattice representation of visual information, and one object (or object category) is cued, the top-down bias that results follows the components or features that define it in the lattice using the same mechanism described in chapter 5.

Inhibition of Return   A bias against returning attention to a previously attended location or object.

All computational attention models include IOR simply because the mathematics of winner-take-all processes demand it. If the 'winner' remains in the competing set of responses, then it is the one found over and over. Only if it is removed from the competing set will the next-strongest response be found. ST is no exception. The main difference between ST and other models is that ST permits task influences to modulate IOR.

Neural Modulation   Attention changes baseline firing rates as well as firing patterns of neurons for attended stimuli.

This functionality is one where ST makes a distinct departure from other theories. The most prominent of the other current theories are the single-neuron theories Biased Competition (Desimone & Duncan, 1995; Reynolds et al., 1999) and the Normalization Models [there are two models named similarly, one due to Reynolds and Heeger (2009) and one due to Lee and Maunsell (2009)]. In each of these cases, the goal was to provide a mathematical model that is able to match recorded neural responses during attentive tasks. All provide strong evidence in their favor. However, what they depend on is an assumed selection process and simple direct manipulation of the neuron's gain; all simply increase gain to simulate attention. Further, they do not easily extend to a hierarchy of neurons let alone to a complex structure such as ST's P-Lattice. In contrast, ST makes a strong statement on the cause of the observed neural changes in an attentive task. In the ST algorithm, the recurrent tracing of connections and accompanying suppression of nonselected connections is sufficient to explain attentive response modulation; there is no mechanism of explicit enhancement.

The suppression of non-selected connections also has an ordering and thus predicts a time course of hierarchical modulation effects. Specifically, modulation will be seen at the highest levels first and at the lowest levels last. This is the opposite to what the Normalization and Biased Competition Models would suggest, These models, by virtue of being based on excitatory and inhibitory input neuron pools, imply an ordering of attentional effects from early visual areas to later ones, and opposite to the experimental data as well (Buffalo, Fries, Landman, Liang, & Desimone, 2010; Fallah et al., 2007; Lauritzen, D'Esposoti, Heger, & Silver, 2009; Mehta et al., 2000; O'Connor, Fukui, Pinsk, & Kastner, 2002; Roelfsema et al., 1998). Following figure 8.4, the leftmost panel illustrates a hypothetical activation for the center element of the input pattern. Selection of the strongest response at the top then triggers the recurrent localization process. At each successive layer of recurrence, part of the input to that selected neuron is suppressed, leading to a change in response for all neurons upstream. The changes in response thus occur in time steps defined by the number of layers in the pathway downward, plus the time it would take for the effect of suppression at one layer to ripple up to the neuron being examined.

Overt Attention   Also known as Orienting—the action of orienting the body, head, and eyes to foveate a stimulus in the 3D world.

Algorithm 4.3 includes computations to enable overt shifts of gaze, but it is beyond the scope of the model to detail the control of any accompanying body or head movements and to provide for fixation in depth (but see Bruce & Tsotsos, 2005).

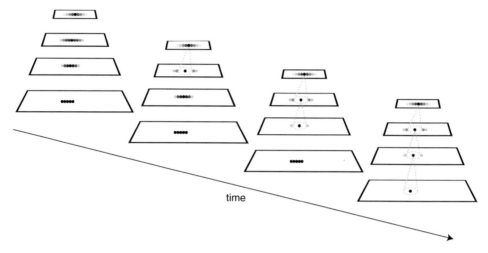

Figure 8.4
The time course of recurrent localization and how it affects neural response modulation.

Postattention The process that creates the representation of an attended item that persists after attention is moved away from it.

A postattentive phase is provided within algorithm 4.3 namely, step 9. An example of this, using Type II Iterative Recurrence Binding, was shown in chapter 7. However, further details such as the higher-order representations that are created and connections to other processes are not within the ST framework at this time.

Preattentive Features The extraction of visual features from stimulus patterns, perhaps biased by task demands.

This element, and similarly in all other computational attention models, is the main connection of attention models to the general vision process. All models require some set of early features, computed in parallel, on which to base attentional computations. ST also requires this but has a more complex setup than other models because it includes separate mechanisms for the input to peripheral fixations and central fixations. ST also addresses the full visual processing hierarchy and not only the early levels of processing because for ST, preattentive means whatever is computed with a single feed-forward pass.

Priming Priming is the general process by which task instructions or world knowledge prepares the visual system for input. **Cueing** is an instance of priming; perception is speeded with a correct cue, whether by location, feature, or complete stimulus. Purposefully ignoring has relevance here also and is termed **Negative Priming**. If one ignores a stimulus, processing of that ignored stimulus shortly afterwards is impaired.

Priming has been a feature of ST since its beginning, and figures 4.1 and 4.2 explicitly include processing elements to achieve this. The section "Task Guidance" in chapter 5 describes how many of the ST variables and parameters can be set by task information. However, ST currently does not include how verbal instructions or instructions about sequences of stimuli or more complex tasks are understood or applied. ST biases processes by suppressing the nonrelevant. In other words, ST ignores what is not relevant. Some degree of Negative Priming is thus included, but to see the Negative Priming experimental effect, it depends on the recovery time of ST neurons; that is, on how long it takes for a biased-against neuron to return to a fully unbiased state. If stimuli are presented during that recovery time, they will be negatively primed.

Recognition   The process of interpreting an attended stimulus, facilitated by attention.

To attend a stimulus within ST means to provide for the best possible conditions for its recognition. Chapter 6 provided more discussion on recognition within ST and how recognition, binding, and attention are tightly interdependent. Attention for ST is the process by which the brain controls and tunes visual processes. The intent is to find a satisficing configuration of processes so that at least the minimum requirements of a behavioral goal can be achieved, and in most if not all instances, recognition of stimuli is necessary. Attention adapts the visual system to its dynamic needs that are dictated by current input and task.

Salience/Conspicuity   The overall contrast of the stimulus at a particular location with respect to its surround.

This element plays an important role in ST in the computation of the Peripheral Priority Map, as described in algorithm 4.3. The method of computation is the AIM algorithm (Bruce & Tsotsos, 2009), an algorithm based in information maximization and shown to have strong predictive power for human gaze patterns. In contrast with a large number of other attention models, ST does not derive all of its attentive performance from a salience representation.

Search   The process that scans the candidate stimuli for detection or other tasks among the many possible locations and features in cluttered scenes.

This is a rather complex 'simple statement.' Search involves perhaps most of the other attentional functionalities listed here. How well ST provides an overall explanation for search depends on how well each element is handled and how they are all put together. It is clear that this was the motivation for the original proofs of the complexity of the process given in chapter 2 and appendix B. Algorithm 4.3 is the extent of the search process ST offers at this time. It is far more than Saliency Map Models or single-neuron models of attention provide but still likely to be insufficient in the general case.

Selection   This is the process of choosing one element of the stimulus over the remainder. Selection can be over locations, over features, for objects, over time, and for behavioral responses, or even for combinations of these.

Chapter 5 provides details on the θ-WTA method ST uses for selection. The selection method differs from the standard Koch and Ullman (1985) winner-take-all process used by most models not only in its formulation but also in its properties.

Shift Attention   The actions involved in moving an attentional fixation from its current to its new point of fixation.

It is difficult to think of why a model of attention might not include this functionality. Yet, some do not: Biased Competition has no method to explicitly shift attention to the next target, Emergent models assume this happens as a property of the dynamical properties of the system, and Temporal Tagging does not address this at all. In ST, the sequence of steps 4 through 8 of algorithm 4.3 define how ST shifts attention.

Time Course   The effects of attention take time to appear, and this is observed in the firing rate patterns of neurons and in behavioral experiments, showing delays as well as cyclic patterns.

In Tsotsos et al. (1995), a timing plot was provided to show the time course of the elements of ST's algorithm. This plot is redrawn here and appears as figure 8.5. The figure shows the time course of the variable ς_{ijxy} defined in chapter 5, equation 5.14, for a four-layer pyramid. In other words, as should be clear from the figure, there is a distinct cycle time or duration to an attentional fixation due to the combined feedforward and recurrent traversals. The gating control signals in the figure, layer by layer, take time to appear and have a clear progression from the highest layers of the system to the lowest. The gating control signals determine the recurrence trajectory.

Update Fixation History   The process by which the system keeps track of what has been seen and processed, and how that representation is maintained and updated that then participates in decisions of what to fixate and when.

Algorithm 4.3 explicitly includes a computation to update fixation history. Several questions remain, however, with respect to how this may occur in the brain. Where

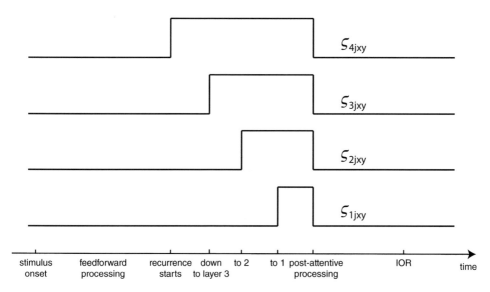

Figure 8.5
Time course of gating signal progression in a hypothetical four-layer pyramid.

could this representation be? What is the extent of the visual world—greater than the visual field—that it represents? How are shifts of gaze and thus visual field integrated and what happens to elements that may no longer be within viewing range? These and other questions remain open, even though within ST, simple assumptions can be made to permit this strategy to be functional.

Summing up the preceding, ST shows good explanatory power for a majority of the attentional elements, but there is still much to be done especially with respect to the executive control functions and how it connects to the rest of an intelligent, behaving brain.

Predictions with Experimental Support

Many predictions have appeared in the Selective Tuning papers, and a significant number have found experimental support. In each case, the prediction was a true one; that is, it was stated well before any evidence for the effect had been observed and was not an explanation of preexisting experimental data. The main predictions that have received supporting experimental evidence, the papers where they are described, the reasoning behind them, and some of those supporting experiments follow.

1. Attention can modify processes at any level where there is a many-to-one neural convergence.

Appeared in: Culhane (1992); Tsotsos et al. (1995).

Supported by: Britten (1996), Kastner, De Weerd, Desimone, and Ungerleider (1998), O'Connor et al. (2002).

Reasoning: Wherever there is a many-to-one convergence of neural signals, there exists the possibility that two or more signals arise from different underlying events (the Context Problem described earlier). As a result, the convergence may lead to interference, and attentional selection can reduce or eliminate that interference.

2. Attentional modulation suppresses irrelevant spatial locations within a receptive field.

Appeared in: Tsotsos (1990a).

Supported by: Caputo and Guerra (1998), Bahcall and Kowler (1999), Mounts (2000a,b), Vanduffel, Tootell, and Orban (2000), Smith, Singh, and Greenlee (2000), Cutzu and Tsotsos (2003), Müller and Kleinschmidt (2004), Schall, Sato, Thompson, Vaughn, and Chi-Hung (2004), Fecteau and Enns (2005), Müller, Mollenhauer, Rosler, and Kleinschmidt (2005), Hopf et al. (2006), Boehler, Tsotsos, Schoenfeld, Heinze, and Hopf (2009).

Reasoning: A typical receptive field may contain more than one stimulus or event, and for a typical task, only a subset may be relevant. If the relevant is considered 'the signal,' then what remains is 'the noise.' Suppression of the noise improves the contrast or signal-to-noise ratio leading to neural responses more closely representing the relevant stimuli.

3. Attentive spatial suppression has a spatial shape similar to a Difference of Gaussians profile.

Appeared in: Tsotsos (1990a).

Supported by: Slotnick, Hopfinger, Klein, and Sutter (2002), Müller and Kleinschmidt (2004), Hopf et al. (2006).

Reasoning: The previous point dealt with suppression of the irrelevant within a receptive field. The current point makes a statement about the kind of suppression. As presented in Tsotsos (1990a), the generalized process of ST's attentional beam would require that the beam have substructure that can be manipulated depending on attended information. The cross section of the beam was modeled with a central portion that represents the pass zone having positive values and with the annulus surrounding this being the inhibit zone with values near zero. This permits easy control of the location, size, and shape of the pass zone. The weighting is applied to the neurons within the beam multiplicatively. This multiplication leads to inhibition of the nonattended signals. A Gaussian profile is a convenient modeling form.

Outside the beam, processing is unaffected. The result of applying this is the Mexican hat profile that has been observed in the above papers.

4. Surround suppression is due to top-down (recurrent) processes.

Appeared in: Tsotsos (1990a).

Supported by: McCarley and Mounts (2007), Boehler, Tsotsos, Schoenfeld, Heinze, and Hopf (2009), Hopf et al. (2010).

Reasoning: The motivation for why surround suppression might be useful appears in the previous paragraphs. But how is the locus of suppression determined (i.e., which neurons are to be affected by this mechanism)? Clearly the neurons that are on the pathways that best represent the attended stimulus are those where the benefit of improved signal-to-noise ratio has the most behavioral utility. The discussions of the Routing Problem and its solution described earlier provide the reason. It cannot be a feed-forward process that makes this decision. Some recent models of vision use a feed-forward maximum operation with the goal of solving the same sort of problem. Although chapter 2 provided a rationale as to why this approach may not find a global maximum, more evidence can be presented as to why this is not likely to be biologically plausible. The experimental evidence against a feed-forward maximum operation is overwhelming. The majority of studies that have examined responses with two non-overlapping stimuli in the classical receptive field have found that the firing rate evoked by the pair is typically lower than the response to the preferred of the two presented alone, inconsistent with a max rule (Chelazzi, Duncan, Miller, & Desimone, 1998; Miller, Gochin, & Gross, 1993; Missal, Vogels, Li, & Orban, 1999; Recanzone, Wurtz, & Schwarz, 1997; Reynolds & Desimone, 1998; Reynolds et al., 1999; Rolls & Tovee, 1995; Zoccolan, Cox, & DiCarlo, 2005). Additional studies have found the response to the preferred stimulus changes when presented along with other stimuli, a pattern inconsistent with a feed-forward max operation (Sheinberg & Logothetis, 2001; Rolls, Aggelopoulos, & Zheng, 2003). A theoretical argument may also be made against a feed-forward max using the equivalence conditions between relaxation labeling processes and max selection (Zucker, Leclerc, & Mohammed, 1981), and especially considering the role of lateral processes in vision (Ben-Shahar, Huggins, Izo, & Zucker, 2003). If lateral interactions are included, time course matters. It has been observed that most V1 response increases due to lateral interactions seem to occur in the latter parts of the response profile. This hints that lateral interaction takes extra time to take effect with V1 responses continuing until about 300 milliseconds after stimulus onset (Kapadia et al., 1995), well after the first feed-forward traversal has completed. As several previous authors have also argued—Milner (1974), Fukushima (1986), Fuster (1990)—ST also argues for a top-down approach to attentional selection, and this now has experimental support.

5. Attentive surround suppression also exists in the feature dimension.

Appeared in: Tsotsos (1990a).

Supported by: Tombu and Tsotsos (2008), Loach, Frischen, Bruce, and Tsotsos (2008), Chen and Tsotsos (2010).

Reasoning: Attentive, and not stimulus-driven lateral, effects are considered here. Suppose the tuning curves for feature neurons—say for orientation—are as shown in figure 8.6a. The figure illustrates a classic conception of a Gaussian-like tuning profile for each of 15 neurons, each tuned to a particular orientation. Figure 8.6b shows what the overall response of this population of neurons might be for a vertically oriented stimulus. A search for the position of the peak of this population response suffices to permit the correct detection of that feature. Noise may make this more difficult, however. Consider what happens if the population as a whole is tuned for the vertical orientation by suppressing neighboring orientations, as shown in figure 8.6c. The response from the neighboring neurons in the orientation dimension is suppressed and, along with it, any responses due to noise in the stimulus from those neurons. As a result, the detection of the correct peak is facilitated. The magnitude and extent of suppression would dictate the amount of improvement. The difference between the overall population response in figure 8.6b [shown in light gray on part (c) of the figure for comparison] and in figure 8.6c exhibits the familiar Difference of Gaussians profile. This neighboring feature suppression is the analogue to the spatial surround suppression described earlier and points to the fact that there is a Context Problem in feature space to contend with as well. Moreover, as is evident in figure 8.6c, the tuning curve of the overall population is sharpened toward the attended orientation, as Haenny and Schiller (1988) and many others since have shown. The experiments cited as support are further detailed below.

6. There are two kinds of attentional effects both appearing with latencies from higher-order visual areas to lower.

Appeared in: Tsotsos (1990a).

Supported by: Mehta et al. (2000), O'Connor et al. (2002), Roelfsema et al. (2007), Lauritzen et al. (2009), Buffalo et al. (2010).

Figure 8.6
The effect of attentional feature surround suppression on tuning curves. (a) A set of hypothetical tuning curves for 15 neurons each tuned to a different orientation. (b) The same set of tunings are shown. The top curve is the overall population response of those neurons for a vertical bar. (c) If attending to vertical, attention suppresses neighboring neurons, and the overall population tuning curve narrows and is more tightly tuned to vertical in comparison with the curve in gray, which is the same as the overall response in (b). The black dots on the curves give the response levels of specific tuning curves for the vertical orientation.

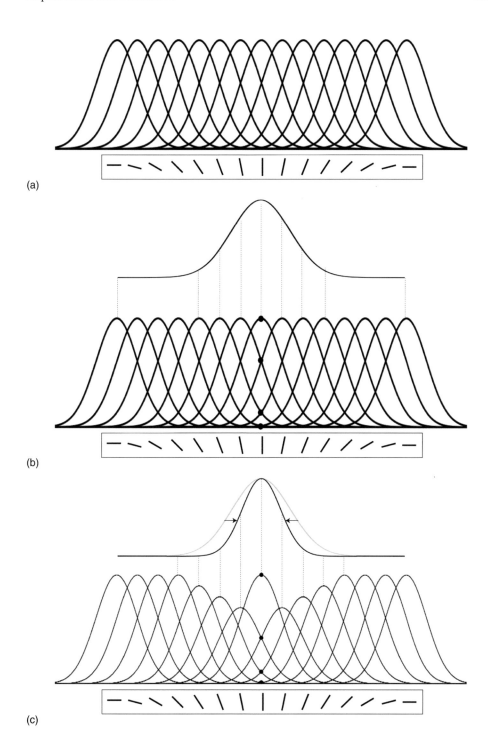

(a)

(b)

(c)

Reasoning: The two processes that have attentional modulation impact on single neurons are priming and recurrent localization. The priming process occurs in advance of stimulus onset and suppresses nonrelevant processing. The signals for this come from executive areas and are top-down with respect to the visual cortex. The localization process selects the neurons and pathways that best represent the attended stimuli and prunes the remainder. The pruning process changes the flow of feed-forward input signals so that neural responses change. As the localization is from higher-order to lower-order visual areas, so too are the modulatory effects. It is important to distinguish these from the other processes that impact a single neuron's response. There are at least three additional processes: feed-forward signal responses, lateral cooperation effects (both within and across columns), and local feedback effects. It is not straightforward to tell these apart (and perhaps there are additional ones as well). However, a start on this appears in at least a couple of sources. Kapadia et al. (1995) show the time course of lateral interactions in V1 neurons. Kondo and Komatsu (2000) have examined the time course of suppression in V4 neurons. Both show that there is a considerable duration to the effects of suppression on these neurons. ST includes processes for each as shown in chapter 5, equation 5.19.

7. Neural baseline modulation—increases for attended location, decreases elsewhere.

Appeared in: Tsotsos (1990a).

Supported by: Kastner, Pinsk, De Weerd, Desimone, and Ungerleider (1999), Luck et al. (1997a)

Reasoning: Suppose there is no stimulus but that a subject is asked to attend to a particular location. ST will suppress signals in all other locations as part of the priming mechanism (figures 7.2, 7.3, and 7.4 demonstrate this). The end result is that any noise in the regions surrounding the attended location is reduced. This means that neurons that receive signals primarily from the suppressed areas may have smaller responses. Neurons within the selected regions might show enhancement following the same argument made in the section "Competition to Represent a Stimulus" of chapter 5.

8. Attentive selection has a cycle time.

Appeared in: Tsotsos et al. (1995).

Supported by: Van Rullen et al. (2007).

Reasoning: The overall ST strategy includes a number of processing stages all of which require time to execute. The control signals for the top-down localization part were presented in figure 8.5. The implication is that if the system is to attend to several items in succession and the task required for each item requires some localization, then there is a limit to how fast this may be done, and thus it appears as if there is a fixed cycle time for accomplishing the task. It is not a new concept; certainly the early visual experiments that concluded conjunction search required a self-terminating serial search imply exactly the same [summarized in Wolfe (1998a), but also see Wolfe (1998b)]. Testing with a challenging detection task, Van Rullen et al. (2007) found that human performance best matched a sampling strategy. They concluded that multiple items of interest were processed in series, and the timing showed a rate of about seven per second. Further, they observed that attention operated in this periodic manner, even when focused on a single target. They concluded that attention might operate in an intrinsically periodic fashion.

9. The suppressive surround does not rely on the existence of distractors.

Appeared in: Tsotsos et al. (1995).

Supported by: Boehler (2006), Boehler et al. (submitted).

Reasoning: The existence of distractors is not the determinant of attention; the task required for the visual input determines attention. Even if there is only a single stimulus in the visual field, if the task requires localization or detailed reports of the stimulus' characteristics, attention will impose the suppressive surround.

10. Suppressive surround is not seen for discrimination tasks.

Appeared in: Tsotsos (1990a), Tsotsos et al. (2005).

Supported by: McCarley and Mounts (2007), Boehler et al. (2009), Hopf et al. (2010).

Reasoning: Following on point 9 above, if the task is discrimination, no localization or detailed reports of the stimulus' characteristics are needed, and thus no top-down attention either. As a result, no suppressive surround is seen.

These 10 predictions not only have experimental support but also, as a group, represent a very broad subset of attentional issues, and the fact that Selective Tuning foreshadowed the observations significantly supports the overall theory.

Some Supporting Experiments

A number of experiments have been carried out with an excellent cadre of students, postdoctoral fellows, and collaborators. They provide direct support for Selective Tuning, testing several predictions, some appearing in the previous section. Each is described in a previous publication, and as a result only a brief summary of the main points and a few key figures appear here. The reader should see the original papers for full details and discussion. Each section is headed by the publication citation. The behavioral experiments will be given first followed by the imaging studies.

Cutzu, F., Tsotsos, J.K. (2003). The selective tuning model of visual attention: Testing the predictions arising from the inhibitory surround mechanism. *Vision Research* 43, pp. 205–219.

The goal for this set of experiments was to map the variation of the attentional field around a target and discriminate between the predictions of the traditional models and of the Selective Tuning model. The principle of the experimental method was the following: Direct the subjects' attention to a reference location in the visual field and concomitantly measure their ability to process visual information (i.e., the intensity of the attentional field) at different probe locations of equal retinal resolution. By systematically varying the reference–probe distance, one can determine the dependence of the attentional field on distance to the focus of attention. The experimental requirements were threefold:

1. Engaging visual attention: The classical *L–T* discrimination task was used. Discrimination accuracy was employed as performance measure.

2. Directing the attention of the subject to one, prespecified reference target location: We resorted to pre-cueing because in this way the Selective Tuning beam structure is supposedly in place before stimulus onset.

3. Ensuring equal retinal resolution for all stimuli: We used a circular array display with fixation point in the center.

A typical experimental sequence, from left to right, consisted of cue image, a test image, and a mask image (see figure 8.7). The cue, a light-gray disk, anticipated the position of the reference target in the following test image. This will be referred to as the peripheral cue condition. It was shown for 180 milliseconds, which is within

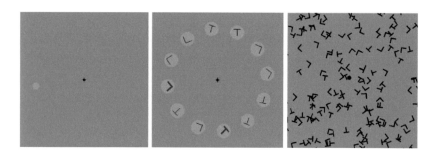

Figure 8.7
The basic trial sequence. (Left) The cue, a light-gray disk, indicated the position of the reference target character in the subsequent test image. The cue was shown for 180 milliseconds. (Middle) Test image, shown for 100 milliseconds. The target characters were red (drawn in this figure with thick lines), and the distractors were black (drawn with thin lines). The task was to decide whether the two targets are identical or different by pressing certain keys on the keyboard. (Right) The mask was shown until the subject responded. (From Cutzu & Tsotsos, 2003, © 2003, with permission from Elsevier.)

the time range of effective cueing. The stimulus set in the test image consisted of six randomly oriented *L*s and six randomly oriented *T*s arranged in random order on a ring. The characters were evenly spaced and were overlaid on light-gray disks as shown (middle panel of the figure). Two of the characters, the reference target and the probe target, were red (shown in the figure in bold), and the rest, the distractors, were black. The orientation of the imaginary line joining the two targets was randomly changed from trial to trial. The radius of the ring was 6°, and character size was 0.6° visual angle. The task of the subject was to decide whether the two red characters were identical or different by pressing one of two keys on the computer keyboard. After 200 milliseconds, the test image is replaced by a mask. The role of the mask was to erase the iconic memory of the target letters in the test display. It was during the mask that the subjects made their response. To ensure that all characters in the ring were perceived at same resolution, the subjects were instructed to always fixate the crosshair in the center of the ring. The main variable of interest in this experiment was intertarget separation, taking on six distinct values, from one, when the two target characters were next neighbors, to six, when the targets were diametrically opposite. Each of the six intertarget separations was tested four times in the same condition and four times in the different condition. Thus, an experimental session included 24 same and 24 different trials.

The result of this is seen in figure 8.8. ST predicts that if the cue stimulus is attended, then the area around it is suppressed. As a result, intertarget separation of 1 would lead to poor performance and separation of 6 should lead to good performance. Figure 8.8 shows exactly this and further provides some indication of the extent of suppression.

The experiment was also performed using an odd-man-out strategy. Instead of a target and probe, the subjects are asked to determine whether or not the ring of rotated *T*s and *L*s contained an odd-man-out, a *T* among *L*s, for example. The position of the odd-man-out was varied with respect to the cue position. In this case, ST would predict that if one attends the cue and the region around it is suppressed, then if the odd-man-out appeared at the cue position, performance should be good. If it appeared nearby, performance should be poor, and if it appeared farther away, performance should improve. Figure 8.9 shows the typical sequence of stimuli, and figure 8.10 shows the resulting performance. Once again, it is clear that the expected performance, predicted by ST, is observed. Further, this experiment samples the attentional field at the point of attention where the first experiment could not.

Tombu, M., Tsotsos, J.K. (2008). Attending to orientation results in an inhibitory surround in orientation space. *Perception & Psychophysics* 70 (1), pp. 30–35.

ST predicts that attention to a given feature value (i.e., to a particular orientation or particular color) results in a suppression of nearby values within that feature

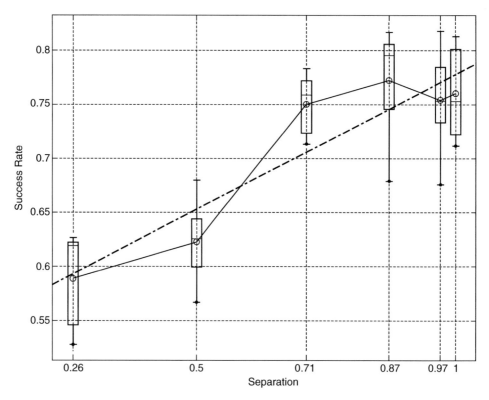

Figure 8.8
Box plot of the dependence of target discrimination accuracy on target separation. The thick dash-dot line represents the linear regression model. Target separation is expressed in fractions of letter ring diameter. The boxes, one per separation value, have lines at the lower quartile, median, and upper quartile values. The whiskers show the extent of the rest of the data. Performance initially improves with inter-target distance, reaches a maximum, and then levels off. (From Cutzu & Tsotsos, 2003, © 2003, with permission from Elsevier.)

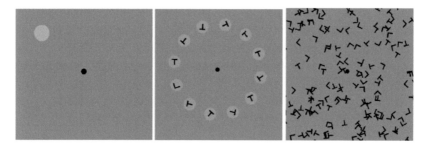

Figure 8.9
A typical trial sequence. (Left) The cue, a light-gray disk, was shown for 180 milliseconds. (Middle) Test screen, shown for 100 milliseconds. The characters were overlaid on light-gray disks identical to the cue. In this case, the target is present: there is an odd *L* among the *T*s in the test image. However, the cue is invalid. The subject's task was to detect the odd letter in the ring. (Right) The mask was always removed after 2 seconds, whether the subject responded or not, and a new trial sequence was initiated. (From Cutzu & Tsotsos, 2003, © 2003, with permission from Elsevier.)

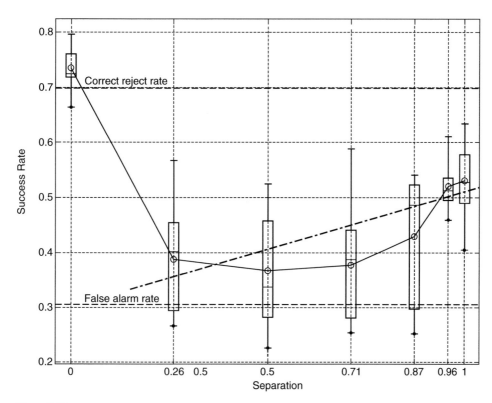

Figure 8.10

Box plot of dependence of target detection accuracy on target–cue distance in the odd-man-out detection experiment. The cue–target distance was defined as the length of the chord joining the cued location on the ring to the target location on the ring. It was expressed in units of ring diameter and ranges from 0 (the odd letter is at the cued location) to 1 diameter (the odd letter is diametrically opposite to the cued location). The interrupted lines represent the false-alarm level (0.31) and the mean correct reject (target absent) rates. The thick dash-dot line represents the linear regression model. The boxes, one per separation value, have lines at the lower quartile, median, and upper quartile values. The whiskers are lines extending from each end of the box and show the extent of the rest of the data. Target detection performance peaks both at the cued location and diametrically opposite to it. (From Cutzu & Tsotsos, 2003, © 2003, with permission from Elsevier.)

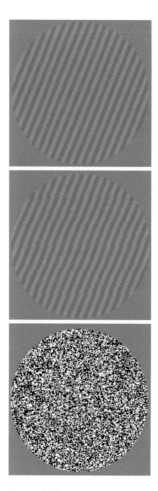

Figure 8.11
(Top) The subjects were instructed to indicate whether the stripes on the disk were straight or jagged. The 22° orientation disk is shown (22°, 67°, 112°, or 157° were used as stimuli). (Middle) An example of a jagged-stripe disk. (Bottom) The mask that followed each trial. (Reprinted with permission from Tombu & Tsotsos, 2008)

dimension. This experiment was designed to demonstrate this. In this experiment, subjects were required to attend to an orientation and make judgments about the stripes on briefly presented disks. It was important that the display was designed so that all location information was eliminated and that a large portion of the visual field was covered. Stripe orientation was varied so that they could be at, near, or far from the attended orientation.

Figure 8.11 shows the stimulus sequence. Striped disks, with stripe orientations (clockwise from vertical) of 22°, 67°, 112°, or 157° (22° orientation disk shown in the figure), were used as stimuli. The subjects were instructed to indicate whether the stripes on the disk were straight or jagged. Stimulus presentation times varied between subjects from 67 to 150 milliseconds, as well as from block to block for each subject, in order to keep performance levels at approximately 80% correct. A 166-millisecond mask preceded and followed stimulus presentation. At the beginning of each block, the subjects were instructed to attend to one orientation. For that block, 70% of the trials were at the attended orientation, with each unattended orientation presented 10% of the time. Within each condition, the stripes on the disk were straight 50% of the time and jagged 50% of the time. Each orientation was the attended orientation for two blocks per session. The straight versus jagged test represented the task that masked (for the subject) the fact that orientation was the key element of the study. The unattended trials provided the controls for the experiment. In line with the prediction of ST, the results revealed an inhibitory surround. As in the spatial domain, attending to a point in orientation space results in an inhibitory surround for nearby orientations as figure 8.12 shows. This is the first demonstration of an attentional modulation along a feature dimension, around a particular feature value.

Loach, D., Frischen, A., Bruce, N., Tsotsos, J.K. (2008). An attentional mechanism for selecting appropriate actions afforded by graspable objects. *Psychological Science* 19 (12), pp. 1253–1257.

An object may afford a number of different actions. If the kind of attentional mechanism ST proposes applies throughout the cortex and not only for vision, then similar suppression of competing perceptions or actions should be observed. Here we show that an attentional mechanism inhibits competing motor programs that could elicit erroneous actions.

To test this hypothesis, we developed a behavioral task that relies on the rationale that a graspable object activates a suitable motor program, which is expressed in facilitated responses with the hand that is compatible with the graspable part of the object. We briefly presented pictures of door handles: a prime handle followed by a probe handle (see figure 8.13). The orientation of the two handles varied by 0°, 20°, 40°, or 60° relative to one another, but the probe handle was always presented

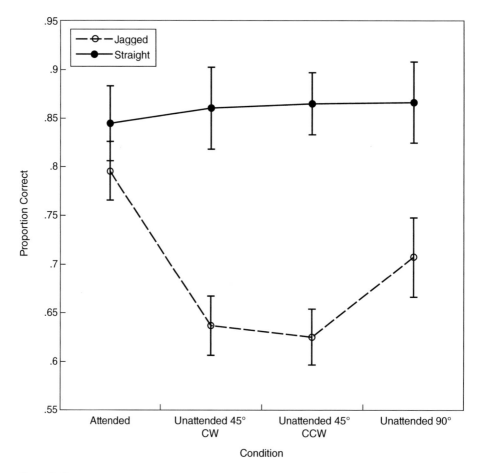

Figure 8.12
Results for eight subjects collapsing across stripe orientation. When the stripes were straight, the ability of subjects to perceive straightness was not affected by orientation tuning. However, when the stripes were jagged, the subjects performed best when the stimulus was at the attended orientation. They performed at an intermediate level when the stimulus was at an orientation far from the attended orientation and performed worst when the stripe orientation was near the attended orientation. Performance when the stripes were near the attended orientation was significantly worse than when the stripe orientation was far from the attended orientation. CW, clockwise; CCW, counterclockwise. (Reprinted with permission from Tombu & Tsotsos, 2008)

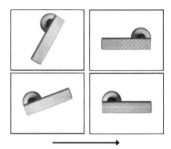

Figure 8.13
Example of prime (left two images) and probe door (right two images) handles in two types of trials. Participants responded either to the texture (experiment 1) or to the color (experiment 2) of the probe handle. The column on the left shows a trial in which the orientation of the prime handle differs from the orientation of the subsequently presented probe handle by 60°. The probe handle (always horizontal) is green and has a diamond-plate metal texture, and the compatible responding hand is the left hand. The column on the right shows a trial in which the orientation of the prime handle differs from the orientation of the subsequently presented probe handle by 20°. The probe handle is blue and has a wood-grain texture, and the compatible responding hand is the right hand. (Adapted from Loach et al., 2008)

in a horizontal orientation. The handles all had a color and a texture. Texture is a tactile, and therefore action-relevant, dimension whereas color is not, as explained in the paper. It would activate a motor program for acting on the handle and color would not. In the first experiment (experiment 1) subjects were asked to respond to the texture and in the second experiment (experiment 2) to the color. Participants made speeded key-press responses to the probe handle. Each responding hand was assigned a response key, so that it was either compatible or incompatible with the door handles, which faced to the right or left. We predicted that presentation of the prime handle for the texture task would elicit the generation of a motor program suitable for a reach of that orientation. Surround inhibition associated with this motor program should inhibit other motor programs coding for slightly dissimilar reaches (i.e., 20° or 40° difference in orientation). Thus, if the subsequently presented probe handle elicits a reach within that range, it would require the activation of a recently inhibited motor program. In contrast, the color task, not being a tactile one, would not show this suppression.

Compatible responses were faster than incompatible responses if the two handles shared an identical orientation but were slower if the two handles were aligned at slightly dissimilar orientations for the texture task. Figure 8.14a gives the response times and clearly shows how the incompatible responses are suppressed. This difference does not appear for the color task, figure 8.14b. Such suppressive surround effects due to attention in the visual domain have been previously demonstrated but have never been observed behaviorally in the motor domain. This finding delineates a common mechanism involved in two of the most important functions of the brain: to process sensory data and to prepare actions based on that information.

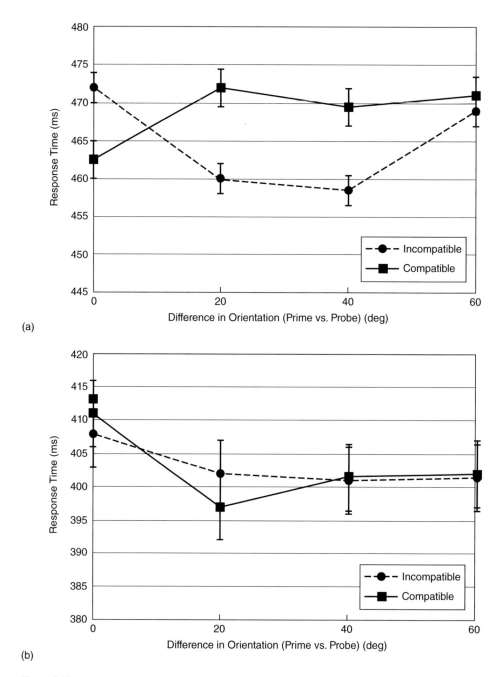

(a)

(b)

Figure 8.14
Response times for (a) the texture task of the first experiment and (b) the color task of the second experiment. Means of median response times (y-axis) are displayed as a function of the difference in orientation between the prime and probe handles (x-axis). Results are shown separately for responses with the compatible hand and responses with the incompatible hand. Error bars indicate within-subjects 95% confidence intervals. (Adapted from Loach et al., 2008)

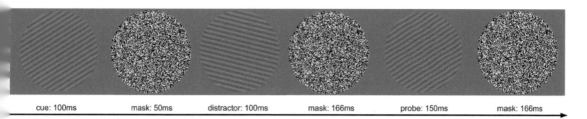

cue: 100ms   mask: 50ms   distractor: 100ms   mask: 166ms   probe: 150ms   mask: 166ms

Figure 8.15
The striped disks used in experiments 1 and 2 and the presentation sequence. The subjects were asked to indicate whether the stripes on the disk were straight or jagged.

Chen, X., Tsotsos, J.K. (2010). Attentional Surround Suppression in the Feature Dimension. Department of Computer Science & Engineering, TR2010-01, York University.

Following up on a previous positive study (Tombu & Tsotsos, 2008), we describe new experiments that test attentive feature surround suppression using a pre-cue paradigm in both orientation and color feature spaces. We observed that orientations or colors near the attended one, in that feature space, are suppressed, but not orientations or colors farther away in feature space.

Three experiments were done using the same stimuli as in Tombu and Tsotsos (2008). The first (experiment 1) sought to replicate those results but with a different experimental paradigm—figure 8.15—that included distractors. We also included a denser sampling in orientation space. The same suppression as in Tombu and Tsotsos was indeed found; however, comparing with those results (suppression occurred at under 45° condition), we found a much nearer inhibition to the attended orientation (5°, 10°, or at most 20°). This difference could result from many factors, such as the different paradigm, finer probes, and even different stimulus size and viewing distance. However, the result was indeed replicated.

In the second experiment (experiment 2), we addressed the question of whether or not the difference between the first experiment and that of Tombu and Tsotsos (2008) came from the presence of distractors. There were no distractors in the experiment of Tombu and Tsotsos (2008). In the current experiment, we modified the paradigm by taking away the distractor presented after the pre-cue. We were also interested in whether or not the orientation attention would be affected by the absence of a competing distractor. As is evident in figure 8.16, this change in paradigm brought the results closer in line to those of Tombu and Tsotsos, and again, the basic suppressive result for nearby orientations is observed. The denser sampling along the orientation dimension better reveals the structure of the response.

Finally, in the third experiment (experiment 3), we wondered if the same feature suppression would be seen in color space. The experimental procedure was exactly

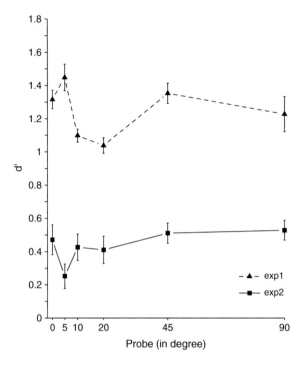

Figure 8.16
The subjects' median d′ (d′ is a measure of the distance between the signal and the signal+noise—see Macmillan and Creelman 2005 for further details) under different orientation probe conditions in experiments 1 and 2. The dotted line represents the results of experiment 1 and the solid line the results of experiment 2. The error bars represent 1 standard deviation error.

the same as in the second experiment. However, this time the color but not orientation of the cues and the probes was manipulated. The 180 kinds of color of the cues and probes were determined in the following way: The saturation and value of all the 180 colors were the same, but the hue of the 180 colors was given by equally dividing the HSV (hue, saturation, value) color wheel into 180 units. The pre-cues could be any of the 180 colors randomized on a trial-by-trial basis. The probes were the same color as the cues for 66% of the trials. For the rest of the trials, the probe's hue could be 5, 10, 20, 45, or 90 units different from the cues. A typical trial is shown in figure 8.17.

Figure 8.18 represents the subjects' median sensitivity, d′, under different probe conditions. The suppression occurred when the probes' color hue was about 20 units different from the attended color's hue. Figure 8.19 shows the raw values for each subject. Although each subject shows a pattern of suppressed response for nearby probes, the exact position of the minimum point and the extent of suppression vary by subject. This is perhaps the reason for the uneven characterization of the

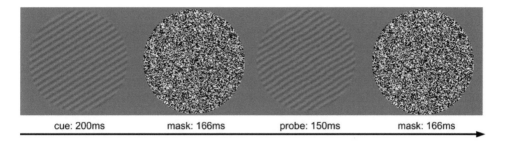

Figure 8.17
Colored, striped circular disks were used, and they are similar to the stimuli used in experiments 1 and 2 (color not shown). But this time the stripes of the disks are of alternating color and dark gray on a medium gray background. Also, as orientation is not our concern any more, all disks are oriented at 70° at this time. The current experiment could be regarded as a color version of experiment 2.

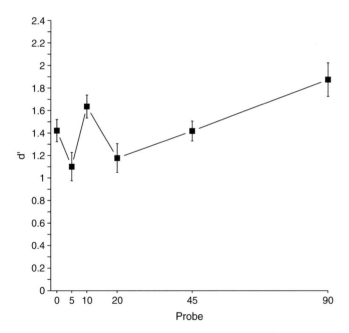

Figure 8.18
The subjects' median d′ under different color probe conditions in experiment 3.

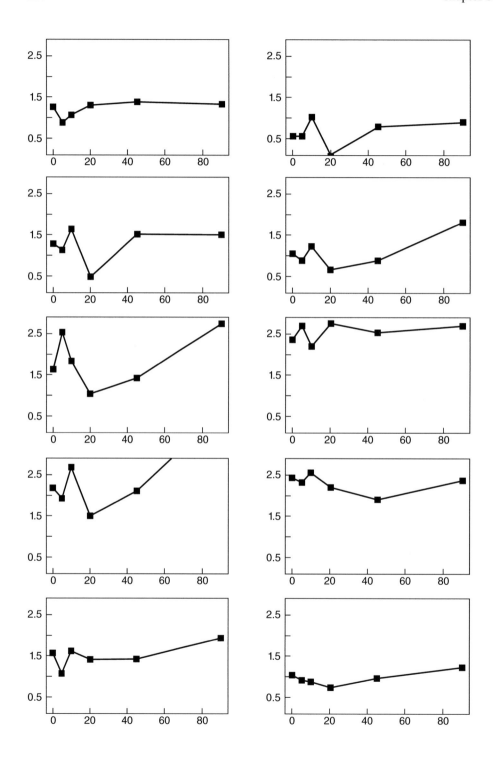

aggregate measure of the previous figure. In summary, we successfully expanded our finding of nearby inhibition from the orientation domain to the color domain.

Hopf, J.-M., Boehler, C.N., Luck, S.J., Tsotsos, J.K., Heinze, H.-J., Schoenfeld, M.A. (2006). Direct neurophysiological evidence for spatial suppression surrounding the focus of attention in vision. *Proceedings of the National Academy of Sciences USA* 103 (4), pp. 1053–1058.

The spatial focus of attention has traditionally been envisioned as a simple spatial gradient, where the attended stimulus is enhanced and that enhancement decays monotonically with distance. Using high-density magneto-encephalographic recordings of human observers, we show that the focus of attention is not a simple monotonic gradient but instead contains an excitatory peak surrounded by an inhibitory region. To demonstrate this center-surround profile, we asked subjects to focus attention onto a color pop-out target and then presented probe stimuli at various distances from the target. This is shown in figure 8.20 (color figure 8.20W). We observed that the electromagnetic response to the probe was enhanced when the probe was presented at the location of the target, but the probe response was suppressed in a zone surrounding the target and then recovered farther away (see

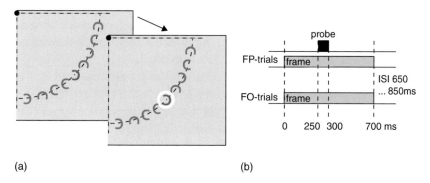

(a)   (b)

Figure 8.20 (color figure 8.20W)
Illustration of the search frame and the timing of the probe presentation. (a) Nine randomly oriented *C*s were presented at an iso-eccentric distance from fixation (black dot with two black dashed lines at the top left) in the lower right visual field. The target item, a red *C*, appeared randomly at one of the nine locations (here at the center position), and observers had to discriminate its gap position (left, right). (b) On 50% of the trials, a probe stimulus (white circle) was flashed (duration 50 milliseconds) around the center position 250 milliseconds after search frame onset. These are the FP (frame plus probe) trials whereas the FO (frame only) trials are those without the probe. (From Hopf et al., 2006; ©2006 National Academy of Sciences, USA)

◀ **Figure 8.19**
Individual d′ values for the 10 subjects, whose median value is plotted in figure 8.18. d′ is plotted against the different probe conditions, as in the previous figure. Although each subject shows a pattern of suppressed response for nearby probes, the exact position of the minimum point and the extent of suppression varies by subject. This is perhaps the reason for the uneven characterization of the aggregate measure of the previous figure.

figure 8.21; color figure 8.21W). When we removed attention from the pop-out target by engaging observers in a demanding foveal task, this pattern was not seen, confirming a truly attention-driven effect. These results indicate that neural enhancement and suppression coexist in a spatially structured manner that is optimal to attenuate the most deleterious noise during visual object identification.

Boehler, C.N., Tsotsos, J.K., Schoenfeld, M., Heinze, H.-J., Hopf, J.-M. (2009). The center-surround profile of the focus of attention arises from recurrent processing in visual cortex. *Cerebral Cortex* 19, pp. 982–991.

The attentive suppressive surround of ST is the result of the Full Recurrence Binding process described in chapter 6. Although there is substantial behavioral evidence for it, there was no neurophysiology to support the recurrent aspect of the prediction. In this set of experiments, we pursued this point. Two experiments based on the experimental paradigm of Hopf et al. (2006) showed that surround suppression appears in search tasks that require spatial scrutiny (experiment 1); that is, the precise binding of search-relevant features at the target's location but not in tasks that permit target discrimination without precise localization (experiment 2). Furthermore, they demonstrate that surround attenuation is linked with a stronger recurrent activity modulation in early visual cortex. Finally, we observed that surround suppression appears with a delay of more than 175 milliseconds; that is, at a time beyond the time course of the initial feed-forward pass in the visual system. These observations together indicate that the suppressive surround is associated with recurrent processing and binding in the visual cortex.

Figure 8.21 gives the experimental setup and details the experiment, and figures 8.22, 8.23, and 8.24 show the evidence supporting the conclusions. In experiment 1, subjects were asked, while fixating, to search for a luminance pop-out target (the letter *C*) among nine items presented at an iso-eccentric distance in the right lower visual quadrant. In 50% of the trials, a white probe ring was presented at the center position with varying delay relative to search frame onset. The frame-probe SOA (stimulus onset asynchrony) was varied in five steps of 75 milliseconds beginning with an SOA of 100 milliseconds. On each trial, the target appeared randomly at any of nine item positions, providing five attention-to-probe distances: attention at probe (PD0) and attention 1–4 items away from the probe toward the horizontal or the vertical meridian (PD1–PD4). Figure 8.23 shows the responses to the probe for each SOA. There is a clear collapse of response at position PD1 for SOA of 250 and 325 milliseconds, not before and not beyond. In experiment 2, subjects searched for a color pop-out (red or green *C* among blue distractor *C*s) and were asked to either discriminate the color (the color task) or the orientation of the letter *C* as the pop-out target (the orientation task). The probe appeared on 50% of the trials as in experiment 1 but with a fixed frame-probe SOA of 250 milliseconds. Items

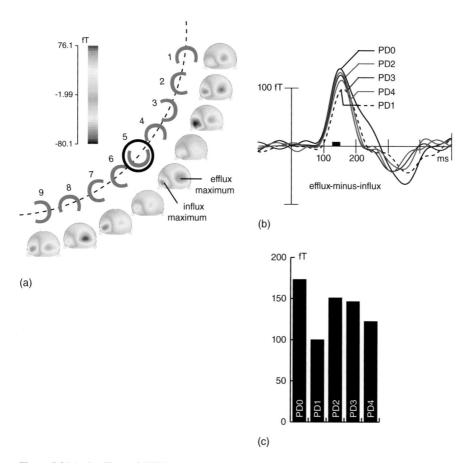

Figure 8.21 (color Figure 8.21W)
Event-related magnetic field (ERMF) distribution and time course of the probe-related response.
(a) Mean ERMF distribution of the probe-related response (FP minus FO difference from 130 to 150 milliseconds, averaged across observers) for all probe-distance conditions. Attending to the *C* next to the probe (positions 4 and 6) reveals a reduced response magnitude in comparison with both the at-probe position (5) as well as the positions farther away from the probe (1–3, 7–9). (b) Time course of the probe-related ERMF response (FP minus FO) for each probe distance collapsed across corresponding conditions toward the horizontal and vertical meridian (4 and 6, 3 and 7, etc.). Shown is the time course of the ERMF difference between corresponding efflux- and influx-field maxima (efflux minus influx; see panel a). (c) Mean size of the probe-related response between 130 and 150 milliseconds, collapsed across corresponding probe-distance conditions. The size of the effect represents the average of the ERMF difference between the observers' individual field maxima and minima. (From Hopf et al., 2006; ©2006 National Academy of Sciences, USA)

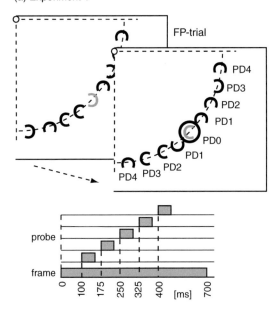

(a) Experiment 1

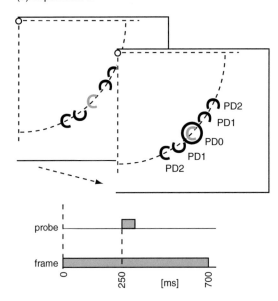

(b) Experiment 2

Figure 8.22
(a) Stimulus setup and presentation sequence of experiment 1. The target is a luminance pop-out target (shown as a gray *C*) among nine items presented at an iso-eccentric distance (8° of visual angle) in the right lower visual quadrant. In 50% of the trials, a white ring (the probe; black in this figure) was presented at the center position with varying delay relative to search frame onset as shown in the lower part the figure. (b) Stimulus setup and presentation sequence of experiment 2. Subjects searched for a color pop-out (red or green *C* among blue distractor *C*s) and were required to discriminate either the color (color task) or the gap orientation of the pop-out target (orientation task). The probe appeared with a fixed frame-probe SOA of 250 milliseconds. (From Boehler et al., 2009, by permission of Oxford University Press)

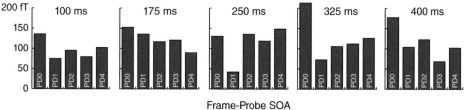

Figure 8.23
ERMF results of experiment 1. Size of the probe-related response for the five different frame-probe SOAs. Each bar graph shows the size of the response at probe distances PD0–PD4. The responses at the same probe distances toward the vertical and horizontal meridian were collapsed. (From Boehler et al., 2009, by permission of Oxford University Press)

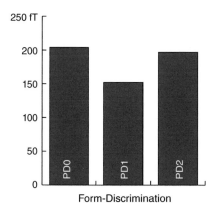

(a)

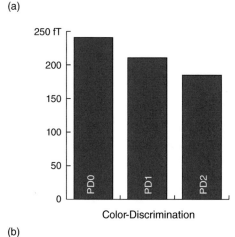

(b)

Figure 8.24
ERMF results of experiment 2. (a) Size of the probe-related response at probe distances PD0–PD2 of the orientation task. Responses at the same PDs toward the vertical and horizontal meridian are collapsed. (b) Size of the probe-related response at probe distances PD0–PD2 of the color task. (From Boehler et al., 2009, by permission of Oxford University Press)

were not presented at positions PD3 and PD4 in this experiment in order to maximize the number of trials per condition. The results of this are shown in figure 8.24. There is no apparent effect for the color task but a clear drop at position PD1 for the orientation task. Finally, a cortical surface-constrained current source analysis of the event-related magnetic field (ERMF) response is given in figure 8.25 for these two tasks. They are easily seen to be different with a major response peak in the early visual cortex area for the orientation task in the time interval, approximately 190–275 milliseconds. Most important, the maximum response in that time interval appeared at approximately the same location in early visual cortex as the maximum of the initial feed-forward response, suggesting recurrent activity.

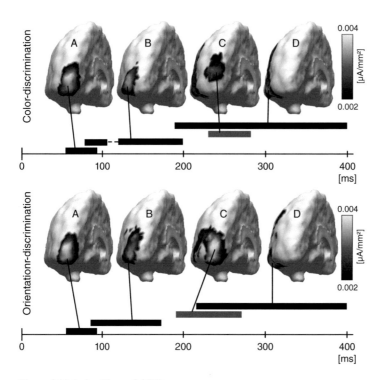

Figure 8.25 (color Figure 8.25W)
Cortical surface-constrained current source analysis of the ERMF response elicited by search frames (no-probe trials only) of the orientation and color discrimination tasks in experiment 2. Estimates were computed in a time range between 0 and 400 milliseconds after search frame onset. (A–D) A sequence of four different distributional patterns was observed, shown here at the time point of their current density maximum. The temporal extension of those distributions is indicated by the horizontal bars below. Whereas (A) the initial feed-forward response in early visual cortex around 75 milliseconds as well as (B) the subsequent extrastriate activity did not differ between the color and the orientation tasks, (C) the following maximum in early visual cortex was substantially larger in the orientation task than in the color task. Notably, for both experimental tasks, the maximum in (C) appeared at approximately the same location in early visual cortex as the maximum of the initial feed-forward response (A), suggesting (C) to represent recurrent activity. (From Boehler et al., 2009, by permission of Oxford University Press)

The results of the two experiments converge on the conclusion that the Mexican hat profile of the focus of attention in visual search is a direct consequence of recurrent processing in the visual system. This notion is suggested by (1) the time course analysis showing that the temporal onset of surround attenuation is significantly beyond the initial feed-forward sweep of processing through the visual hierarchy and (2) the observation that surround attenuation does not appear when target identification can be achieved without recurrence binding. Further, figure 8.25 clearly indicates that there is strong feedback to early visual areas in the raw response for the gap discrimination task compared with the color task. These observations are in line with predictions of ST according to which the suppressive surround arises from a top-down propagating WTA process that prunes away feed-forward connections from distractor locations not contributing to the search target. Finally, because this pruning operation attenuates competitive influences from distractor units in the surround, it should cause a subsequent relative enhancement of units in the attended pass zone as ST predicts.

Summary

The above are not the full extent of what Selective Tuning has to say about vision and visual attention. For example, in Tsotsos et al. (1995), an explanation of the results in Moran and Desimone (1985) was presented, and in Tsotsos et al. (2001), an explanation of Motter (1993) was given. The Motter demonstration highlighted the fact that the inhibitory process within ST can lead to both enhancement and suppression of neural responses. It was also evident that the suppressive surround concept applies not only to locations in the input stimulus but also to each corresponding location throughout the visual processing hierarchy. Thus, attentional modulation suppresses irrelevant spatial locations within a receptive field at all levels of processing (Tsotsos, 1990a, 1999, Tsotsos, Culhane and Cutzu 2001). This means that attentional modulation has a nontrivial physical structure within the processing network.

In the previous paragraph, the word 'explanation' was used rather than 'prediction.' This is because the experimental observations had appeared prior to the explanation. The word 'prediction' as used in this chapter applies only to statements that precede experimental observation.

The main conclusion for this chapter is that there is a great deal of experimental support for Selective Tuning. The support comes from the breadth of explanation ST provides for the many elements of attention and existing experimental data. Support also comes from the significant body of new experimental observations that followed ST's published predictions. This breadth and depth of verification is an important aspect of the scientific method.

9 Wrapping Up the Loose Ends

Eight chapters beyond those classic words regarding attention, *we all know what it is*, we can perhaps hope to be closer to knowing. And if we are not close enough, perhaps ideas for the next few steps appeared in the preceding pages. The theory underlying the Selective Tuning model presents a means of overcoming the computational complexity issues inherent in vision and proposes a unifying view of attention, recognition, and binding. The model itself provides explanations for a broad set of attentional observations, perhaps broader than any other model. It also shows interesting performance in a wide variety of attentional tasks and has made (and makes) many predictions regarding attentional function that have now been strongly supported over the course of 20 years of experimental work.

Chapter 1 introduced attention from the historical and primarily biological point of view and included some of the main findings and general statements about attention. The chapter then moved on to make a connection between biology and computation with the goal of providing a very general definition of attention that applies to both biological and computational systems.

Chapter 2 introduces computational complexity, provides computational foundations, and dives into extensions such as active vision and visual search. The set of theorems and proofs contribute to a sound theoretical foundation for vision science and specifically for visual attention. The basic problem of Visual Match was claimed to be a ubiquitous building block of any vision system. It was proved that in a pure feed-forward version, Visual Match is computationally intractable, whereas a task-directed version of it has linear complexity. A number of theorems building on these two results were presented. Attempting to deal with this intractability led to several constraints on the architecture of a vision system. While solving some of the complexity issues, the constraints in turn led to a number of additional representational problems. These were identified and defined, setting up the next chapters that begin to suggest solutions. The chapter concluded with a definition of attention that was more specific than that in the previous chapter as a result of the computational theory that was laid out. That definition is repeated here:

Attention is a set of mechanisms that help tune and control the search processes inherent in perception and cognition.

The main point by far is that the brain cannot be solving the most general statement of the vision problem and that it necessarily is solving some approximation to it. Unfortunately, formal characterization of this altered problem is not easy. It is, however, possible to say something about the difference between instances of visual problems that can be solved at a glance and those that cannot. Instances of Visual Match that can be solved using only a single feed-forward pass through the visual processing machinery of the brain are those that correspond with the 'at a glance' problems (call this set of problems the AG set). This implies that any visual quantities that require computation are available at the end of that pass—or within 150 milliseconds or so of stimulus onset [consistent with the Marr (1982) theory, with Bullier (2001), Lamme and Roelfsema (2000), and with Thorpe et al. (1996), among many others]. The only action required is to select from those quantities the subset that may satisfy the task at hand and to verify that they in fact do satisfy the task. It is implied by the time course that the selection is clear (in the Marr sense); that is, there are no other potential subsets that may compete for task satisfaction, so the first selected is the correct one. It is important to note that the vast majority of modern computer vision limits consideration to exactly this scenario (see, e.g., Dickinson, Leonardis, Schiele, & Tarr, 2009).

There are many vision tasks that fall outside the above limitation; we may call them the 'more than a glance' (MG) problems. The way to specify them can be guided by the shortcomings of the overall strategy described in the previous paragraph. A partial specification would include scenes where selection is not immediately clear. Such scenes may contain more than one copy of a given feature each at different locations, contain more than one object/event each at different locations, or contain objects/events that are composed of multiple features and share at least one feature type. It is not sufficient to characterize only the image: one must also consider the task. MG problems would include those tasks where simple detection or naming of a single item in a scene do not suffice. For exampling, tracking objects in time-varying scenes requires more than a glance. The questions Yarbus asked subjects about image contents require more than a glance (Yarbus, 1967). Non-pop-out visual search requires more than a glance (Treisman & Gelade, 1980; Wolfe, 1998a). Tasks where a behavior is required such as an eye movement or a manipulation require more than a glance. From Macmillan and Creelman (2005), it is clear to see that all N-interval scenarios with $N \geq 2$ are MG; even some one-interval problems are MG if localization is required for a subject's response. There are many more, and it is not too much of a stretch to suggest that the majority of vision tasks we face in our everyday lives are not of the single-glance variety. It is for all of these that dynamic tuning is needed.

In chapter 3, the body of past work on visual attention is the star, both from computational and biological viewpoints. A particular decomposition of the elements of attention, how they are related (within a specific taxonomy), and how the differing approaches to the problem are related (again within a taxonomy of approaches) are presented. The goal is to begin to organize the diversity and enormity of the literature and ideas. The particular decomposition and organization is just a beginning; it is likely to be refined and enhanced with time and understanding. The key is that the process of organization has started. Overall, a complete (as much as possible) review of the main models of visual attention and their general features is presented. Chapter 3 also presents a set of three main classes of attentional processing mechanisms: Selection, Restriction, and Suppression, and their subtypes. Also, the four major modeling hypotheses—Selective Routing, Saliency Map, Emergent Attention, Temporal Tagging—are described and are diagrammed in such a way as to highlight research gaps that might be fruitful research directions.

Chapter 4 begins the main thrust of the book, namely the description of the Selective Tuning model. The basic algorithms and concepts that underpin the model are included with some brief comparisons with other models. The algorithms may be considered to be the precursor to a complete executive controller for attention.

The details of the ST model appear in chapter 5. The basic equations that govern the model's performance (within the algorithms of chapter 4) are derived and some important properties proved theoretically. The chapter also includes a detailed comparison of the mathematical formulations of five other major models against ST.

Chapter 6 proposes that attention, binding, and recognition are intimately connected and provides definitions for recognition and binding processes to join the definition of attention, attempting to reconcile a conflicting literature. Importantly, none of the terms *attention*, *recognition*, or *binding* are monoliths; each has subelements decomposing them into specific, better-defined concepts. They are thus more amenable to further study and analysis. A set of four novel binding processes— Convergence Binding, Partial Recurrence Binding, Full Recurrence Binding, and Iterative Recurrence Binding (two types)—are proposed that act to supplement basic recognition (feed-forward processing) using the glue of attentional mechanisms. For the AG problems, Convergence Binding suffices; the MG problems require one of the forms of Recurrence Binding.

The focus of chapter 7 is to give many examples of ST's performance for different tasks. The reader is encouraged to look at the accompanying Web pages for the color and animated versions of the figures. Although the examples provide convincing evidence, they are far from complete, and much further work is needed. The main outstanding task is to test the full model as described in figure 4.2. Secondary issues include procedures for setting of parameter values and quantitative performance evaluation on larger sets of stimuli.

Finally, chapter 8 offers some explanations and predictions of the ST tuning model. The breadth of explanations for the main elements of visual attention laid out in chapter 3 is evident. A set of 10 major model predictions—true predictions stated before any experimental observations existed—are detailed with pointers to subsequent supporting works. The chapter concludes with a set of summaries of the various experiments performed in our lab to test some of the predictions. The case seems quite strong in ST's favor.

But even after all this detail, a good deal remains unaddressed. It is easy to enumerate the many important issues that were not addressed, and this is where the next section begins.

The Loose Ends

Although it should be evident that the Selective Tuning model covers a great many elements of attention to some degree, it certainly does not cover all of them, and it remains a challenge for any theory to do so. In this section, a number of missing elements will be highlighted.

Task Memory, Priming, and Decision Making

Priming has been included as one of the major elements of attention, and it is clear how it has played an important role in experiments. In models, it is included mostly as a simple prior bias on early processing. Questions about how the priming signals are derived from instructions, where those task details are stored, and how they are used to determine that a task is complete are certainly outside the scope of ST at the moment and similarly in most other models.

What Is Extracted and Remembered in a Fixation?

This refers to **working memory** and how it is populated. Working memory is believed to store information that supports the processing of current tasks. But what exactly is stored there? What is the time course or sequence of events that accompany this? After a visual stimulus is attended, what is extracted and placed into working memory? Is working memory location-specific or is it location-independent? Is there any side-effect to the act of fixating and extracting? ST makes no statement on any of these questions. Raymond et al. (1992) discovered an attentional blink—probes are poorly detected if presented in the time interval following a target of 180–450 milliseconds. In other words, as a result of attending to a target, there is an interference produced for a second item—a side-effect of attention. ST's process of recurrent localization and necessary subsequent IOR may be relevant to this even though it has not been fully explored at this time. Change blindness (Rensink, O'Regan, & Clark, 1997) is a well-known example of where there is a manipulation of what is extracted and remembered by a single fixation. Certainly ST is silent on how it might explain change blindness. Ester, Serences, and Awh (2009) performed human imaging experiments to test the location specificity of working memory and concluded that visual details are held in working memory as a result of a spatially global recruitment from early sensory cortex. This does not address the process by which this might occur but points to interesting avenues for future modeling efforts.

Learning to Attend

Is attention learned or is it innate? Can the ability to attend be improved with specific training? The nature versus nurture debate will not be solved here. However, given the importance of a developmental side to a theory of attention, these are good questions. There is no component of ST that deals with learning; however, the addition of a simple learning strategy is not difficult. There are a variety of parameters described in chapter 5 that could be dynamically modified with experience and thus demonstrate adaptive behavior. Both modeling and experimental work exists to inform such future ST enhancements. The section "Other Relevant Ideas" of chapter 3 provided several pointers to past work on this, and more are given here. Weber and Triesch (2006) look at saccade learning and develop models to test whether a reward that takes advantage of the foveal magnification might guide the adaptation of saccades. Triesch, Teuscher, Deak, and Carlson (2006) also developed a model based on the idea that infants learn that monitoring their caregiver's direction of gaze allows them to predict the locations of interesting objects or events in their environment. Amit and Geman (1998) learn to determine what input patterns are salient. Della Libera and Chelazzi (2009) use an experimental approach involving rewards. Using variable monetary rewards as feedback on performance, they tested whether acts of attentional selection and the resulting after-effects can be modulated by their consequences. They found that what is learned regarding selecting or ignoring particular visual objects is strongly biased by the circumstances of rewards during previous attentional interactions with those objects.

Mozer et al. (1992) looked at a closely related issue, how does a system learn to bind visual features. Their system MAGIC (mentioned in chapter 3) learns how to group features, discovering grouping heuristics from a set of presegmented examples. They use a relaxation network to bind related features dynamically. Binding is represented by phase-locking relationships among features. The overall scheme is a generalization of back-propagation learning.

What Is the Neural Locus for the Elements of Figure 4.2?

Rather little has been included in the description of ST regarding the neural locus of any of its components with the following exceptions: the Fixation History Map may be linked with the frontal eye fields, and the Peripheral Priority Map may be linked with the parieto-occipital area PO. In addition, the specific implementation on which examples were developed did use visual areas V1, V4, IT, MT, MST, and 7a, but this is rather common in such models. In contrast, other models are quite specific regarding neural loci. Shipp (2004) develops his model by piecing together the brain areas that have shown some involvement in attentional activity. Knudsen (2007) takes a more functional approach than Shipp, providing a flow diagram of what he believes to be the elements of attention. He also provides a flow diagram of how the visual areas are connected and how they communicate to accomplish the required attentional tasks. These are examples of how a theory may develop using the data as starting point, whereas ST was developed beginning with the desire to quantify the capacity question computationally. ST is less specific on neural loci, and Shipp, Knudsen, and others are less specific on mechanisms and computational details. At this point, both are viable and important approaches. To hazard a speculation, the time when they converge onto the correct model is not likely too far in the future.

Eye Movements

Although the third algorithm of chapter 4 suggests a method for how ST deals with overt attention, it is far from an adequate model of eye movements in general. The kinds of eye movements are many including saccades, torsion, vergence and version, and smooth pursuit. Some of our past work has considered a variety of these (Jenkin & Tsotsos, 1994; Jenkin, Tsotsos, & Dudek, 1994; Milios et al., 1993), but that work was just a beginning. It is easy to appreciate that, in general, these are beyond the scope of ST. Many have studied the oculomotor system. The edited volume of Carpenter (1991) provides a superb collection of papers dealing with many if not all aspects of this. More recent surveys are those by Schall and Thompson (1999) and Sommer and Wurtz (2004a,b). Detailed models of several aspects of the oculomotor system are many, and only a few examples follow. Corbetta et al. (1998) provide detailed discussion of the kinds of networks in frontoparietal cortex that might be involved directing attention and eye movements. Zelinsky, Rao, Hayhoe, and Ballard (1997), Rao, Zelinsky, Hayhoe, and Ballard (2002), and Pomplun, Shen, and Reingold (2003) describe models of saccadic movements in visual search. The issue of integration across scenes obtained by each saccade is addressed by Prime, Tsotsos, Keith, and Crawford (2007). Hayhoe and Ballard (2005) look at the role of eye movements when performing natural visuomotor tasks. Then there is a different scale of consideration as well. Hafed and Clark (2002) suggest microsaccades—rapid eye movements that reorient gaze but are so small that they do not cause the foveation of new visual targets—occur because of subliminal activation of the oculomotor system by covert attention. Moore and Fallah (2001) showed that spatial attention can be enhanced by altering oculomotor signals within the brain. Monkeys performed a spatial attention task while neurons within the frontal eye field were electrically stimulated below the level at which eye movements are evoked. The monkey's performance improved with microstimulation only when the object to be attended was positioned in the space represented by the cortical stimulation site. Jie and Clark (2005) studied microsaccades during pursuit eye movements and show that covert attention leads pursuit movements. Certainly, there is much here to inspire future developments of ST.

How Is High Spatial Resolution Information Communicated?

The need for an attentional mechanism that enables access to high spatial resolution data within the visual cortex has played an important role in the development of ST. But at this point, ST does not provide a mechanism for that data to be communicated to the other brain areas that may require it to further their processing. Can we speculate about what such a mechanism might be? The most important requirement perhaps is that whatever the mechanism, there must be appropriate neural connectivity to provide a conduit for that access. This means that for whichever visual area attention localizes a stimulus, there must be connections to other brain areas. This is not a feasible requirement as it stands; it was shown in Tsotsos (1990a) that such complete connectivity is not possible. Some other less 'brute force' solution is needed.

The next requirement is that the brain areas involved be those found experimentally to be involved in a wide variety of attentional tasks. The thalamus—and its several components, the LGN, the pulvinar, thalamic nuclei—has long been implicated in attention. Singer (1977) proposed that top-down connections between cortex and thalamus played a role in regulating thalamic processes. Crick (1984) was an early proponent focusing on the role of the reticular nuclei, but more recently, many including Shipp (2003), Sillito, Cudiero, and Jones (2006), Cudiero and Sillito (2006), Weng, Jones, Andolina, Salt, and Sillito (2006), McAlonan, Cavanaugh, and Wurtz (2008), Mayo (2008), and Kastner, Saalmann, and Schneider (2011) have all discussed the role of thalamus in attention. The thalamus has been called the guardian, gatekeeper, switchboard, integrator, or coordinator of attention and assigned the roles of controller and regulator of transmission. The LGN, pulvinar, and thalamic nuclei have all been implicated in one way or another, and the cited authors do a good job of detailing the experimental evidence. These functions are described using colorful but not too specific metaphors and remain mostly undefined. But perhaps the two stated requirements, plus these metaphors, can point to a potential extension of Selective Tuning for this problem.

Suppose that the thalamic areas, specifically the pulvinar, did not 'control' attention. After all, what does it mean to control? The experimental evidence does not point to control or any other particular mechanism. The control aspect is the interpretation that various authors have proposed as explanation. This is not to say that the sum of those metaphors is not useful, far from it. But they must be defined in a different manner. Here, it is proposed that the pulvinar acts as a *blackboard* (another colorful metaphor!) but with specific characteristics. An early AI system, the HEARSAY-II system for speech understanding (Erman et al., 1980) mentioned in chapter 1, pioneered such a representational structure. A blackboard is a representation that can be written by some set of processes and read by some set of processes. For a neural network, one could imagine that some set of neural areas provide afferents for that representation, and for some other set of neural areas the resulting representation provides afferents. The function is similar to one's intuitive notion of a blackboard—someone writes on it, anyone can read it, and the information stays as it was written unless someone erases or alters it. In particular, a blackboard does not alter the information written on it, and here this means we do not assume any processing by the pulvinar at all.

What kind of information should the blackboard encode? Really, the right question is what information would other visual areas need from earlier (or perhaps even later) ones in the hierarchy? Likely, neural selectivity is important, coded for each location. In other words, a retinotopic representation that can code neural type is needed. This would provide the 'what' and 'where' for the visual features in a scene [note how different these uses of the terms 'what' and 'where' are from those of Ungerleider and Mishkin (1982)]. The inferior and lateral part of the pulvinar have clearly organized retinotopic maps and are reciprocally connected with at least cortical areas V1, V2, V4, and MT [Kastner et al. (2011) provide an excellent review of the data]. All that remains is for these retinotopic areas to code neuron selectivity, and there currently appears to be no evidence for such a coding. It would be interesting to examine this prediction of the blackboard structure.

Next, we must think about how information about a selected subset of neurons can be routed to the blackboard. Imagine a mechanism—related to but different than shifter circuits (Anderson & Van Essen, 1987)—that acts as a switch (the switchboard metaphor used earlier is relevant; Guillery, Feig, & Lozsádi, 1998). This would be a mechanism that permits signals from a subset of many sources to be transmitted over a single channel. The selection is the easy part; the attentional mechanism of ST does that for each representational layer. How many connections are needed? It is a reasonable assumption that spatial resolution cannot be more precise than the size of the receptive field of the neuron in question. So for example, if human area V1 has about 2100 columns on average (Stensaas et al., 1974), and all the neurons in each column have roughly the same receptive field, then location can be coded by 2100 connections in a binary fashion—lack of signal means an unselected location. Each of the other higher visual areas would have no more than this number. This would not yield an unmanageable number of connections. They would require registration onto the retinotopic blackboard of course; but the wiring pattern would seem to be sufficient in the same manner that it is for the retinal registration in LGN for binocular vision. To read this representation, no more than this number of outgoing connections would be needed to cover the available location specificity.

Do all the areas need to read the blackboard? Clearly, if the point is to allow access to the attended representations, then the higher-order layers seem to have a greater need, whereas the early layers have less use for the higher-order information because they are indirect recipients of it through the recurrent tracing functionality of ST's attentive mechanism.

When ST's attentional beam selects a stimulus, the act of selection (winning the competition) could also activate the appropriate connection to the blackboard. What remains then is how to code for feature type. One might imagine all manner of schemes—phase, firing rates, and more—that may be decoded into a feature type. We will not further speculate on these because computationally, many may be made to work properly, but there is no evidence to inform the development one way or another.

Figure 9.1 is a caricature of this scheme. It shows a subset of the visual areas and a subset of their connections, abstracted from Felleman and Van Essen (1991), Shipp (2003), May (2006), and Orban (2008). Many areas and their connections are not included; the goal of this figure is to illustrate the nature of the blackboard function and not to be a complete depiction of areas and their connections. Further, the laminar structure of the pulvinar is not shown (see May, 2006). The connections to and from the pulvinar are of different types. The afferent connections result in writing to the blackboard, and they are depicted as terminating on this hypothetical blackboard. The efferent connections are shown beginning on the border of the blackboard to signify that the whole blackboard can be read. The lighter-gray connections identify those that are likely less important.

This proposal also is relevant for observed multisensory integration. Location and type information from other sensory modalities may also be registered here and 'seen' by the remaining kinds of sensory processes. A clear test of this proposal would be to see if there is pulvinar involvement in visual tasks that do not involve localization. Without localization, there is no recurrent process of attention and thus no selection within layers. Without recurrent selection, there is no writing on the blackboard. More specifically, no involvement of the pulvinar is expected for tasks

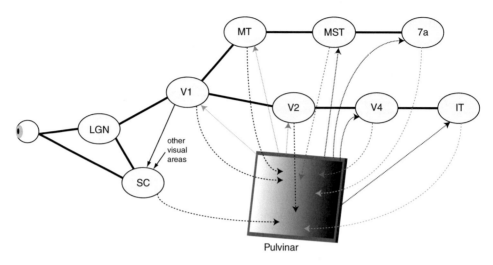

Figure 9.1
The pulvinar as a *blackboard*, magnified in this pulvinar-centered depiction to show its blackboard nature. Dotted lines are 'read' connections; dashed lines are 'write' connections. Lines between the main visual areas represent both feed-forward and recurrent neural connectivity. Their shading reflects the importance of the function as detailed in the text. Pulvinar shading highlights connection visibility only.

where Convergence Binding suffices. This is not to say the pulvinar may not be involved in other functions; just that this particular function will be absent without attention.

Among all the previous proposals for the function of the pulvinar, the current one seems closest to that of Shipp (2003). There, he writes that cortico-pulvinar-cortico circuits tend to mirror direct local cortical connections between areas, and he terms this the **replication principle**. He continues to suggest that the pulvinar replicates the pattern of cortical circuitry but not its function, acting to coordinate cortical information processing by facilitating and sustaining the formation of synchronized trans-areal assemblies. We do not require this synchronization function; it may be a side-effect of the overall process, but ST has no mechanism that imposes or detects synchronization. The replication is part of our proposal but for a very different purpose; perhaps a marriage of Shipp's replication principle and Guillery and colleagues' (1998) switchboard function is a more reasonable comparison.

This blackboard idea has surfaced before in exactly this context. Mumford (1991) suggested that each area of the cortex carries on its processing with the active participation of a thalamic nucleus with which it is reciprocally and topographically connected. Each cortical area is responsible for maintaining and updating knowledge of a specific aspect of the world, ranging from low-level raw data to high-level abstract representations. Multiple sources of expertise and potentially conflicting hypotheses are integrated by the thalamic neurons and then sent back. He proposed that this part of the thalamus plays the role of an 'active blackboard' on which the current best reconstruction of some aspect of the world is always displayed. The function then is a 'data fusion' one with the thalamus performing substantial computation. Although sounding similar to the proposal here, the differences are important. The main difference is the fact that for Mumford the thalamus is 'active,' integrating information into a reconstruction of the visual world, where in ST the pulvinar (not the full thalamus) is used in a 'passive' manner. ST has the specific requirement of relaying higher-resolution visual information to other visual areas, and for this, 'passive' suffices. Similar to Mumford, connectivity needs to be topographically registered and reciprocal; however, the directionality has a definite gradient of importance. Writing on to the blackboard is more important for the earlier areas, whereas reading from it is more important for the later areas. Distinctly different from Mumford, there is no reconstruction assumed by ST; this is a concept he borrowed from Marr (1982), and here it is rejected implicitly for the early visual areas because of the complexity arguments in chapter 2. To represent a full reconstruction and categorized version of the visual world—like Marr's 3D model—even for a static fixation is implausible for even the full cortex. Mumford suggests this reconstruction is maintained and updated over time. This seems to be a massive task that certainly requires more than ST assumes for the pulvinar. In ST, the pulvinar is only responsible for the dynamic representation of attended information. Perhaps most important, the explicit connection to attentional selection and localization is the largest difference of all. Mumford suggests a possible attentional gating plus active blackboard role for the thalamus. In ST, attentional selection occurs elsewhere, and the pulvinar only provides a means for communicating those results. The contents of the pulvinar's representation are determined by current attentional selection only.

The information represented on the pulvinar can be used in the same way that any other representation is used. Elements of it can be considered inputs to the selectivity of a neuron. This would allow the early portion (in time) of the response of a higher-layer neuron to reflect the primary hierarchical response (V1 through to IT, for example) and the later portions of response to reflect the attended version through both the V1 to IT paths that ST would identify via recurrent localization and the additional details of the stimulus attended to and passed through the pulvinar.

Executive Control

It has already been stated that ST is rather weak with respect to executive control functions. Although there is enough to make the overall system function, this does not really address the right questions. Recent authors, including Yantis and Serences (2003), Corbetta and Shulman (2002), Posner and DiGirolamo (1998), and Yantis (1998), review the issues involved. Fuster (2008) nicely summarizes the three main functions of executive attention, which itself is one of the three main executive functions of prefrontal cortex (executive attention, planning, and decision making):

• Set: selection of motor actions and the supporting sensory and motor preparation.

• Working Memory: attention focused on an internal representation for a purposive action. The representation consists of recent sensory events and their context.

• Interference Control: the exclusion or suppression to protect behavioral structures from external or internal interference (such as distractors).

Fuster goes on to describe the complex overall structure of prefrontal executive actions, but this is clearly outside the scope of the current work. Nevertheless, some of Fuster's elements are indeed covered in Selective Tuning.

Where Do Those Attentional Signals Come From?

Throughout the presentation of the Selective Tuning model, a variety of top-down signals were used, but the neural source for them was never discussed. Szczepanski, Konen, and Kastner (2010) present evidence that topographic frontal and parietal cortex are possible attentional signal sources, and notably, the areas of one hemisphere affect processing in the contralateral visual field. Phillips and Segraves (2009) argue that the frontal eye fields exhibit cell activity whose timing during natural visual search suggests target selection for future saccades in search. That FEF participates in saccade selection is also argued for by Armstrong, Chang, and Moore (2009). However, they add that FEF also maintains spatial information in the absence of saccade preparation. FEF is also claimed to play a role in covert search. Monosov and Thompson (2009) present data to support this suggesting that spatial signals from FEF directly affect visual processing during stimulus selection. The lateral intraparietal area (LIP) is proposed by Mirpour, Arcizet, Ong, and Bisley (2009) to represent all the data needed to guide visual search and saccades. Still, more brain areas are argued to be involved in generating attentional signals. Lauritzen et al. (2009) point out that two regions within the intraparietal sulcus of posterior parietal cortex, IPS1 and IPS2, transmit signals to early visual cortex. They lead activity in comparison with early visual areas by several hundred milliseconds. The question that heads this section is an important one, and it is a challenge to ST to include a theoretical counterpart for these experimental conclusions.

Neural Details

Although the mathematics of neuron response in chapter 5 was specified, there are loose ends here, too. First of all, most parameter values are left unspecified, and the weights for most of the processes are not given (although clearly for the examples of chapter 7 they do have values; it is just that those values are not ones that would apply for all possible stimuli and tasks). This is a shortcoming that learning procedures may correct. Still, in such a complex network, learning procedures may not yet be able to find ways of dealing with the many layers of the network and the many different kinds of connections between them. A second loose end concerns the issue of timing. That is, there is no reason to think that all visual areas compute their results with the same delay, receive all information at the same time, and so on. The overall system seems highly asynchronous. The latency figures for the feed-forward pathways given in Bullier (2001) suffice to convince of this. Proper consideration of timing throughout the network is a source of constraint that has not been exploited. Finally, a thorough analysis of neural responses in direct comparison with experimental ones is needed. These issues require further study.

A different sort of loose end concerns the issue of neural connection type. There is no reason to think that all connections among neurons have the same meaning, the same semantics. To be sure, in chapter 5 different kinds of connections were shown, for bias, for lateral computation, for classic neural response, and for gating. There are likely more, and borrowing from Tsotsos (1980), we may make suggestions as to what these might be. In Tsotsos (1980), a network representation was presented for the interpretation of visual motion. Connections between motion category nodes in the network were of four types: generalization/specification, part/whole, competition/similarity, and temporal precedence. These connection types are illustrated in figure 9.2.

If the concept, B, that a neuron represents is a specialization of some other concept, A, then the relationship is as shown is figure 9.2a. Concept A could prime concept B, and concept B could activate concept A. If the concept is a component of another, then the example of figure 9.2b applies. The five neurons B, C, D, E, and F are all components of the concept that A represents. The parts contribute to the whole. In figure 9.2c, five neurons that are all related to each other are shown. If all are in competition, then the connection is inhibitory; if they are similar, then the connection is excitatory. Finally, if several concepts are ordered in time, figure 9.2d shows the connectivity. Concept B could prime concept C, and so on in time. Of course, these patterns may be combined. It is easy to imagine a network where some concept has components, but one of those components has options; that is, it may be one of a number of other concepts. All the parts could be ordered in time to

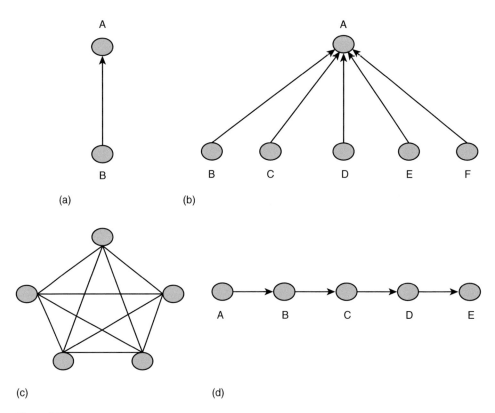

Figure 9.2
Connection types: (a) generalization/specialization; (b) part/whole; (c) competition/similarity; (d) temporal precedence. The connections depict semantic relationships.

represent some time-varying concept. The combinations are quite broad. Tsotsos (1980) made good use of these connection types, developing a network with several hundred concepts that represent the dynamics of human heart wall motion. The mathematics of relaxation labeling extended to time-varying events and with empirically defined compatibility functions for these representational connections rounded out the theory. Competition and cooperation are common concepts in neural modeling. These were not only representational constructs; they also served as pathways for specific kinds of search or decision-making. For example, in the Within-Category Identification task of chapter 6, following connections from a category (the 'whole') to the feature elements that comprise it (the 'parts') seems to be a sensible strategy for executing that task. Each node may be a component of several concepts (feed-forward neural divergence), and each concept receives a number of input components (feed-forward neural convergence). The generalization connectivity may permit categories and subcategories to be related. The interactions among connection types leads to even greater possibilities, and it remains for future research to determine whether or not these kinds of connection classes have value for real neural circuits.

Vision as Dynamic Tuning of a General-Purpose Processor

The importance of generality in computer vision systems whose goal is to achieve near-human performance was emphasized early in the field's development (Barrow & Tenenbaum, 1981; Zucker, Rosenfeld, & Davis, 1975). To be specific, Zucker et al. write:

How can computer vision systems be designed to handle unfamiliar or unexpected scenes? Many of the current systems cope quite well with limited visual worlds, by making use of specialized knowledge about these worlds. But if we want to expand these systems to handle a wide range of visual domains, it will not be enough to simply employ a large number of specialized models. It will also be important to make use of what might be called 'general-purpose models.'

With similar thinking, Barrow and Tenenbaum say:

Like relaxation, hierarchical synthesis is conceptually parallel, with plausible hypotheses emerging from a consensus of supporting evidence. When resources are finite (the extreme case being a conventional serial computer), control can be allocated among processes representing various levels of hypotheses in accordance with strength of support, goals, expectations, and so forth. In this way, data-driven and goal-driven operation can be integrated as suggested earlier . . . . the principles and techniques brought together in this paper represent a significant step beyond current special-purpose computer vision systems, towards systems approaching the generality and performance of human vision.

Yet this generality in practice has been elusive. Here, a proposal is made in this direction. Using formal methods from complexity theory, we have shown what an architecture for vision might be that has two main properties:

· It can solve a particular class of vision problems very quickly.

· It can be tuned dynamically to adapt its performance to the remaining subclasses of vision problems but at a cost of greater time to process.

Further, we have shown that a major contributor in this dynamic tuning process is the set of mechanisms that have come to be known as attention. Importantly, the data-driven processes of Barrow and Tenenbaum are the same as the feed-forward ones described herein, but goal-driven processing is not the only top-down mechanism. The top-down and recurrent mechanisms here include both goals as well as top-down attention mechanisms not specific to tasks or goals. This is a significant difference and one that seems to be missing from current computational vision works as well. The combined application of elements from the set of attentional mechanisms of chapter 2 provides for a means to tune the general-purpose, but limited in functionality, processing network to enable a far broader set of visual tasks to be solved albeit at the expense of greater processing time.

Final Words

After tens of thousands of words and dozens of figures and animations, theorems and proofs, and equations and algorithms, it would be very satisfying to be able to say we now know:

what attention is,

why the brain as well as computer systems need it,

how to construct a theory to formalize it, and

how to build mechanisms to embody that theory.

Maybe! But things are definitely not as bad as Sutherland had said—there is a bit of a glimmer in the center of that black hole! By providing structure to the elements of the field, by giving concrete definitions to many previously vague concepts, by adding a formal mathematical foundation to attention and vision, perhaps some small steps have been made in the right direction.

Three main conclusions have been drawn:

1. Attention is a set of mechanisms that tune and control the search processes inherent in perception and cognition, with the major types of mechanisms being Selection, Suppression, and Restriction.

2. Attention, recognition, and binding are neither monolithic nor separable concepts, each having many subelements interconnected in subtle ways in order to enable visual perception.

3. Vision as we know it seems to involve a general purpose processor that can be dynamically tuned to the task and input at hand. This general purpose processor can solve a class of visual perception problems (AG) very quickly but for more difficult problems time is the major cost factor, that is, those problems take longer to solve using that same general processor but tuned for specific subproblems that together solve the MG problems.

It is clear that in order for our understanding to increase, the language of computation must play a central role, even for studies that may be currently considered purely experimental. Whenever experimentalists attempt to provide an explanation for observed phenomena, they are using the language of computation, and the more precise, detailed, and computational an explanation is, the less it adds to the confusion we currently see. Similarly, the importance of experiment should not be ignored by theorists or modelers. Tying model development to existing knowledge and clearly stating a model's consequences as bases for future experimentation is the only way that theories evolve. There is room around the cycle of scientific discovery, shown in chapter 8, for all types of attention researchers. If nothing else, the exercise of completing this volume has shown that only through determined collaboration around the cycle will a comprehensive understanding of attention emerge.

Appendix A: A Few Notes on Some Relevant Aspects of Complexity Theory

What follows is a supplement to the very brief introduction to the theory of computational complexity given in chapter 2. Readers interested in more background on the theory of computational complexity, on NP-Completeness, and on related topics should consult Garey and Johnson (1979) or Papadimitriou (1994). The birth of this area may be traced back to the famous proof of Cook's theorem in 1971.

The set of problems P contains all decision problems that can be solved by a deterministic Turing Machine using a polynomial amount of computation time, (the "P" here simply stands for "polynomial"). The polynomial function is in terms of the size of the input. NP is the set of decision problems solvable in polynomial time by a nondeterministic Turing Machine. The "NP" stands for nondeterministic polynomial time. In other words, the problem can be solved in polynomial time by an oracle (the nondeterministic part). A nondeterministic Turing Machine may embody an algorithm where there might be more than one action for a given situation. It always picks the transition that eventually leads to a successful state, if there is such a transition, by guessing correctly (or asking an oracle for help!). In other words, a deterministic machine would have a single computation path rather than a computation tree. A nondeterministic Turing Machine would accept its input if any branch halts with an accept result.

A decision problem (defined in chapter 2) C is NP-Complete if:

C is in NP, and

Every problem in NP is reducible to C in polynomial time.

C can be shown to be in NP by demonstrating that a candidate solution to C can be verified in polynomial time.

A problem K is reducible to C if there is a polynomial-time reduction, a deterministic algorithm that transforms any instance $k \in K$ into an instance $c \in C$, such that the answer to c is yes if and only if the answer to k is yes. To prove that an NP problem C is indeed an NP-Complete problem, it suffices to show that a known NP-Complete problem reduces to C.

A problem satisfying the second condition is said to be NP-hard, whether or not it satisfies the first condition. NP-hard problems may be of any type: decision problems, search problems, or optimization problems. If an optimization problem has an NP-Complete decision version, then it is NP-hard.

If we had a polynomial time algorithm for C, we could solve all problems in NP in polynomial time. The class of NP problems includes as a proper subset the set of problems in P (assuming $P \neq NP$). The class of problems that are NP-hard has members that are in NP and others that are not in NP (but none in P). The ones in NP are known as the NP-Complete problems.

Although any particular solution can be verified quickly, there is no known efficient way to locate a solution in the first place; no fast solution to NP-Complete problems is currently known. As a result, the time required to solve even moderately large versions of many of these problems becomes enormous, as the example given in chapter 2 by Stockmeyer and Chandra demonstrates. As a result, determining whether or not it is possible to solve these problems is one of the major unsolved problems in computer science.

It is additionally important to note that such problems are not rare nor are they only of theoretical interest. When developing a computational model, theory, or solution, it is imperative that one be able to determine whether or not the nature of the solution proposed is equivalent to one of the known NP-Complete problems. If it is, it is potentially not a useful—nor realizable—solution. NP-Complete problems are often addressed by approximation algorithms or in limited form only; for the problem of interest, that would have to suffice. Even if one religiously follows Marr's three levels of analysis, for example, proposing a solution that is computationally intractable is a potentially useless exercise. For this reason, it was proposed that a fourth—complexity—level of analysis always accompany Marr's three levels (Tsotsos, 1987, 1988a, 1990a).

NP-Complete problems are studied because the ability to quickly verify solutions to a problem (NP) seems to correlate with the ability to quickly solve that problem (P). It is not known whether every problem in NP can be quickly solved. In other words, it is not known whether the set of problems in NP is the same as the set of problems in P (that can be solved in polynomial time). But if any single problem in NP-Complete can be solved quickly, then every problem in NP can also be quickly solved, because the definition of an NP-Complete problem states that every problem in NP must be quickly reducible to every problem in NP-Complete (i.e., it can be reduced in polynomial time). Because of this, it is often said that the NP-Complete problems are harder or more difficult than NP problems in general.

Parallelism does not necessarily help. A problem can be solved by an efficient parallel algorithm if inputs of size m can be solved using a parallel computer with $m^{O(1)}$ processors and in time $\log^{O(1)} m$. $O(1)$ as an exponent is equivalent to saying the exponent is some constant. NC is the name of the class of efficiently paralleliz-able problems. The theory of P-Completeness delineates which problems are likely to be in NC and which are not. Currently, it is not known if P = NC, but this is believed not to be the case. Problems such as integer multiplication and division, computing the product or matrices, determining rank or inverse of a matrix, and some graph theoretic algorithms such as shortest path and minimum spanning tree all have been shown to have fast parallel implementations. However, problems such as minimum matching and linear programming are not known to have any good parallel implementations, and current belief is that they do not have any. The inter-ested reader can consult Papadimitriou (1994).

Appendix B: Proofs of the Complexity of Visual Match

The following proofs were first presented at the International Conference on Artificial Intelligence, Detroit, August 20–25 1989, and appeared in those proceedings, pp. 1571–1577.

Preliminaries

Recall the description of the Visual Search algorithm in the section "The Computational Complexity of Vision" of chapter 2. This begins where that discussion left off. The main elements of the Visual Match problem are

A test image I

A goal image G, modified using a 2D spatial transformation

A difference function $diff(p)$ for $p \in I$, $diff(p) \in R_\rho^0$

A correlation function $corr(p)$ for $p \in I$, $corr(p) \in R_\rho^0$

Two thresholds, θ and ϕ, both positive integers.

R_ρ^0 is the set of non-negative real numbers of fixed precision ρ; that is, ρ is the distance between adjacent floating point numbers in the set R_ρ^0.

A test image I is the set of pixel/measurement quadruples (x,y,j,m_j). $p = (x,y)$ specifies a location in a Euclidean coordinate system with a given origin. M_i is the set of measurement types in the image, such as color, motion, depth, and so forth, each type coded as a distinct positive integer. m_j is a measurement token of type j, represents scene characteristics, and is a non-negative real number of fixed precision, that is, with positive error due to possible truncation of at most ρ. (Only a finite number of bits may be stored.) I' is a subimage of I (i.e., an arbitrary subset of quadruples). It is not necessary that all pixel locations contain measurements of all types. Further, it is not necessary that the set of pixels be spatially contiguous. For ease of notation, $i_{x,y,j}$ has value m_j. If $j \notin M_i$ or if the (x,y) values are outside the image array, then $i_{x,y,j} = 0$.

A goal image G is a set of pixel/measurement quadruples defined in the same way as I. The set of (x,y) locations is not necessarily contiguous. M_g is the set of measurement types in the goal image. The types correspond between I and G (i.e., type 3 in one image is the same type 3 in the other). The two sets of measurement types, however, are not necessarily the same. The coordinate system of the goal image is the same as for the test image, and the origin of the goal image coincides with the origin of the test image. $g_{x,y,j}$ has value m_j. If $j \notin M_g$ or if the (x,y) values are outside the image array, then $g_{x,y,j} = 0$.

For purposes of the proof, the *diff* function will be the sum of the absolute values of the point-wise differences of the measurements of a subset of the test image with the corresponding subset of the goal image. The constraint that results, for an arbitrary subset I' of the test image, is

$$\sum_{p \in I'} diff(p) = \sum_{p \in I'} \sum_{j \in M_i} \left| g_{x,y,j} - i_{x,y,j} \right| \leq \theta.$$

This sum of differences must be less than a given threshold θ in order for a match to be potentially acceptable. Note that other specific functions that could find small-enough values of some other property may be as suitable. The threshold is a positive integer. The number of operations required to compute this is on the order of $\|I'\|$ $\|M_i\|$ additions and comparisons for each subset I'.

Because a null I' satisfies any threshold in the above constraint, we must enforce the constraint that as many figure matches must be included in I' as possible. Two-dimensional spatial transforms that do not align the goal properly with the test items must also be eliminated because they would lead to many background-to-background matches. One way to do this is to find large-enough values of the point-wise product of the goal and image. This is also the cross-correlation commonly used in computer vision to measure similarity between a given signal and a template. A second threshold, ϕ, provides a constraint on the acceptable size of the match. Therefore,

$$\sum_{p \in I'} corr(p) = \sum_{p \in I'} \sum_{j \in M_i} \left| g_{x,y,i} \times i_{x,y,j} \right| \geq \phi.$$

The number of operations required to compute this is on the order of $\|I'\|$ $\|M_i\|$ multiplications and comparisons for each subset I'. The above assumes that the full set of measurements of the test image are always considered regardless of which features exist in the goal image. This could be reformulated to include a search for the correct subset of features for matching; this is straightforward and not further elaborated here (but is reflected in chapter 2). Note that there is no claim here that the algorithm necessarily corresponds with human performance. The function definitions are given primarily for purposes of the proof and are claimed to be reasonable ones. It is possible to provide other functions for difference and correlation and reconstruct similar proofs using them.

Unbounded (Bottom-up) Visual Match

The task posed by Bottom-Up Visual Match is as follows: Given a test image, a difference function, and a correlation function, is there a subset of pixels of the test image such that the difference between that subset and the corresponding subset of pixels in the goal image is less than a given threshold and such that the correlation between the two is at least as large as another specified threshold? In other words, is there a set $I' \subseteq I$ such that it simultaneously satisfies

$$\sum_{p \in I'} diff(p) \leq \theta \text{ and } \sum_{p \in I'} corr(p) \geq \phi?$$

$2\|I'\|$ operations are required to compute this for each subset I'. The number of subsets for each possible value of $\|I'\|$, $0 \leq \|I'\| \leq \|I\|$, is given by

$$\binom{\|I\|}{\|I'\|},$$

the total number of subsets is given by

$$\sum_{\mu=0}^{\|I\|} \binom{\|I\|}{\mu} = 2^{\|I\|},$$

and thus the total number of operations is

$$\sum_{\mu=0}^{\|I\|} 2\mu \binom{\|I\|}{\mu} = \|I\|(\|I\|+1)2^{\|I\|}.$$

This reflects the cost of a brute-force solution; this does not prove that there is no more efficient solution. The proof below will provide this. One point regarding the above specification of visual matching must be emphasized. This definition is one that forces a bottom-up approach to the solution of visual matching. The goal image is not permitted to provide direction to any aspect of the computation other than in the computation of the *diff* and *corr* functions. The constraints given must be satisfied with subsets of the input image. It is not unexpected that this definition involves two constraints to be simultaneously satisfied and that the two constraints represent error and size satisfaction criteria. Note that this definition does not force acceptance of only the 'best' match but accepts any 'sufficiently good' match. This is very similar to many other kinds of recognition definitions. For example, the standard definition of region growing involves the maximal contiguous subset of

pixels that satisfies a given property (Ballard & Brown, 1982) Moreover, this definition should not be interpreted as a template-matching operation. Although template
matching may be posed in the above manner, there is nothing inherent in the definition to exclude other matching forms—the notions of image points, measurements,
and constraints representing large-enough size and low-enough error are ubiquitous
in visual matching definitions.

The Bottom-up Visual Match problem as stated has exactly the same structure as
a known NP-Complete problem, namely the Knapsack problem (Garey & Johnson,
1979) Therefore, it would seem that a direct reduction (by local replacement) of
Knapsack to Visual Match is the appropriate proof procedure.

Theorem B.1   *Unbounded (Bottom-up) Visual Match is NP-Complete.*

It must be clear that this problem is NP-Complete because it shares with the
Knapsack problem the following characteristics: an arbitrary subset of the input
may be the correct solution; and, two constraints must be satisfied simultaneously.
Other aspects of the problem statement such as the specific form of the functions
or the fact that real numbers of fixed precision are used do not lead to the
NP-Completeness.

One problem must first be solved before proceeding to the reduction. The statement of Visual Match involves images whose measurements may be non-negative
real numbers (of finite precision ρ as stated in the original problem). By stating a
precision ρ, we mean that the significant digits whose value is less than ρ are not
represented. Therefore, a fixed number of bits are required to represent each value.
This is easily solved by first proving that Knapsack with non-negative real numbers
is NP-Complete. It should be stressed that the use of real numbers versus integers
in no way leads to the NP-Completeness of the problem—the inherent structure of
the problem is the same as that of Knapsack, regardless of the representation.

Knapsack-R_f^0

instance: Finite set A
    for each $a \in A$ there is a function $w(a) \in R_f^0$ (the set of non-negative real numbers
    of fixed precision f)
    a function $z(a) \in R_f^0$
    and positive integers C, D
question: Find a subset $A' \subseteq A$ such that

$$\sum_{a \in A'} w(a) \leq C \ \text{ and } \ \sum_{a \in A'} z(a) \geq D?$$

The proof of NP-Completeness is trivial because the structure is identical to the
traditional Knapsack problem (Garey & Johnson, 1979). Now we are ready to prove
the main theorem of this section.

Proof Let the set A, the functions w and z, and the integers C and D specify an arbitrary instance of Knapsack-R_f^0. Set $M_i = M_g = \{1\}$. Define a test image and a goal image to be of size $\lceil \|A\|^{1/2} \rceil \times \lceil \|A\|^{1/2} \rceil$. Because $\|A\| \le \lceil \|A\|^{1/2} \rceil^2$, $\lceil \|A\|^{1/2} \rceil^2 - \|A\|$ elements of each image will be of value 0 (i.e., they join the background in the image). Therefore, $\|I\| = \lceil \|A\|^{1/2} \rceil^2$. The elements of the set A will be used to determine values for the elements of the goal and test images in the following way. Set

$$diff(p) = \sum_{M_i} |g_{x,y,j} - i_{x,y,j}| = |g_{x,y,1} - i_{x,y,1}| = w(a)$$

and

$$corr(p) = \sum_{M_i} g_{x,y,j} \times i_{x,y,j} = g_{x,y,1} \times i_{x,y,1} = z(a)$$

for each $a \in A$. p is the point with location (x, y) within both images, and the location is set arbitrarily, as long as each position is used and each unique position is associated with a unique element of A. It is clear from the above why the number 0 must be included as possible values for the functions w and z (it is not in Knapsack), because the difference function may have value zero, and because the background has value zero and thus the correlation function may be zero as well. A correspondence has now been set up between pixels in the test and goal image and elements of the set A. A subset of A has an associated subset of I, and the values of the difference and correlation functions correspond directly with values of the functions w and z for the corresponding element of A. Now one can solve for the values of g and i given the above pair of equations, for each spatial position. For ease of notation, g will represent $g_{x,y,1}$ and similarly for i. Because i must be non-negative, if we wish $g \ge i$, then

$$i = \frac{-w(a) + \sqrt{w(a)^2 + 4z(a)}}{2},$$

and $g = w(a) + i$, or if $g < i$,

$$i = \frac{-w(a) + \sqrt{w(a)^2 + 4z(a)}}{2},$$

and $g = i - w(a)$.

It does not matter which assumption is made. The problem with this is the square root may be irrational and thus require an infinite number of bits to represent. This is solved by using the precision ρ, as given above, thus explaining the need to include this precision in the original definition. Thus, if each value is truncated, then the error ε in each would be less than ρ. The value of ρ can be anywhere within the open interval:

$$0 < \rho < \frac{-\sum_A w(a) + \sqrt{\left(\sum_A w(a)\right)^2 + 4f\|I\|}}{2\|I\|}.$$

This expression will be derived shortly. The error in the values can be stated explicitly as:

$$i_{correct} = i_{computed} + \varepsilon, g_{correct} = g_{computed} + \varepsilon, 0 \le \varepsilon < \rho.$$

The error for g is the same as for i as no further approximations are necessary.

Next we must address the effect of this approximation on the *diff* and *corr* functions. It should be clear that if there were no truncation error, then the correspondence between the Visual Match problem and Knapsack-R_f^0 is complete and the proof is also complete. In fact, the approximations do not affect the *diff* function at all, only the *corr* function. The diff function becomes

$$diff = |g_{computed} - i_{computed}| = |g_{correct} - \varepsilon - i_{correct} + \varepsilon| = |g_{correct} - i_{correct}|.$$

The errors cancel out because they are due to a single source. Therefore, the sums are the same, and if θ is set to C, the difference constraint will be satisfied by exactly those subsets that would satisfy it for the Knapsack-R_f^0 problem. On the other hand, the *corr* function becomes:

$$corr = g_{computed} \times i_{computed} = (g_{correct} - \varepsilon) \times (i_{correct} - \varepsilon)$$
$$= g_{correct} \times i_{correct} - \varepsilon \times (g_{correct} + i_{correct} - \varepsilon)$$

There is an error term of $\varepsilon \times (g_{correct} + i_{correct} - \varepsilon)$. In an exact representation, it is clear that the values of *corr* are exactly those of the function z for corresponding subsets. So, we need to show that as ε goes to zero, the error in the sum of the *corr* values also goes to zero. The largest possible value of ε is ρ. In the Knapsack-R_f^0 problem, the sums of the values of the function $z(a)$ for the subsets of A are ordered, and each is separated from the other by at least the value of f, by definition. It would then be sufficient to show that for ρ sufficiently small,

$$\sum_{I'} \rho \times (i_{correct} + g_{correct} - \rho) < f$$

for all subsets I' (i.e., the precision of values is higher than in Knapsack-R_f^0). The largest possible subset is the entire image, so if this inequality is true for the entire image, then it is also true for all other subsets. As we do not know the correct values of i and g and we only have the computed values, substitute those into the above expression, giving:

$$\sum_{I} \rho \times \left(\left(i_{\text{computed}} + \rho \right) + \left(g_{\text{computed}} + \rho \right) - \rho \right) = \|I\| \times \rho^2 + \rho \sum_{I} \left(i_{\text{computed}} + g_{\text{computed}} \right) < f.$$

It remains to be shown that there exists some nonzero value of ρ that satisfies the above inequality. The value of ρ that satisfies the inequality is less than the root of

$$\|I\| \times \rho^2 + \rho \sum_{I} \left(i_{\text{computed}} + g_{\text{computed}} \right) - f = 0.$$

The values of i_{computed} and g_{computed} are not known before their computation, but the value of ρ is part of the problem definition and must be known before computation. Therefore, we can replace them with smaller known values and not affect the end result. Because $w(a) = g - i$, then $w(a)$ is less than $g + i$, and

$$\sum_{A} w(a) \le \sum_{I} \left(i_{\text{computed}} + g_{\text{computed}} \right).$$

Substituting this into the quadratic equation above and solving for ρ:

$$\rho' = \frac{-\sum_{A} w(a) + \sqrt{\left(\sum_{A} w(a) \right)^2 + 4f \|I\|}}{2\|I\|}.$$

As the solution must be positive, there is only one possible root (and it is real). All variables have values that are known before the computation of the image elements. The value of precision for the problem can then be stated as any value of ρ such that $0 < \rho < \rho'$. Given this precision, which is less than that of the original Knapsack-R_f^0 problem, and if ϕ is set to D, it follows directly that the subsets of the image that satisfy the second constraint are exactly those corresponding with the subsets of A that satisfy the second constraint of the Knapsack-R_f^0 problem. Therefore, set A' exists if and only if I' exists and Unbounded (Bottom-up) Visual Match is NP-Complete.   ∎

Because Visual Match is a subproblem of Visual Search, then

Theorem B.2   *Unbounded (Bottom-up) Visual Search is NP-Complete.*

Even though the Visual Search algorithm allows Visual Match to have a starting point in terms of location in the test image, the target extent is still not known and as a result the search remains exponential.

Bounded (Task-directed) Visual Match

The next theorem considers the version of visual matching that includes guidance using task information. The bottom-up version prohibits any use of such information for solution.

Theorem   B.3   *Bounded   (Task-directed)   Visual   Match   has   linear   time complexity.*

If we consider task-directed optimizations using the goal item, it is easy to show that the problem has linear time complexity. The key is to direct the computation of the difference and correlation functions using the goal rather than the test image. However, we still seek the appropriate subset of the test image. If there is a match that satisfies the constraints, then its extent can be predicted in the test image; all locations are possible. The Bounded Visual Match task is stated as follows: Given a test image, a goal image, a difference function, and a correlation function, is there a subset of pixels of the test image such that the difference between that subset and the corresponding subset of pixels in the goal image is less than a given threshold and such that the correlation between the two is as large as possible? In other words, is it true that

$$\sum_{p \in G} diff(p) \le \theta \ \text{ and } \ \sum_{p \in G} corr(p) \ge \phi$$

where

$$\sum_{p \in G} diff(p) = \sum_{p \in G} \sum_{j \in Mg} \left| g_{x,y,j} - i_{x,y,j} \right| \ \text{ and } \ \sum_{p \in G} corr(p) = \sum_{p \in G} \sum_{j \in Mg} \left| g_{x,y,j} - i_{x,y,j} \right|?$$

Proof   Note that the definition of *diff* and *corr* have changed slightly in that the pixel locations and measurement set used are that of the goal rather than the test image. The computation of the *diff* and *corr* functions is driven by the goal image and the measurements present in the goal. A simple algorithm is apparent. First, center the goal item over a candidate pixel of the test image; compute the *diff* and *corr* measures between the test and goal image at that position. The Visual Search algorithm then considers all the positions possible, and chooses the solution that satisfies the constraints. The resulting time complexity function for Visual Match would be

$$O(\|G\| \times \|M_g\|) .$$

In other words, the worst-case number of computations of the *diff* and *corr* functions is determined by the product of the size of the goal image in pixels and the number of measurements in the goal image. If the complexity of visual search (within which Visual Match is embedded) is considered, this would add only a multiplicative term to represent the total number of possible locations, rotations, and scalings. If display items can be localized, (via attentional selection, for example), the complexity is linear in the number of items in the display, but all rotations and scalings must still be considered. As at least one linear algorithm exists, the proof is complete.   ∎

The bounded problem is constrained to find subsets that are the same size and shape as the goal, whereas the unbounded version can find subsets of arbitrary sizes and shapes. As a result, the problems are not directly comparable in their results.

These theorems were proved independently by Ron Rensink shortly afterwards using a completely different proof procedure, thus cementing their validity (Rensink, 1989).

Appendix C: The Representation of Visual Motion Processes

The domain that was chosen to demonstrate many of the capabilities of Selective Tuning is visual motion. Note that this is a pure motion representation—there is no concept of edge or texture or depth or luminance and so on. The input is a video stream in the form of a sequence of images, and ST is able to detect, localize, and classify the motions of moving objects in the scene.

Four cortical visual areas are simulated: V1, MT, MST, and 7a. These four areas are known to participate in the processing of visual motion (Felleman & Van Essen, 1991). The model consists of 694 feature maps each of which encodes the entire visual field with a given neural selectivity. These feature maps are organized into areas based on their properties, and areas are structured in a pyramid with information flowing from the input at the bottom to the top of the pyramid (feed-forward, data-driven process) and from the top back to the bottom (recurrent process). There are no connections that skip layers, and there are no lateral cooperation connections with one exception that will be described below. The full P-Lattice is depicted in figure 7.2. Details are now presented on what is computed by each area.

Area V1

Area V1 receives visual input as a temporal sequence of images. Spatiotemporal filters are used to model the selectivity of V1 neurons for speed and direction of local motion (Orban, Kennedy, & Bullier, 1986). V1 neurons are selective to motion direction and motion speed. For simplicity, only 12 directions spaced at 30° increments ($0°, 30°, ... , 330°$), are used to model direction selectivity, although cells in the macaque visual cortex may distinguish more directions (Orban et al., 1986). For speed selectivity, we consider three different speed bands with means at 0.5, 1, and 2 pixels/frame, a bit differently from Orban et al. (1986), who report four types of velocity-sensitive neurons. The reduction in quanta along each of these two dimensions was made simply for computational efficiency of the implementation. In the current implementation, V1 neurons are divided into two types. The first type performs spatiotemporal filtering on the raw image sequence. We refer to this first type as a filtering neuron, or VF. The second type integrates the local activation of filtering neurons within its receptive field. We refer to this second type as an integrating neuron, or VI. Subscripts will be introduced below that qualify tuning properties and position for each.

The filtering neurons have spatiotemporal receptive fields (RFs) that provide access to the intensity values of T images in the most recent subsequence. For the examples in chapter 7, T is set to 5. We will refer to the intensity value at position p in the image taken at time t as $I(p\,t)$, where $t = 1$ and $t = T$ indicate the first and the most recent image in the sequence, respectively. The image sequence forms a three-dimensional image cube, a spatiotemporal volume as in Adelson and Bergen (1985). In this volume, the RF of a filtering neuron is oriented in such a way that local motion at position i in direction α with speed s_v would induce constant intensity across the RF.

For a preferred direction α and a preferred speed s, the spatial offset $\delta(\alpha,s,t)$ of the line of constant intensity in the image taken at time t can be computed as follows:

$$\delta(\alpha,s,t) = s\left(t - \frac{T+1}{2}\right)\left(\frac{\cos\alpha}{\sin\alpha}\right). \tag{C.1}$$

In practice, because in most cases this function will not yield integer values, up to four inputs (pixels) per image are included in the RF for each line of constant intensity. Figure C.1 is a visualization of a sequence of one-dimensional motion

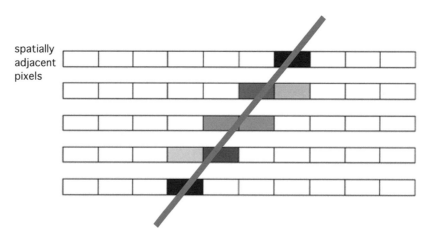

Figure C.1
In a one-dimensional image sequence—each row of pixels is an image and time proceeds from the bottom upward—the line of constant intensity for a neuron's preferred motion may intercept at most two pixels in each image layer.

images, where two inputs per image are necessary. The darker a pixel, the larger its weight will be in the subsequent computation of the input from its image (because the line is passing through it more centrally). Assuming the spatial offset is x, the weights for these two inputs are $1 - (x - \lfloor x \rfloor)$ and $x - \lfloor x \rfloor$, respectively. It is straightforward to generalize to two-dimensional motion images. In the following quantitative description, we will simply use the real-valued function $\delta(\alpha, s, t)$.

A filtering neuron receives input from each temporal layer and computes an intensity value IC that decreases as the standard deviation of the intensity across the layers increases:

$$IC_{\alpha, s_v} = M_{VF} - \sqrt{\frac{1}{T} \sum_{t=1}^{T} \left\{ I[p(i) + \delta(\alpha, s_v, t), t] - \frac{\sum_{k=1}^{T} I[p(i) + \delta(\alpha, s_v, k), k]}{T} \right\}^2}, \qquad (C.2)$$

where M_{VF} is the maximum activation of the neuron. With intensities ranging from 0 to 255, we choose the value of M_{VF} to be 128. In the current implementation, to compensate for noise in the visual input, the RF of each filtering neuron consists of multiple ($N = 20$) such linear arrangements of inputs. V1 neurons are selective to three speeds (0.5, 1, and 2 pixels/frame) and 12 directions (30° increments). Every filtering neuron obtains one $IC_{\alpha_n s_n}$ value for each linear arrangement of inputs, and the activation is given by

$$VF_{\alpha, v, i} = \max_{1 \leq n \leq N} IC_{\alpha_n s_n}. \qquad (C.3)$$

Obviously, the filtering neurons reach a state of maximum activation if motion of their preferred orientation and speed is present in their RFs. However, maximum activation can also be induced if there is no motion in a region of homogeneous intensity in the image sequence. Therefore, the role of the integrating neurons is not only to integrate the raw filtering neuron activations but also to eliminate such pseudo-motion detected by the filtering neurons. This is achieved by implementing lateral inhibition between integrating neurons with identical positions and speed selectivity but different preferred directions of motion:

$$VI_{\alpha, v, j} = \frac{1}{|R_j|} \sum_{i \in R_j} W_j \cdot VF_{\alpha, v, i} - \frac{1}{(n_\alpha - 1)|R_j|} \sum_{\beta, \beta \neq \alpha} \sum_{i \in R_j} W_j \cdot VF_{\beta, v, i}, \qquad (C.4)$$

where R_j is the set of neurons in the RF of the integrating neuron j, and n_α denotes the number of implemented preferred directions of motion; in the current model, $n_\alpha = 12$. Here, α and β assume only these directions. W_j denotes a Gaussian weighting of all filtering neurons. It is determined by a 2D Gaussian function as follows:

$$W_j = \frac{e^{\frac{(x_j-x_c)^2+(y_j-y_c)^2}{2\sigma^2}}}{\sum_{k \in R(j)} W_k} . \qquad\qquad\qquad (C.5)$$

(x_c, y_c) is the center coordinate of the RF, and $\sigma = 2.5$. The closer the filtering neuron is to the center of the RF, the more it contributes to the response.

To achieve the V1 computation, the model uses one hypercolumn of filtering neurons for each pixel in the visual field. Each hypercolumn comprises one neuron for each combination of preferred speed and direction. Because there are three different preferred speeds and 12 different preferred directions of motion, there are 36 neurons in each hypercolumn. There is also a 64×64 array of integrating neuron hypercolumns (also 36 neurons per hypercolumn) that are evenly spatially distributed and receive input from local filtering neurons.

Area MT

Neurons in MT are tuned toward a particular local speed and direction of movement, similar to V1 neurons (Lagae, Maes, Raiguel, Xiao, & Orban, 1994; Maunsell & Van Essen, 1983; Perrone & Thiele, 2002). In addition, MT neurons are selective for a particular angle between the direction of movement and the speed gradient (Treue & Andersen, 1996; Xiao, Marcar, Raiguel, & Orban, 1997). Our model of area MT contains two different types of neurons. MT compartment MT-t contains neurons with selectivity identical to V1 neurons but with larger RFs (detectors of translational motion). MT compartment MT-g contains neurons selective for the local speed and direction of motion and the angle between the direction of movement and the speed gradient. MT-t is a 32×32 array of hypercolumns with 36 neurons in each, as in V1, whereas MT-g is a 32×32 array of hypercolumns of 432 neurons each, one for each of three speeds, 12 directions, and 12 direction/gradient angles. Each MT-t neuron receives input from a 4×4 field of V1 neurons with the same direction and speed tuning as the MT-t neuron. The activation of translation selective MT-t neurons is computed as:

$$MT_{\alpha,v,i} = \sum_{j \in R_i} W_j VI_{\alpha,v,j}. \qquad\qquad\qquad (C.6)$$

Speed gradient detecting MT-g neurons are selective for angles between the directions of movement and speed gradient. For each motion direction, 12 direction/gradient angles are modeled. The activation is computed as the product of the activation of V1 neurons in the RF with the same speed and direction tuning, and the gradient response. The gradient is determined by oriented RFs (e.g., RF for detecting upward gradient): For a speed gradient neuron i with preferred direction of motion α, preferred angle δ between the motion, and gradient speed selectivity MG of type v:

$$MG_{\alpha,\delta,v,i} = \begin{cases} 0, & if\left(\sum_{j \in R_i} W_j VI_{\alpha,v,i}\right)\left(A_0 + \sum_{k=1}^{3} c_k \Delta(\alpha, \alpha+\delta, k, i)\right) < 0 \\ \left(\sum_{j \in R_i} W_j VI_{\alpha,v,i}\right)\left(A_0 + \sum_{k=1}^{3} c_k \Delta(\alpha, \alpha+\delta, k, i)\right), & \text{otherwise.} \end{cases} \quad \text{(C.7)}$$

The c_k, $k = \{1,2,3\}$, are coefficients for the linear reconstruction of absolute speed from the activation of the three types of speed-selective neurons, $A_0 = 40$ is a baseline activation for preferred direction, W is a 4×4 Gaussian filter with $\sigma = 1.0$, and $\Delta(\alpha,\beta,v,i)$ specifies the activation increase in direction β in the receptive field of neuron i for speed selectivity type v and direction α:

$$\Delta(\alpha,\beta,v,i) = \sum_{j \in R_i} O_{\beta,j} VI_{\alpha,v,j}. \quad \text{(C.8)}$$

Here, $O_{\beta,j}$ is an orientation selective configuration of weights that leads to a maximum activation of the target neuron if the inputs increase in direction β. If we weight, for example, the connections in the upper half of a receptive field with 1 and in the lower half with –1, the resulting activation will be maximal if the inputs in the upper half are strong and the ones in the lower half are weak. These weights would be selective for an activation gradient pointing upward. We refer to the receptive fields assigned with these weights as oriented RFs. Therefore, we can design configurations of weights that prefer any of the 12 gradient directions in question. Figure C.2 shows the 12 kinds of oriented RFs considered in our implementation.

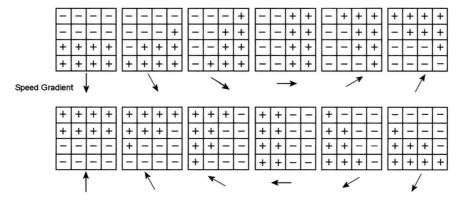

Figure C.2
Oriented RFs corresponding with $O_{\beta,j}$ in the equation.

Area MST

Similar to area MT, two different types of neurons are modeled in area MST. The first type of neuron populates compartment MST-t and responds to translation motion, in the same manner as V1 neurons, but with larger receptive fields. The second type of neuron, in compartment MST-s, responds to spiral motion (clockwise and counterclockwise rotation, expansion, contraction, and combinations) (Duffy & Wurtz, 1991; Graziano, Andersen, & Snowden, 1994; Saito et al., 1986; Sakata, Shibutani, Ito, & Tsurugai, 1986). MST is modeled as an 8×8 array of hypercolumns with 72 neurons in each hypercolumn (36 for translation as in MT and three speeds and 12 types of pattern selectivity for motion patterns). Each MST neuron receives input from an 11×11 field of MT neurons that have the same tuning as the MST neuron. Similar to V1 and MT, in the implementation and visualization, neurons with the same tuning are grouped into one layer. In total, area MST has 36 sheets for translation detection and 36 sheets for spiral motion detection.

The activation of $ST_{\alpha,v,i}$ that is tuned to motion in direction α with speed v is computed as:

$$ST_{\alpha,v,i} = \sum_{j \in R_i} W_j MT_{\alpha,v,j}. \tag{C.9}$$

Here, W_j is an 11×11 Gaussian filter with $\sigma = 11/3$. In area MT, neurons that are tuned to the angles between the moving directions and speed gradients are modeled. The angle between moving direction and the speed gradient is very important to motion pattern understanding. If the angle is $0°$, it is expansion; if the angle is $90°$, the motion pattern is counterclockwise rotation; if the angle is $180°$, the motion pattern is contraction; and if the angle is $270°$, the motion pattern is clockwise rotation. If the angle lies between, the motion pattern is a combination of the two patterns it lies between. Responses for a spiral neuron i selective for a pattern δ (a coherent angle between the direction and the speed gradient of motion) and of speed selectivity type v receives input from MT neurons in its receptive field with the same direction/gradient angle selectivity. Because 12 moving directions are modeled, there are 12 such neurons in each MT hypercolumn. The activation of this type of MST neuron, SS, is given by:

$$SS_{\delta,v,i} = \sum_{j \in R_i} \sum_{\alpha} W_j MG_{\alpha,\delta,v,j}. \tag{C.10}$$

Area 7a

Area 7a seems to be involved in at least four different types of computations (Read & Siegel, 1997; Siegel & Read, 1997): translation and spiral motion, as in MST but with larger RFs; rotation, regardless of direction; and radial motion, regardless of direction (perhaps participating in egomotion computations). Two types of 7a neurons are modeled; the latter two types are described in Tsotsos et al. (2005) but are not included here. The first two types are similar to neurons in MST layers, one tuned to translation, AT (compartment 7a-t), and the other tuned to spiral motion, AS (compartment 7a-s). The activations of these two types of neurons are just the Gaussian weighted sum of the MST neurons in their receptive field:

$$AT_{\alpha,v,i} = \sum_{j \in R_i} W_j ST_{\alpha,v,j} \tag{C.11}$$

$$AS_{\delta,v,i} = \sum_{j \in R_i} W_j SS_{\delta,v,j}. \tag{C.12}$$

Here, W_j is a 3×3 Gaussian filter with $\sigma = 1.0$.

Spatial Derivatives of Velocity

Our representation has one major unique component; that is, the representation of gradients. Our gradient computation corresponds with the spatial derivatives of the affine motion model, and evidence for its neural correlate can be found in monkey and human (Martinez-Trujillo et al., 2005; Sunaert, Van Hecke, Marchal, & Orban, 1999; Treue & Andersen, 1996).

It is important to put this motion process into context, starting with Koenderink and Van Doorn (1976) and Longuet-Higgins and Prazdny (1980) who made the suggestion that such motion channels may exist in the brain. On the assumptions that a moving object can be modeled (at least piecewise) by rigid planar patches, and that there is a fixation point on the surface in question, the motion may be estimated using an affine transformation. The affine model can be described on the basis of four quantities: image translation, image rotation, divergence, and shear. The first two terms specify respectively a rigid 2D translation and rotation of the fixated object. The third term describes an isotropic expansion (or contraction) that specifies a change in scale or a pure deformation. The shear term yields a distortion of the image pattern and corresponds with an expansion in a specified direction and a simultaneous contraction in the perpendicular one so that the area of the pattern is preserved. Under perspective projection, the velocity vector at each point of an image is given by computing the time derivative of the gray value changes at each point (x,y) and yields (u, v). This represents translational motion. Spatial derivatives are taken of each velocity component u and v in the x and y directions (u_x, u_y, v_x, v_y). Combinations of derivatives provide definitions of each of the remaining three affine motions, rotation, deformation, and divergence. Divergence is represented by $l = u_x + v_y$. Deformation or shear has two components θ and ρ, and these are expressed as $\theta = u_x - v_y$ and $\rho = u_y + v_x$. Rotation is given as $k = u_y - v_x$. The extraction of the affine estimates has essentially two components: the identification of an appropriate set of 2D spatial patches to represent each surface in a scene, and the tracking of the patches through the image sequence. The point here is that the setting of a fixation point or the identification of the 2D patches to track is central to the definition, and the majority if not all past uses of affine estimation make assumptions about where this fixation comes from. In this system, attention plays this central role. The above specified gradient operations provide initial estimates of the spatial derivatives of the affine definition, MST-s neurons provide estimates of homogeneous patterns of those gradients, and the attentive process selects regions of strong response for further analysis.

The motion processes described here do have weaknesses, among them that they include little cooperative or competitive processing among units within a layer other than V1. On the other hand, there is one major strength as well. The use of gradients within the representation solves a rather difficult connectivity problem. Suppose an MST-s neuron needs to be wired up to detect, say, rotation. Consider how that may be accomplished by connecting the neuron to an optic flow representation. This would not be straightforward because it needs precise alignment of flow direction and speed with location for a small number of connections from each of the full set of possible directions and speeds. By comparison, rotation has a gradient response that is uniform over the entire extent of the rotating object. Neurons need no special connectivity—they can be connected uniformly to an entire representation—and need only seek regions of homogeneity within that representation. This resolves the problem very simply. Perhaps this may be a general neural computation principle whenever representational and connectivity issues become too difficult. The strategy would be to transform complex spatial (or temporal) patterns of neural responses into intermediate representations for which simple filters that are tuned to homogeneous patterns suffice in subsequent computation stages.

Summary

This representation of motion processes has many elements common to several past works. Most other models of biological motion perception focus on a single cortical area. For instance, the models by Zemel and Sejnowksi (1998), Simoncelli and

Heeger (1998), and Beardsley and Vaina (1998) are biologically relevant approaches that explain some specific functionality of MT or MST neurons but do not include the embedding hierarchy in the motion pathway. On the other hand, there are hierarchical models for the detection of motion. Meese and Anderson (2002) argue that a minimum of eight spiral detecting mechanisms with direction bandwidths around ±45° are necessary for the computation of generalized spiral motions but do not provide a computationally plausible version of the motion processing hierarchy that may include these. Giese and Poggio (2003) describe a sophisticated, biologically motivated, and complex hierarchy for processing human movement patterns. However, they did not include any attentional influences. Further, they provide early input to their algorithm manually. Hand-tracked body joint positions were manually converted to stick figures where optic flow is easily computed. They cannot handle complex, overlapping, dense flow or discontinuous motions and certainly cannot process real image sequences directly. Lu and Sperling (1995) present a motion hierarchy as well as attentive processes, but the model is not a computational one. However, it has strong biological plausibility in its function. They proposed that human visual motion perception is served by three separate motion systems: a first-order system that responds to moving luminance patterns, a second-order system that responds to moving modulations of feature types, and a third-order system that computes the motion of marked locations in a Saliency Map. This third-order system of Lu and Sperling seems to be similar to the process of attending to motion in ST, but without the computational details, it is difficult to draw too close a comparison.

Our model is not the first to be developed with explicit connection to attentive processes. The earliest ones are due to Nowlan and Sejnowski (1995) and Daniilidis (1995). In Nowlan and Sejnowski, processing is much in the same spirit as ours but very different in form. They compute motion energy with the goal of modeling MT neurons. This energy is part of a hierarchy of processes that include softmax (a neural activation function whose output lies between zero and one) for local velocity selection. They suggest that the selection permits processing to be focused on the most reliable estimates of velocity. There is neither top-down component nor a full processing hierarchy nor binding for complex patterns. Attentional modulation in motion neurons was described experimentally in Treue and Maunsell (1996) after their model was presented; thus, of course it is not developed and does not appear to be within the scope of their model. Based on the optical flow, Daniilidis (1995) computed 3D motion and structure. He fixated on an object to estimate egomotion in the presence of translation and rotation of the observer from the flow in the log-polar periphery. Computation of time to collision was a goal, not the definition of an attentive motion hierarchy. Although he used attentive fixations to advantage, the motion processing there was quite specific and based on log-polar representations, and the connection to affine motion, implicated by the need to fixate, was not recognized. Finally, Grossberg, Mingolla, and Viswanathan (2001) present an integration and segmentation model for motion capture. Called the Formotion BCS model, their goal is to integrate motion information across the image and segment motion cues into a unified global percept. They employ models of translational processing in areas V1, V2, MT, and MST and do not consider motion patterns. Competition determines local winners among neural responses, and the MST cells encoding the winning direction have an excitatory influence on MT cells tuned to the same direction. A variety of motion illusions are illustrated, but no real image sequences are attempted. This model seems to be closest to ST here in goal and methodology.

Although our motion model seems to cover many different motion classes, it is not complete by any means. A key missing set of motion categories is that of motion change. That is, there is no representation for discontinuities of motion such as start and stop. There is no representation for accelerations such as changes in speed or in direction. There seems little experimental work to inform the development of such representations [but we are making a start with Martinez-Trujillo, Cheyne, Gaetz, Simine, and Tsotsos (2007)]. Finally, there is no representation for abrupt onset and onsets [although one was proposed in Wai and Tsotsos (1994) and Tsotsos et al. (1995), it is not included in the model of this chapter].

References

Adelson, E., & Bergen, J. (1985). Spatiotemporal energy models for the perception of motion. *Journal of the Optical Society of America. A, Optics and Image Science, 2*(2), 284–299.

Adesnik, H., & Scanziani, M. (2010). Lateral competiton for cortical space by layer-specific horizontal circuits. *Nature, 464*, 1155–1160.

Ahissar, M., & Hochstein, S. (1997). Task difficulty and the specificity of perceptual learning. *Nature, 387*, 401–406.

Aloimonos, Y. (1992). Purposive and qualitative active vision. *CVGIP: Image Understanding, 56*(1), 840–850.

Amit, Y., & Geman, D. (1998). A Computational Model for Visual Selection. TR no. 469. Department of Statistics, University of Chicago.

Anderson, C. (2008). The End of Theory: The Data Deluge Makes the Scientific Method Obsolete. *WIRED Magazine,* 16:07, June 23.

Anderson, C., & Van Essen, D. (1987). Shifter circuits: A computational strategy for dynamic aspects of visual processing. *Proceedings of the National Academy of Sciences of the United States of America, 84*, 6297–6301.

Anderson, J. (1976). *Language, memory and thought.* Hillsdale, NJ: Erlbaum Associates.

Arbib, M. A. (ed.), (1995). *The handbook of brain theory and neural networks.* Cambridge, MA: MIT Press.

Ardid, S., Wang, X.-J., & Compte, A. (2007). An integrated microcircuit model of attentional processing in the neocortex. *Journal of Neuroscience, 27*(32), 8486–8495.

Armstrong, K., Chang, M., & Moore, T. (2009). Selection and maintenance of spatial information by frontal eye field neurons. *Journal of Neuroscience, 29*(50), 15621–15629.

Bahcall, D., & Kowler, E. (1999). Attentional interference at small spatial separations. *Vision Research, 39*(1), 71–86.

Bajcsy, R. (1985). Active Perception vs Passive Perception. In L. Shapiro and A. Kak (eds.), Proc. 3rd IEEE Workshop on Computer Vision: Representation and Control (pp. 55–62). October 13–16, Bellaire, MI. Washington DC: IEEE Computer Society Press.

Ballard, D. (1991). Animate vision. *Artificial Intelligence, 48*, 57–86.

Ballard, D., & Brown, C. (1982). *Computer vision.* Englewood Cliffs, NJ: Prentice-Hall.

Barlow, H. B. (1972). Single units and sensation: a neuron doctrine for perceptual psychology? *Perception, 1*(4), 371–394.

Barrow, H., & Popplestone, R. (1971). Relational descriptions in picture processing. In B. Meltzer & D. Michie (eds.), *Machine intelligence 6* (pp. 377–396). UK: Edinburgh University Press.

Barrow, H., & Tenenbaum, J. (1981). Computational vision. *Proceedings of the IEEE, 69*(5), 572–595.

Barstow, D. R. (1979). *Knowledge-based program construction.* New York: North-Holland.

Beardsley, S. A., & Vaina, L. M. (1998). Computational modeling of optic flow selectivity in MSTd neurons. *Computation and Neural Systems, 9*, 467–493.

Ben-Shahar, O., Huggins, P., Izo, T., & Zucker, S. W. (2003). Cortical connections and early visual function: Intra- and inter-columnar processing. *Journal of Physiology (Paris), 97*(2), 191–208.

Berlyne, D. E. (1974). Attention. In E. C. Carterette and M. P. Friedman (eds.), *Handbook of perception.* Vol.1, *Historical and philosophical roots of perception.* New York: Academic Press.

Bichot, N. P., & Schall, J. D. (1999). Saccade target selection in macaque during feature and conjunction visual search. *Visual Neuroscience, 16*, 81–89.

Biederman, I. (1987). Recognition-by-components: A theory of human image understanding. *Psychological Review, 94*, 115–147.

Birkoff, G. (1967). *Lattice theory* (3rd ed.). Providence, RI: American Mathematical Society.

Boehler, C. N. (2006). The Spatiotemporal Profile of Visual Attention. Doctoral Dissertation, Der Fakultät für Naturwissenschaften der Otto-von-Guericke-Universität, Magdeburg, Germany.

Boehler, C. N., Tsotsos, J. K., Schoenfeld, M., Heinze, H.-J., & Hopf, J.-M. (2009). The center-surround profile of the focus of attention arises from recurrent processing in visual cortex. *Cerebral Cortex, 19*, 982–991.

Boehler, C. N., Tsotsos, J. K., Schoenfeld, M. A., Heinze, H.-J., & Hopf, J.-M. (in press). Neural mechanisms of surround attenuation and distractor competition in visual search. *Journal of Neuroscience.*

Boussaoud, D., & Wise, S. P. (1993). Primate frontal cortex: Neuronal activity following attentional versus intentional cues. *Experimental Brain Research, 95*(1), 15–27.

Boynton, G. (2005). Attention and visual perception. *Current Opinion in Neurobiology, 15*, 465–469.

Braun, J. (1998a). Vision and attention: The role of training. *Nature, 393*, 424–425.

Braun, J. (1998b). Divided attention: Narrowing the gap between brain and behavior. In R. Parasuraman (ed.), *The attentive brain.* Cambridge, MA: MIT Press.

Brentano, F. (1874). *Psychologie vom Empirischen Standpunkt.* Leipzig: Meiner.

Britten, K. (1996). Attention is everywhere. *Nature, 382*, 497–498.

Broadbent, D. (1958). *Perception and communication.* New York: Pergamon Press.

Bruce, N. D. B. (2008). Saliency, Attention and Visual Search: An Information Theoretic Approach. PhD Thesis, Department of Computer Science and Engineering, York University, Canada.

Bruce, N. D. B., & Tsotsos, J. K. (2005). Saliency Based on Information Maximization. In Y. Weiss, B. Schölkopf, & J. Platt (eds.), Proceedings of the 19th Annual Conference on Neural Information Processing Systems, December 5–10, Vancouver, BC. La Jolla, CA: Neural Information Processing Systems Foundation.

Bruce, N. D. B., & Tsotsos, J. K. (2008). Spatiotemporal Saliency: Towards a Hierarchical Representation of Visual Saliency. 5th International Workshop on Attention in Cognitive Systems, May 12, Santorini, Greece.

Bruce, N. D. B., & Tsotsos, J. K. (2009). Saliency, attention, and visual search: An information theoretic approach. *Journal of Vision (Charlottesville, Va.), 9*(3), 1–24.

Buffalo, E., Fries, P., Landman, R., Liang, H., & Desimone, R. (2010). A backward progression of attentional effects in the ventral stream. *Proceedings of the National Academy of Sciences of the United States of America, 107*, 361–365.

Buia, C., & Tiesinga, P. (2006). Attentional modulation of firing rate and synchrony in a model cortical network. *Journal of Computational Neuroscience, 20*(3), 247–264.

Bullier, J. (2001). Integrated model of visual processing. *Brain Research. Brain Research Reviews, 36*, 96–107.

Bundesen, C. (1990). A theory of visual attention. *Psychological Review, 97*, 523–547.

Burt, P. (1988). Attention Mechanism for Vision in a Dynamic World. IEEE Proc. 9th Int. Conf. on Pattern Recognition, pp. 977–987, Nov. 14–17, Rome Italy. International Association for Pattern Recognition.

Burt, P., Adelson, E. (1983). The Laplacian Pyramid as a Compact Image Code. *IEEE Transactions on Communications COM-3l(4)* 532–540.

Buschman, T., & Miller, E. (2007). Top-down versus bottom-up control of attention in the prefrontal and posterior parietal cortices. *Science, 315*(5820), 1860–1862.

Caputo, G., & Guerra, S. (1998). Attentional selection by distractor suppression. *Vision Research, 38*(5), 669–689.

Carpenter, R. H. S. (ed.) (1991). *Vision and visual dysfunction (8): Eye movements.* Boca Raton, FL: CRC Press.

Cave, K. (1999). The featuregate model of visual selection. *Psychological Research, 62,* 182–194.

Chelazzi, L. (1999). Serial attention mechanisms in visual search: a critical look at the evidence. *Psychological Research, 62,* 195–219.

Chelazzi, L., Duncan, J., Miller, E. K., & Desimone, R. (1998). Responses of neurons in inferior temporal cortex during memory-guided visual search. *Journal of Neurophysiology, 80,* 2918–2940.

Chen, X., & Tsotsos, J. K. (2010). Attentional Surround Suppression in the Feature Dimension. TR2010–01. Department of Computer Science & Engineering, York University.

Cherry, E. C. (1953). Some experiments on the recognition of speech, with one and with two ears. *Journal of the Acoustical Society of America, 2595,* 975–979.

Churchland, P., Koch, C., & Sejnowski, T. (1990). What is computational neuroscience? In E. L. Schwartz (ed.), *Computational neuroscience.* Cambridge, MA: MIT Press.

Clark, J. J., & Ferrier, N. (1988). Modal Control of an Attentive Vision System. In R. Bajcsy & S. Ullman (eds.), Proc. IEEE 2nd International Conference on Computer Vision (pp. 514–523). December 5–8, Tarpon Springs, Florida. Washington DC: IEEE Computer Society Press.

Clowes, M. (1971). On seeing things. *Artificial Intelligence, 2,* 79–116.

Colby, C., Gattass, R., Olson, C., & Gross, C. (1988). Topographical organization of cortical afferents to extrastriate visual area PO in the macaque: A dual tracer study. *Journal of Comparative Neurology, 269*(3), 392–413.

Colby, C., & Goldberg, M. (1999). Space and attention in parietal cortex. *Annual Review of Neuroscience, 22,* 319–349.

Corbeil, J. C. (1986). *The Stoddart visual dictionary.* Toronto: Stoddart Publishing Co.

Corbetta, M., & Shulman, G. L. (2002). Control of goal-directed and stimulus-driven attention in the brain. *Nature Review Neuroscience, 3,* 201–215.

Corbetta, M., Akbudak, E., Conturo, T., Snyder, A., Ollinger, J., Drury, H., et al. (1998). A common network of functional areas for attention and eye movements. *Neuron, 21,* 761–773.

Corchs, S., & Deco, G. (2001). A neurodynamical model for selective visual attention using oscillators. *Neural Networks, 14,* 981–990.

Coull, J., & Nobre, A. (1998). Where and when to pay attention: The neural systems for directing attention to spatial locations and to time intervals as revealed by both PET and fMRI. *Journal of Neuroscience, 18*(18), 7426–7435.

Cowan, N., Elliott, E., Saults, J., Morey, C., Mattox, S., Hismjatullina, A., et al. (2005). On the capacity of attention: Its estimation and its role in working memory and cognitive aptitudes. *Cognitive Psychology, 51,* 42–100.

Crick, F. (1984). Function of the thalamic reticular complex: The Searchlight Hypothesis. *Proceedings of the National Academy of Sciences of the United States of America, 81,* 4586–4590.

Crick, F., & Koch, C. (1990). Some reflections on visual awareness. In J. Watson & J. A. Witkowski (eds.), *Cold Spring Harbor symposia on quantitative biology* (Vol. LV, pp. 953–962). Cold Spring Harbor, NY: Cold Spring Harbor Laboratory Press.

Cudiero, J., & Sillito, A. (2006). Looking back: Corticothalamic feedback and early visual processing. *Trends in Neurosciences, 29*(6), 298–306.

Culhane, S. (1992). An Implementation of an Attentional Beam for Early Vision. MSc Thesis, Department of Computer Science, University of Toronto.

Culhane, S., & Tsotsos, J. K. (1992). An Attentional Prototype for Early Vision. In G. Sandini (ed.), Computer Vision—ECCV'92. Second European Conference on Computer Vision Santa Margherita Ligure, Italy, May 19–22, 1992. Lecture Notes in Computer Science 588, pp. 551–560. Springer-Verlag.

Curcio, C., & Allen, K. (1990). Topography of ganglion cells in human retina. *Journal of Comparative Neurology*, *300*, 5–25.

Curcio, C. A., Sloan, K. R., Kalina, R. E., & Hendrickson, A. E. (1990). Human photoreceptor topography. *Journal of Comparative Neurology*, *292*, 497–523.

Cutzu, F., & Tsotsos, J. K. (2003). The selective tuning model of visual attention: Testing the predictions arising from the inhibitory surround mechanism. *Vision Research*, *43*, 205–219.

Daniel, P. M., & Whitteridge, D. (1961). The representation of the visual field on the cerebral cortex in monkeys. *Journal of Physiology*, *159*, 203–221.

Daniilidis, K. (1995). Attentive visual motion processing: Computations in the log-polar plane. *Computing*, *11*(Suppl.), 1–20.

Davis, M. (1958). *Computability and unsolvability*. New York: McGraw-Hill.

Davis, M. (1965). *The undecidable*. New York: Hewlett Raven Press.

Deco, G., & Zihl, J. (2001). A neurodynamical model of visual attention: feedback enhancement of spatial resolution in a hierarchical system. *Journal of Computational Neuroscience*, *10*(3), 231–253.

Deco, G., Pollatos, O., & Zihl, J. (2002). The Time course of selective visual attention: theory and experiments. *Vision Research*, *42*, 2925–2945.

Della Libera, C., & Chelazzi, L. (2009). Learning to attend and to ignore is a matter of gains and losses. *Psychological Science*, *20*(6), 778–785.

Denning, P. J. (2007). Computing is a natural science. *Communications of the ACM*, *50*(7), 13–18.

Descartes, R. (1649). *Les Passions de l'âme*. Paris: Le Gras.

Desimone, R. (1990). Complexity at the neuronal level. *Behavioral and Brain Sciences*, *13*(3), 446.

Desimone, R., & Duncan, J. (1995). Neural mechanisms of selective attention. *Annual Review of Neuroscience*, *18*, 193–222.

Deutsch, J., & Deutsch, D. (1963). Attention: Some theoretical considerations. *Psychological Review*, *70*, 80–90.

Dickinson, S. (2009). The evolution of object categorization and the challenge of image abstraction. In S. Dickinson, A. Leonardis, B. Schiele, & M. Tarr (eds.), *Object categorization* (pp. 1–37). New York: Cambridge University Press.

Dickinson, S., Christensen, H., Tsotsos, J., & Olofsson, G. (1997). Active object recognition integrating attention and viewpoint control. *Computer Vision and Image Understanding*, *67*(3), 239–260.

Dickinson, S., Leonardis, A., Schiele, B., & Tarr, M. (eds.), (2009). *Object categorization*. New York: Cambridge University Press.

Dickinson, S., Wilkes, D., & Tsotsos, J. (1999). A computational model of view degeneracy. *IEEE Transactions on Pattern Analysis and Machine Intelligence*, *21*(8), 673–689.

Dolson, D. (1997). Hierarchical, Attentive Object Recognition. MSc Thesis, Department of Computer Science, University of Toronto.

Duffy, C. J., & Wurtz, R. H. (1991). Sensitivity of MST neurons to optic flow stimuli: mechanisms of response selectivity revealed by large-field stimuli. *Journal of Neurophysiology*, *65*, 1329–1345.

Duhamel, J., Colby, C., & Goldberg, M. (1992). The updating of the representation of visual space in parietal cortex by intended eye-movements. *Science*, *255*(5040), 90–92.

Duncan, J. (1979). Divided attention: The whole is more than the sum of its parts. *Journal of Experimental Psychology. Human Perception and Performance*, *5*(2), 216–228.

Duncan, J. (1984). Selective attention and the organization of visual information. *Journal of Experimental Psychology: General*, *113*(4), 501–517.

Duncan, J., Ward, J., & Shapiro, K. (1994). Direct measurement of attentional dwell time in human vision. *Nature*, *369*, 313–315.

Egeth, H., & Dagenbach, D. (1991). Parallel versus serial processing in visual search: further evidence from subadditive effects of visual quality. *Journal of Experimental Psychology. Human Perception and Performance, 17*, 551–560.

Egeth, H. E., & Yantis, S. (1997). Visual attention: control, representation, and time course. *Annual Review of Psychology, 48*, 269–297.

Egly, R., & Homa, D. (1984). Sensitization of the visual field. *Journal of Experimental Psychology: Human Perception and Performance, 10*, 778–793.

Eriksen, C., & St. James, J. (1986). Visual attention within and around the field of focal attention: A zoom lens model. *Perception & Psychophysics, 4*, 225–240.

Erman, L., Hayes-Roth, F., Lesser, V., & Reddy, R. (1980). The hearsay-II speech-understanding system: Integrating knowledge to resolve uncertainty. *ACM Computing Surveys, 12*, 213–253.

Ester, E., Serences, J., & Awh, E. (2009). Spatially global representations in human primary visual cortex during working memory maintenance. *Journal of Neuroscience, 29*(48), 15258–15265.

Evans, K., & Treisman, A. (2005). Perception of objects in natural scenes: Is it really attention free? *Journal of Experimental Psychology: Human Perception and Performance, 31*(6), 1476–1492.

Fallah, M., Stoner, G. R., & Reynolds, J. H. (2007). Stimulus-specific competitive selection in macaque extrastriate visual area V4. *Proceedings of the National Academy of Sciences of the United States of America, 104*(10), 4165–4169.

Fecteau, J., & Enns, J. (2005). Visual letter matching: Hemispheric functioning or scanning biases. *Neuropsychologia, 43*, 1412–1428.

Fecteau, J., & Munoz, D. (2006). Salience, relevance, and firing: A priority map for target selection. *Trends in Cognitive Sciences, 10*(8), 382–390.

Feldman, J., & Ballard, D. (1982). Connectionist models and their properties. *Cognitive Science, 6*, 205–254.

Felleman, D., & Van Essen, D. (1991). Distributed hierarchical processing in the primate visual cortex. *Cerebral Cortex, 1*, 1–47.

Fidler, S., & Leonardis, A. (2007). Towards Scalable Representations of Object Categories: Learning a Hierarchy of Parts. In S. Baker, J. Matas, R, Zabih, T. Kanade, & G. Medioni (eds.), IEEE Proc. Conference on Computer Vision and Pattern Recognition (pp. 18–23). June 19–21, Minneapolis, MN. Washington DC; IEEE Computer Society Press.

Fidler, S., Boben, M., & Leonardis, A. (2009). Learning hierarchical compositional representations of object structure. In S. Dickinson, A., Leonardis, B. Schiele, & M. Tarr (eds.), *Object categorization computer and human perspectives* (pp. 196–215). New York: Cambridge University Press.

Freuder, E. (1976). A Computer System for Visual Recognition Using Active Knowledge. PhD Thesis, AI-TR-345, Artificial Intelligence Lab, MIT.

Fries, P., Reynolds, J. H., Rorie, A. E., & Desimone, R. (2001). Modulation of oscillatory neuronal synchronization by selective visual attention. *Science, 291*, 1560–1563.

Frintrop, S., Rome, E., Christensen, H. (2010). Computational visual attention systems and their cognitive foundations: A survey. *ACM Transactions on Applied Perception* 7(1), article 6, 1–39.

Fukushima, K. (1986). A neural network model for selective attention in visual pattern recognition. *Biological Cybernetics, 55*(1), 5–15.

Fuster, J. M. (1990). Inferotemporal units in selective visual attention and short-term memory. *Journal of Neurophysiology, 64*, 681–697.

Fuster, J. M. (2008). *The prefrontal cortex*. San Diego: Academic Press.

Gao, D., Mahadevan, V., Vasconcelos, N. (2008). On the Plausibility of the Discriminant Center-Surround Hypothesis for Visual Saliency. *Journal of Vision* 8(7): article 13, 1–18.

Garey, M., & Johnson, D. (1979). *Computers and intractability: A guide to the theory of NP-completeness*. San Francisco: Freeman.

Gattass, R., Sousa, A. P., & Gross, C. G. (1988). Visuotopic organization and extent of V3 and V4 of the macaque. *Journal of Neuroscience, 8*, 1831–1845.

Ghose, G., & Maunsell, J. (2008). Spatial summation can explain the attentional modulation of neural responses to multiple stimuli in area V4. *Journal of Neuroscience, 28*(19), 5115–5126.

Gibson, J. J. (1979). *The ecological approach to visual perception.* Boston: Houghton, Mifflin and Company.

Gilbert, C. D., & Sigman, M. (2007). Brain states: Top-down influences in sensory processing. *Neuron, 54*, 677–696.

Giese, M., & Poggio, T. (2003). Neural mechanisms for the recognition of complex movements and actions. *Nature Reviews Neuroscience, 4*, 179–192.

Gottlieb, J. P., Kusunoki, M., & Goldberg, M. E. (1998). The representation of visual salience in monkey parietal cortex. *Nature, 391*, 481–484.

Grätzer, G. (1978). *General lattuce theory.* New York: Academic Press.

Graziano, M. S., Andersen, R. A., & Snowden, R. J. (1994). Tuning of MST neurons to spiral motions. *Journal of Neuroscience, 14*, 54–67.

Grill-Spector, K., & Kanwisher, N. (2005). Visual recognition: As soon as you know it is there, you know what it is. *Psychological Science, 16*, 152–160.

Grimson, W. E. L. (1990). The combinatorics of object recognition in cluttered environments using constrained search. *Artificial Intelligence, 44*(1–2), 121–165.

Groos, K. (1896). *Die Spiele der Thiere.* Jena: Fischer.

Gross, C. G., Bruce, C., Desimone, R., Fleming, J., & Gattass, R. (1981). Cortical visual areas of the temporal lobe. In C. N. Woolsey (ed.), *Cortical sensory organization.* Vol. 2, *Multiple visual areas* (pp. 187–216). Englewood Cliffs, NJ: Humana.

Grossberg, S. (1975). A neural model of attention, reinforcement, and discrimination learning. *International Review of Neurobiology, 18*, 263–327.

Grossberg, S. (1980). Biological competition: decision rules, pattern formation and oscillations. *Proceedings of the National Academy of Sciences of the United States of America, 77*, 2338–2342.

Grossberg, S. (1982). A psychophysiological theory of reinforcement, drive, motivation, and attention. *Journal of Theoretical Neurobiology, 1*, 286–369.

Grossberg, S., Mingolla, E., & Viswanathan, L. (2001). Neural dynamics of motion integration and segmentation within and across apertures. *Vision Research, 41*, 2521–2553.

Gueye, L., Legalett, E., Viallet, F., Trouche, E., & Farnarier, G. (2002). Spatial orienting of attention: a study of reaction time during pointing movement. *Neurophysiologie Clinique, 32*, 361–368.

Guillery, R. W., Feig, S. L., & Lozsádi, D. A. (1998). Paying attention to the thalamic reticular nucleus. *Trends in Neurosciences, 21*, 28–32.

Haenny, P. E., & Schiller, P. H. (1988). State dependent activity in monkey visual cortex. I. single cell activity in V1 and V4 on visual tasks. *Experimental Brain Research, 69*(2), 225–244.

Hafed, Z. M., & Clark, J. J. (2002). Microsaccades as an overt measure of covert attention shifts. *Vision Research, 42*(22), 2533–2545.

Hallett, P. (1978). Primary and Secondary Saccades to Goals Defined by Instructions. *Vision Research, 18*, 1279–1296.

Hamker, F. H. (1999). The Role of Feedback Connections in Task-Driven Visual Search. In D. Heinke, G. W. Humphreys & A. Olson (eds.), *Connectionist Models in Cognitive Neuroscience* (Proceedings of the 5th Neural Computation and Psychology Workshop London) (pp. 252–261). Berlin: Springer-Verlag.

Hamker, F. H. (2000). Distributed Competition in Directed Attention. In G. Baratoff & H. Neumann (eds.), Proceedings in Artificial Intelligence, Vol. 9. Dynamische Perzeption (Workshop der GI-Fachgruppe 1.0.4 Bildverstehen) (pp. 39–44). Berlin: AKA, Akademische Verlagsgesellschaft.

Hamker, F. H. (2005). The emergence of attention by population-based inference and its role in distributed processing and cognitive control of vision. *Computer Vision and Image Understanding, 100*, 64–106.

Hamker, F. H., & Zirnsak, M. (2006). V4 receptive field dynamics as predicted by a systems-level model of visual attention using feedback from the frontal eye field. *Neural Networks, 19*, 1371–1382.

Hamilton, W. (1859). *Lectures on metaphysics and logic*. Vol. 1, *Metaphysics*. Edinburgh: Blackwood.

Hanson, A. R., & Riseman, E. M. (1978). *Computer vision systems*. New York: Academic Press.

Hayhoe, M. M., & Ballard, D. H. (2005). Eye movements in natural behavior. *Trends in Cognitive Sciences*, *9*(4), 188–194.

Hebart, J. F. (1824). *Psychologie als Wissenschaft neu Gegründet auf Erfahrung. Metaphsyik und Mathematik*. Konigsberg: Unzer.

Heeger, D. (1992). Half-squaring in responses of cat simple cells. *Visual Neuroscience*, *9*, 181–197.

Heinke, D., & Humphreys, G. W. (1997). SAIM: A Model of Visual Attention and Neglect. 7th International Conference on Artificial Neural Networks, October 8–10, Lausanne, Switzerland. Berlin: Springer-Verlag.

von Helmholtz, H. (1860/1962). *Physiological optics*, Vol. 3 (3rd ed.) (translated by J. P. C. Southall). New York: Dover.

von Helmholtz, H. (1896/1989). Physiological optics (1896–2nd German Edition, translated by M. Mackeben. In K. Nakayama & M. Mackeben, Sustained and transient components of focal visual attention. *Vision Research*, *29*(11), 1631–1647.

Hernández-Peón, R., Scherrer, H., & Jouvet, M. (1955). Modification of electrical activity of cochlear nucleus during "attention" in unanesthetized cats. *Science*, *123*, 331–332.

Hillyard, S. A., Vogel, E. K., & Luck, S. J. (1998). Sensory gain control (amplification) as a mechanism of selective attention: electrophysiological and neuroimaging evidence. *Philosophical Transactions of the Royal Society of London. Series B, Biological Sciences*, *353*, 1257–1270.

Hobbes, T. (1655). *Elementorum Philosophiae Sectio Prima de Corpore*. London: Crook.

Hopf, J.-M., Boehler, C. N., Luck, S. J., Tsotsos, J. K., Heinze, H.-J., & Schoenfeld, M. A. (2006). Direct neurophysiological evidence for spatial suppression surrounding the focus of attention in vision. *Proceedings of the National Academy of Sciences of the United States of America*, *103*(4), 1053–1058.

Hopf, J.-M., Boehler, C. N., Schoenfeld, M. A., Heinze, H.-J., & Tsotsos, J. K. (2010). The spatial profile of the focus of attention in visual search: Insights from MEG recordings. *Vision Research*, *50*, 1312–1320.

Horwitz, G. D., & Newsome, W. T. (1999). Separate signals for target selection and movement specification in the superior colliculus. *Science*, *284*, 1158–1161.

Hubel, D., & Wiesel, T. (1962). Receptive fields, binocular interaction and functional architecture in the cat's visual cortex. *Journal of Physiology*, *160*(1), 106–154.

Hubel, D., & Wiesel, T. (1965). Receptive fields and functional architecture in two nonstriate visual areas (18 and 19) of the cat. *Journal of Neurophysiology*, *28*, 229–289.

Hubel, D., & Wiesel, T. (1969). Anatomical demonstration of columns in the monkey striate cortex. *Nature*, *221*(5182), 747–750.

Huffman, D. (1971). Impossible objects as nonsense sentences. In B. Meltzer & D. Michie (eds.), *Machine intelligence 6* (pp. 295–323). Edinburgh: Edinburgh University Press.

Hummel, J. E., & Biederman, I. (1992). Dynamic binding in a neural network for shape recognition. *Psychological Review*, *99*, 480–517.

Hummel, R. A., & Zucker, S. W. (1983). On the foundations of relaxation labeling processes. *IEEE Transactions on Pattern Analysis and Machine Intelligence*, *5*, 267–287.

Humphreys, G., & Muller, H. (1993). Search via recursive rejection (SERR): A connectionist model of visual search. *Cognitive Psychology*, *25*, 45–110.

Itti, L., & Baldi, P. (2006). Bayesian surprise attracts human attention. *Advances in Neural Information Processing Systems*, *18*, 547–554.

Itti, L., & Koch, C. (2000). A saliency-based search mechanism for overt and covert shifts of visual attention. *Vision Research*, *40*(10–12), 1489–1506.

Itti, L., & Koch, C. (2001). Computational modeling of visual attention. *Nature Reviews Neuroscience*, *2*, 1–11.

Itti, L., Koch, C., & Niebur, E. (1998). A model for saliency-based visual attention for rapid scene analysis. *IEEE Transactions on Pattern Analysis and Machine Intelligence*, *20*, 1254–1259.

Itti, L., Rees, G., & Tsotsos, J. K. (eds.) (2005). *Neurobiology of attention*. Amsterdam: Elsevier Press.

Izhikevich, E. M. (2003). Simple model of spiking neurons. *IEEE Transactions on Neural Networks*, *14*, 1569–1572.

Izhikevich, E. M. (2004). Which model to use for cortical spiking neurons? *IEEE Transactions on Neural Networks*, *5*, 1063–1070.

James, W. (1890). *Principles of psychology*. New York: Holt.

Jenkin, M., Tsotsos, J. (1994). Active Stereo Vision and Cyclotorsion. In K. Bowyer, L. Shapiro, & S. Tanimoto (eds.), Proceedings Computer Vision and Pattern Recognition (pp. 806–811). Seattle, June 21–23. Washington DC: IEEE Computer Society Press.

Jenkin, M., Tsotsos, J., & Dudek, G. (1994). The Horoptor and Active Cyclotorsion. In *IAPR Conference on Pattern Recognition* (Vol. A, pp. 707–710). Jerusalem. International Association for Pattern Recognition.

Jie, L., & Clark, J. J. (2005). Microsaccadic eye movements during ocular pursuit. [abstract]. *Journal of Vision*, *5*(8), 697a.

Johnson, D. (1990). A Catalog of Complexity Classes. In J. van Leeuwen (ed.), *A Handbook of theoretical computer science* (Vol. A). Amsterdam: Elsevier Science Publishers.

Jolion, J.-M., & Rosenfeld, A. (1994). *A pyramid framework for early vision*. Dordrecht: Kluwer.

Jordan, H., Tipper, S. (1998). Object-based inhibition of return in static displays. *Psychonomic Bulletin & Review*, *5*(3), 504–509.

Kahneman, D. (1973). *Attention and effort*. Engelwood Cliffs, NJ: Prentice-Hall.

Kant, E. (1979). Efficiency Considerations in Program Synthesis: A Knowledge-Based Approach. PhD Thesis, Stanford University.

Kapadia, M., Ito, M., Gilbert, C. D., & Westheimer, G. (1995). Improvement in visual sensitivity by changes in local context: parallel studies in human observers and in V1 of alert monkeys. *Neuron*, *15*, 843–856.

Kastner, S., De Weerd, P., Desimone, R., & Ungerleider, L. (1998). Mechanisms of directed attention in the human extrastriate cortex as revealed by functional MRI. *Science*, *282*, 108–111.

Kastner, S., Pinsk, M., De Weerd, P., Desimone, R., & Ungerleider, L. (1999). Increased activity in human visual cortex during directed attention in the absence of visual stimulation. *Neuron*, *22*, 751–761.

Kastner, S., Saalmann, Y. B., & Schneider, K. A. (2011). Thalamic control of visual attention. In R. Mangun (ed.), *Neuroscience of attention*. New York: Oxford University Press.

Kelly, M. (1971). Edge detection in pictures by computer using planning. *Machine Intelligence*, *6*, 397–409.

Khayat, P., Niebergall, R., & Martinez-Trujillo, J. (2010). Attention differentially modulates similar neuronal responses evoked by varying contrast and direction stimuli in area MT. *Journal of Neuroscience*, *30*(6), 2188–2197.

Kirsch, R., Cahn, L., Ray, C., & Urban, G. (1957). Experiments in Processing Pictorial Information with a Digital Computer. In Proc. Eastern Joint Computer Conference (pp. 221–229). New York: Spartan Books.

Kirousis, L., & Papadimitriou, C. (1988). The complexity of recognizing polyhedral scenes. *Journal of Computer and System Sciences*, *37*, 14–38.

Klein, R. M. (1980). Does oculomotor readiness mediate cognitive control of visual attention? In R. Nickerson (ed.), *Attention and performance* (Vol. 8, pp. 259–276). New York: Academic Press.

Klein, R. M. (2000). Inhibition of return. *Trends in Cognitive Sciences*, *4*, 138–147.

Klein, R. M. (2004). On the control of visual orienting. In M. I. Posner (ed.), *Cognitive neuroscience of attention* (pp. 29–44). New York, London: The Guilford Press.

Koch, C. (1984). A Theoretical Analysis of the Electrical Properties of an X-cell in the Cat's LGN: Does the Spine-Triad Circuit Subserve Selective Visual Attention? Artificial Intelligence Memo 787, February. Artificial Intelligence Laboratory, MIT.

Koch, C. (1999). *Biophysics of computation: Information processing in single neurons*. New York: Oxford University Press.

Koch, C., & Ullman, S. (1985). Shifts in selective visual attention: Towards the underlying neural circuitry. *Human Neurobiology, 4,* 219–227.

Koenderink, J. J., & van Doorn, A. J. (1976). Local structure of movement parallax of the plane. *Journal of the Optical Society of America, 66,* 717–723.

Köhler, W. (1929). *Gestalt psychology.* London: Liveright.

Kondo, H., & Komatsu, H. (2000). Suppression on neural responses by a metacontrast masking stimulus in monkey V4. *Neuroscience Research, 36,* 27–53.

Knudsen, E. (2007). Fundamental components of attention. *Annual Review of Neuroscience, 30,* 57–78.

Kulpe, O. (1902). Uber die objectivirung und subjectivirung von sinneseindruken. *Philosophische Studien, 19,* 508–536.

Kustov, A. A., & Robinson, D. L. (1996). Shared neural control of attentional shifts and eye movements. *Nature, 384,* 74–77.

Lagae, L., Maes, H., Raiguel, S., Xiao, D. K., & Orban, G. A. (1994). Response of macaque STS neurons to optic flow components: a comparison of areas MT and MST. *Journal of Neurophysiology, 71*(5), 1597–1626.

Lai, Y. (1992). Experiments with Motion Grouping. MSc Thesis, Department of Computer Science, University of Toronto.

Lamme, V., & Roelfsema, P. (2000). The distinct modes of vision offered by feedforward and recurrent processing. *Trends in Neurosciences, 23,* 571–579.

Lanyon, L. J., & Denham, S. L. (2004). A model of active visual search with object-based attention guiding scan paths. *Neural Networks, 17,* 873–897.

LaBerge, D., & Brown, V. (1989). Theory of attentional operations in shape identification. *Psychological Review, 96*(1), 101–124.

Lauritzen, T., D'Esposti, M., Heeger, D., Silver, M. (2009). Top-down flow of visual spatial attention signals from parietal to occipital cortex. *Journal of Vision, 9*(13):18, 1–14.

Lawler, E., & Wood, D. (1966). Branch-and-bound methods: A survey. *Operations Research, 14*(4), 699–719.

Lee, D. K., Itti, L., Koch, C., & Braun, J. (1999). Attention activates winner-take-all competition among visual filters. *Nature Neuroscience, 2*(4), 375–381.

Lee, J., & Maunsell, J. H. (2009). A normalization model of attentional modulation of single unit responses. *PLoS ONE, 4,* e4651.

Lee, J., & Maunsell, J. H. (2010). Attentional modulation of MT neurons with single or multiple stimuli in their receptive fields. *Journal of Neuroscience, 30*(8), 3058–3066.

Lavie, N. (1995). Perceptual load as a necessary condition for selective attention. *Journal of Experimental Psychology, 21*(3), 451–468.

Lehky, S. R., & Sejnowski, T. J. (1988). Network model of shape-from-shading: neural function arises from both receptive and projective fields. *Nature, 333,* 452–454.

Leibnitz, G. W. (1765). Nouveaux essais sur l'entendement humain. In R. E. Raspe (ed.), *Oeuvres Philosophiques de feu M. Leibnitz.* Amsterdam, Leipzig: Screuder.

Lennie, P. (2003). The cost of cortical computation. *Current Biology, 13,* 493–497.

Li, Z. (2002). A saliency map in primary visual cortex. *Trends in Cognitive Sciences, 6*(1), 9–16.

Liu, Y. (2002). Localizing and Labelling Simple Motion Patterns in Image Sequences. MSc Thesis, Department of Computer Science, York University.

Loach, D., Frischen, A., Bruce, N., & Tsotsos, J. K. (2008). An attentional mechanism for selecting appropriate actions afforded by graspable objects. *Psychological Science, 19*(12), 1253–1257.

Logan, G. D. (1996). The CODE theory of visual attention: an integration of space-based and object-based attention. *Psychological Review, 103,* 603–649.

Logan, G. D. (2002). An instance theory of attention and memory. *Psychological Review, 109*(2), 376–400.

Longuet-Higgins, H. C., & Prazdny, K. (1980). The interpretation of a moving retinal image. *Proceedings of the Royal Society of London. Series B. Biological Sciences*, *208*(1173), 385–397.

Lowe, D. (1990). Probability theory as an alternative to complexity. *Behavioral and Brain Sciences*, *13*(3), 451–452.

Lu, Z. L., & Sperling, G. (1995). The functional architecture of human visual motion perception. *Vision Research*, *35*(19), 2697–2722.

Luck, S., Chelazzi, L., Hillyard, S., & Desimone, R. (1997a). Neural mechanisms of spatial selective attention in areas V1, V2, and V4 of macaque visual cortex. *Journal of Neurophysiology*, *77*, 24–42.

Luck, S., Girelli, M., McDermott, M., & Ford, M. (1997b). Bridging the gap between monkey neurophysiology and human perception: an ambiguity resolution theory of visual selective attention. *Cognitive Psychology*, *33*, 64–87.

Lünnenburger, L., & Hoffman, K.-P. (2003). Arm movement and gap as factors influencing the reaction time of the second saccade in a double-step task. *European Journal of Neuroscience*, *17*, 2481–2491.

MacKay, D. (1973). Aspects of the theory of comprehension, memory and attention. *Quarterly Journal of Experimental Psychology*, *25*, 22–40.

Mackworth, A. K., & Freuder, E. C. (1985). The complexity of some polynomial network consistency algorithms for constraint satisfaction problems. *Artificial Intelligence*, *25*, 65–74.

Macmillan, N. A., & Creelman, C. D. (2005). *Detection theory: A user's guide*. New York: Lawrence Erlbaum Associates.

Marr, D. (1982). *Vision: A computational investigation into the human representation and processing of visual information*. New York: Henry Holt and Co.

Maunsell, J. H. R., & Van Essen, D. C. (1983). Functional properties of neurons in middle temporal visual area of the macaque monkey. I. Selectivity for stimulus direction, speed and orientation. *Journal of Neurophysiology*, *49*, 1127–1147.

Maunsell, J. H. R., & Treue, S. (2006). Feature-based attention in visual cortex. *Trends in Neurosciences*, *29*, 317–322.

Martinez-Trujillo, J., & Treue, S. (2004). Feature-based attention increases the selectivity of population responses in primate visual cortex. *Current Biology*, *14*(9), 744–751.

Martinez-Trujillo, J. C., Cheyne, D., Gaetz, W., Simine, E., & Tsotsos, J. K. (2007). Activation of area MT/V5 and the right inferior parietal cortex during the discrimination of transient direction changes in translational motion. *Cerebral Cortex*, *17*(7), 1733–1739.

Martinez-Trujillo, J. C., Tsotsos, J. K., Simine, E., Pomplun, M., Wildes, R., Treue, S., et al. (2005). Selectivity for speed gradients in human area MT/V5. *Neuroreport*, *16*(5), 435–438.

May, P. (2006). The mammalian superior colliculus: laminar structure and connections. *Progress in Brain Research*, *151*, 321–378.

Mayo, O. (2008). Intra-thalamic mechanisms of visual attention. *Journal of Neurophysiology*, *101*, 1123–1125.

McAlonan, K., Cavanaugh, H. J., & Wurtz, R. (2008). Guarding the gateway to cortex with attention in visual thalamus. *Nature*, *456*(7220), 391–394.

McCarley, J. S., & Mounts, J. (2007). Localized attentional interference affects object individuation, not feature detection. *Perception*, *36*, 17–32.

McCullough, W. S., & Pitts, W. (1943). A logical calculus of ideas immanent in nervous activity. *Bulletin of Mathematical Biophysics*, *5*, 115–133.

McPeek, R. M., & Keller, E. L. (2002). Saccade target selection in the superior colliculus during a visual search task. *Journal of Neurophysiology*, *88*, 2019–2034.

Meese, T. S., & Anderson, S. J. (2002). Spiral mechanisms are required to account for summation of complex motion components. *Vision Research*, *42*, 1073–1080.

Mehta, A., Ulbert, I., & Schroeder, C. (2000). Intermodal selective attention in monkeys. i: distribution and timing of effects across visual areas. *Cerebral Cortex*, *10*(4), 343–358.

Melcher, D., Papathomas, T. V., & Vidnyánsky, Z. (2005). Implicit attentional selection of bound visual features. *Neuron, 46*, 723–729.

Merriam-Webster's medical dictionary. (2007). Springfield, MA: Merriam-Webster.

Metzger, W. (1974). Consciousness, perception and action. In E. C. Carterette and M. P. Friedman (eds.), *Handbook of perception*. Vol. 1, *Historical and philosophical roots of perception*. New York: Academic Press.

Milios, E., Jenkin, M., & Tsotsos, J. (1993). Design and performance of trish, a binocular robot head with torsional eye movements. (Special Issue on Active Robot Vision: Camera Heads, Model Based Navigation and Reactive Control.) *International Journal of Pattern Recognition and Artifici*al Intelligence, *7*(1), 51–68.

Miller, E. K., Gochin, P. M., & Gross, C. G. (1993). Suppression of visual responses of neurons in inferior temporal cortex of the awake macaque by addition of a second stimulus. *Brain Research, 616*(1–2), 25–29.

Milner, P. (1974). A model for visual shape recognition. *Psychological Review, 81*, 521–535.

Mirpour, K., Arcizet, F., Ong, W. S., & Bisley, J. W. (2009). Been there, seen that: a neural mechanism for performing efficient visual search. *Journal of Neurophysiology, 102*, 3481–3491.

Missal, M., Vogels, R., Li, C.-Y., & Orban, G. (1999). Shape interactions in macaque inferior temporal neurons. *Journal of Neurophysiology, 82*(1), 131–142.

Monosov, I., & Thompson, K. (2009). Frontal eye field activity enhances object identification during covert visual search. *Journal of Neurophysiology, 102*, 3656–3672.

Moore, T., & Fallah, M. (2001). Control of eye movements and spatial attention. *Proceedings of the National Academy of Sciences of the United States of America, 98*(3), 1273–1276.

Moore, T., & Fallah, M. (2004). Microstimulation of the frontal eye field and its effects on covert spatial attention. *Journal of Neurophysiology, 91*, 152–162.

Moran, J., & Desimone, R. (1985). Selective Attention Gates Visual Processing in the Extrastriate Cortex. *Science, 229*, 782–784.

Moravec, H. (1981). Rover Visual Obstacle Avoidance. In P. Hayes & R. Schank (eds.), Proc. 7th Int. J. Conference on Artificial Intelligence (pp. 785–790). August 24–28, Vancouver, BC.

Moray, N. (1969). *Attention: Selective processes in vision and hearing*. London: Hutchinson.

Motter, B. C. (1993). Focal attention produces spatially selective processing in visual cortical areas V1, V2, and V4 in the presence of competing stimuli. *Journal of Neurophysiology, 70*, 909–919.

Motter, B. C., & Belky, E. J. (1998a). The zone of focal attention during active visual search. *Vision Research, 38*, 1007–1022.

Motter, B. C., & Belky, E. J. (1998b). The guidance of eye movements during active visual search. *Vision Research, 38*, 1805–1815.

Mounts, J. R. (2000a). Attentional capture by abrupt onsets and feature singletons produces inhibitory surrounds. *Perception & Psychophysics, 62*, 1485–1493.

Mounts, J. R. (2000b). Evidence for suppressive mechanisms in attentional selection: feature singletons produce inhibitory surrounds. *Perception & Psychophysics, 62*, 969–983.

Mozer, M. C. (1991). *The perception of multiple objects: A connectionist approach*. Cambridge, MA: MIT Press.

Mozer, M. C., & Sitton, M. (1998). Computational modeling of spatial attention. In H. Pashler (ed.), *Attention* (pp. 341–393). London: UCL Press.

Mozer, M. C., Zemel, R. S., Behrmann, M., & Williams, C. (1992). Learning to segment images using dynamic feature binding. *Neural Computation, 4*, 650–665.

Muerle, J. L., & Allen, D. C. (1968). Experimental evaluation of techniques for automatic segmentation of objects in a complex scene. In G. C. Cheng, R. S. Ledley, D. K. Pollock, & A. Rosenfeld (eds.), *Pictorial pattern recognition* (pp. 3–13). Washington, DC: Thompson Book Co.

Müller, N., & Kleinschmidt, A. (2004). The attentional spotlights penumbra: Center-surround modulation in striate cortex. *Neuroreport, 15*(6), 977–980.

Müller, N. G., Mollenhauer, M., Rosler, A., & Kleinschmidt, A. (2005). The attentional field has a Mexican hat distribution. *Vision Research*, *45*, 1129–1137.

Mumford, D. (1991). On the computational architecture of the neocortex i. the role of the thalamo-cortical loop. *Biological Cybernetics*, *65*, 135–145.

Nagy, A., & Sanchez, R. (1990). Critical color differences determined with a visual search task. *Journal of the Optical Society of America. A, Optics and Image Science*, *7*, 1209–1217.

Nakayama, K. (1990). The iconic bottleneck and the tenuous link between early visual processing and perception. In C. Blakemore (ed.), *Vision: Coding and efficiency* (pp. 411–422). Cambridge, UK: Cambridge University Press.

Navalpakkam, V., & Itti, L. (2005). Modeling the influence of task on attention. *Vision Research*, *45*(2), 205–231.

Navalpakkam, V., & Itti, L. (2007). Search goal tunes visual features optimally. *Neuron*, *53*(4), 605–617.

Neisser, U. (1964). Visual search. *Scientific American*, *210*(6), 94–102.

Neisser, U. (1967). *Cognitive psychology*. New York: Appleton-Century-Crofts.

Niebur, E., & Koch, C. (1994). A model for the neuronal implementation of selective visual attention based on temporal correlation among neurons. *Journal of Computational Neuroscience*, *1*(1), 141–158.

Niebur, E., Koch, C., & Rosin, C. (1993). An oscillation-based model for the neural basis of attention. *Vision Research*, *33*, 2789–2802.

Norman, D. (1968). Toward a theory of memory and attention. *Psychological Review*, *75*, 522–536.

Norman, D. A., & Shallice, T. (1980). *Attention to action: Willed and automatic control of behavior (CHIP Rep. No. 99)*. San Diego: University of California.

Nowlan, S., & Sejnowski, T. (1995). A selection model for motion processing in area mt of primates. *Journal of Neuroscience*, *15*(2), 1195–1214.

O'Connor, D., Fukui, M., Pinsk, M., & Kastner, S. (2002). Attention modulates responses in the human lateral geniculate nucleus. *Nature Neuroscience*, *5*(11), 1203–1209.

Oliva, A., Torralba, A., Casthelano, M., & Henderson, J. (2003). Top-Down Control of Visual Attention in Object Detection. In Proceedings of the IEEE International Conference Image Processing, Vol. 1 (pp. 253–256). September 14–18, Barcelona, Spain. Washington DC: IEEE Computer Society Press.

Olshausen, B., Anderson, C., & Van Essen, D. (1993). A neurobiological model of visual attention and invariant pattern recognition based on dynamic routing of information. *Journal of Neuroscience*, *13*(11), 4700–4719.

Olson, G. M., & Sherman, T. (1983). Attention, learning and memory in infants. In M. Haith and J. Campos (eds.), *Handbook of child psychology*. Vol. 2, *Infancy and the biology of development* (pp. 1001–1080). New York: Wiley.

Orban, G. A. (2008). Higher order visual processing in macaque extrastriate cortex. *Physiological Reviews*, *88*, 59–89.

Orban, G. A., Kennedy, H., & Bullier, J. (1986). Velocity sensitivity and direction selectivity. *Journal of Neurophysiology*, *56*(2), 462–480.

Østerberg, G. A. (1935). Topography of the layer of rods and cones in the human retina. *Acta Ophthalmologica*, *6*(Suppl), 1–102.

Palmer, J. (1995). Attention in visual search: distinguishing four causes of setsize effects. *Current Directions in Psychological Science*, *4*, 118–123.

Palmer, J., & Moore, C. (2009). Using a filtering task to measure the spatial extent of selective attention. *Vision Research*, *49*, 1045–1064.

Palmer, S. E. (1999). *Vision science—Photons to phenomenology*. Cambridge, MA: MIT Press.

Panum, P. L. (1858). *Physiologische Untersuchungen ueber das Sehen mit zwei Augen*. Kiel, Germany: Schwers.

Papadimitriou, C. (1994). *Computational complexity*. Reading, MA: Addison-Wesley.

Papalambros, P. Y., & Wilde, D. J. (2000). *Principles of optimal design: Modeling and computation.* New York: Cambridge University Press.

Parodi, P., Lanciwicki, R., Vijh, A., & Tsotsos, J. K. (1996). Empirically-Derived Estimates of the Complexity of Labeling Line Drawings of Polyhedral Scenes. RBCV-TR-96–52. Department of Computer Science, University of Toronto.

Parodi, P., Lanciwicki, R., Vijh, A., & Tsotsos, J. K. (1998). Empirically-derived estimates of the complexity of labeling line drawings of polyhedral scenes. *Artificial Intelligence, 105,* 47–75.

Pashler, H. (1998a). *The psychology of attention.* Cambridge, MA: The MIT Press.

Pashler, H. (ed.), (1998b). *Attention.* East Sussex, UK: Psychology Press.

Pastukhov, A., Fischer, F., & Braun, J. (2009). Visual attention is a single, integrated resource. *Vision Research, 49,* 1166–1173.

Perona, P. (2009). Visual recognition circa 2008. In S. Dickinson, A. Leonardis, B. Schiele, & M. Tarr (eds.), *Object categorization* (pp. 55–68). New York: Cambridge University Press.

Perrone, J. A., & Thiele, A. (2002). A model of speed tuning in MT neurons. *Vision Research, 42,* 1035–1051.

Petermann, B. (1929). *Die Wertheimer-Koffka-Köhlerische Gestalttheorie und das Gestaltproblem.* Liepzig: Barth.

Petersen, S. E., Robinson, D. L., & Morris, J. D. (1987). Contributions of the pulvinar to visual spatial attention. *Neuropsychologia, 25,* 97–105.

Phillips, A., & Segraves, M. (2009). Predictive activity in macaque frontal eye field neurons during natural scene searching. *Journal of Neurophysiology, 103,* 1238–1252.

Pillsbury, W. B. (1908). *Attention.* New York: MacMillan.

Poggio, T. (1984). Vision By Man And Machine: How The Brain Processes Visual Information May Be Suggested by Studies in Computer Vision (and Vice Versa). Artificial Intelligence Memo 776, March. Artificial Intelligence Laboratory, MIT.

Pomerantz, J. R., & Pristach, E. A. (1989). Emergent features, attention, and perceptual glue in visual form perception. *Journal of Experimental Psychology. Human Perception and Performance, 15*(4), 635–649.

Pomplun, M., Shen, J., & Reingold, E. M. (2003). Area activation: A computational model of saccadic selectivity in visual search. *Cognitive Science, 27,* 299–312.

Posner, M. I. (1980). Orienting of attention. *Quarterly Journal of Experimental Psychology, 32*(1), 3–25.

Posner, M. I., & DiGirolamo, G. J. (1998). Executive attention: Conflict, Target detection, and cognitive control. In R. Parasuraman (ed.), *The attentive brain.* Cambridge, MA: MIT Press.

Posner, M. I., & Petersen, S. E. (1990). The attention system of the human brain. *Annual Review of Neuroscience, 13,* 25–42.

Posner, M. I., & Snyder, C. R. R. (1975). Attention and cognitive control. In R. Solso (ed.), *Information processing and cognition: The Loyola symposium.* Hillsdale, NJ: Lawrence Erlbaum.

Posner, M. I., Nissen, M., & Ogden, W. (1978). Attended and unattended processing modes: the role of set for spatial locations. In H. L. Pick Jr. & E. Saltzman (eds.), *Modes of perceiving and processing information* (pp. 137–158). Hillsdale, NJ: Erlbaum.

Posner, M. I., Petersen, S. E., Fox, P. T., & Raichle, M. E. (1988). Localization of cognitive operations in the human brain. *Science, 17*(240-4859), 1627–1631.

Posner, M. I., Rafal, R. D., Choate, L. S., & Vaughan, J. (1985). Inhibition of return: neural basis and function. *Cognitive Neuropsychology, 2*(3), 211–228.

Posner, M. I., Snyder, C., & Davidson, B. (1980). Attention and the detection of signals. *Journal of Experimental Psychology. General, 109,* 160–174.

Postma, E. O., et al. (1997). SCAN: A scalable model of attentional selection. *Neural Networks, 10*(6), 993–1015.

Prime, S. L., Tsotsos, L., Keith, G. P., & Crawford, J. D. (2007). Capacity of transsaccadic integration. *Experimental Brain Research, 180*(4), 609–628.

Pylyshyn, Z. (1973). What the mind's eye tells the mind's brain: A critique of mental imagery. *Psychological Bulletin, 80*(1), 1–24.

Rao, R., Zelinsky, G., Hayhoe, M., & Ballard, D. (2002). Eye movements in iconic visual search. *Vision Research, 42*(11), 1447–1463.

Raymond, J. E., Shapiro, K. L., & Arnell, K. M. (1992). Temporary suppression of visual processing in an RSVP task: an attentional blink?, *Journal of Experimental Psychology: Human Perception and Performance 18* (3), 849–860.

Read, H. L., & Siegel, R. M. (1997). Modulation of responses to optic flow in area 7a by retinotopic and oculomotor cues in monkey. *Cerebral Cortex, 7*, 647–661.

Recanzone, G., Wurtz, R., & Schwarz, U. (1997). Responses of MT and MST neurons to one and two moving objects in the receptive field. *Journal of Neurophysiology, 78*(6), 2904–2915.

Rensink, R. (1989). A New Proof of the NP-Completeness of Visual Match. Technical Report 89–22. Department of Computer Science, University of British Columbia.

Rensink, R. A., O'Regan, J. K., & Clark, J. J. (1997). To see or not to see: The need for attention to perceive changes in scenes. *Psychological Science, 8*(5), 368–373.

Reynolds, J., & Chelazzi, L. (2004). Attentional modulation of visual processing. *Annual Review of Neuroscience, 27*, 611–647.

Reynolds, J., & Desimone, R. (1998). Interacting roles of attention and visual salience in V4. *Journal of Neurophysiology, 80*, 2918–2940.

Reynolds, J., & Desimone, R. (1999). The role of neural mechanisms of attention in solving the binding problem. *Neuron, 24*, 19–29.

Reynolds, J., & Heeger, D. (2009). The normalization model of attention. *Neuron, 61*, 168–185.

Reynolds, J., Chelazzi, L., & Desimone, R. (1999). Competitive mechanisms subserve attention in macaque areas V2 and V4. *Journal of Neuroscience, 19*(5), 1736–1753.

Reynolds, J. H., Alborzian, S., & Stoner, G. R. (2003). Exogenously cued attention triggers competitive selection of surfaces. *Vision Research, 43*(1), 59–66.

Reynolds, J. H., Pasternak, T., & Desimone, R. (2000). Attention increases sensitivity of V4 neurons. *Neuron, 26*, 703–714.

Rizzolatti, G., Riggio, L., Dascola, I., & Umilta, C. (1987). Reorienting attention across the horizontal and vertical meridians—Evidence in favor of a premotor theory of attention. *Neuropsychologia, 25*, 31–40.

Roberts, L. G. (1965). Machine perception of three-dimensional solids. In J. T. Tippett et al., (eds.), *Optical and electro-optical information processing*. Cambridge, MA: MIT Press.

Robinson, D. L., & Petersen, S. E. (1992). The pulvinar and visual salience. *Trends in Neurosciences, 15*(4), 127–132.

Rodríguez-Sánchez, A. J., Simine, E., & Tsotsos, J. K. (2007). Attention and visual search. *International Journal of Neural Systems, 17*(4), 275–288.

Roelfsema, P. R., Lamme, V. A., & Spekreijse, H. (1998). Object-based attention in the primary visual cortex of the macaque monkey. *Nature, 395*(6700), 376–381.

Roelfsema, P. R., Tolboom, M. &Khayat, P. S. (2007). Different processing phases for features, figures, and selective attention in the primary visual cortex. *Neuron, 56*, 785–792.

Rolls, E. T., & Deco, G. (2002). *Computational neuroscience of vision*. New York, NY: Oxford University Press.

Rolls, E., & Tovee, M. (1995). The responses of single neurons in the temporal visual cortical areas of the macaque when more than one stimulus is present in the receptive field. *Journal of Experimental Brain Research, 103*(3), 409–420.

Rolls, E., Aggelopoulos, N., & Zheng, F. (2003). The receptive fields of inferior temporal cortex neurons in natural scenes. *Journal of Neuroscience, 23*(1), 339–348.

Rosenblatt, F. (1961). *Principles of neurodynamics: Perceptions and the theory of brain mechanisms*. Washington, DC: Spartan Books.

Rosenfeld, A., Hummel, R. A., & Zucker, S. W. (1976). Scene labeling by relaxation operations. *IEEE Transactions on Systems, Man, and Cybernetics*, *6*(6), 420–433.

Roskies, A. (1999). The binding problem—Introduction. *Neuron*, *24*, 7–9.

Rothenstein, A., & Tsotsos, J. K. (2008) Attention links sensing with perception. *Image & Vision Computing Journal* (Special Issue on Cognitive Vision Systems; H. Buxton, ed.), *26*(1), 114–126.

Rothenstein, A., Rodríguez-Sánchez, A., Simine, E., & Tsotsos, J. K. (2008). Visual feature binding within the selective tuning attention framework. *International Journal of Pattern Recognition and Artificial Intelligence* (Special Issue on Brain, Vision and Artificial Intelligence), *22*(5), 861–881.

Saito, H., Yukie, M., Tanaka, K., Hikosaka, K., Fukada, Y., & Iwai, E. (1986). Integration of direction signals of image motion in the superior temporal sulcus of the macaque monkey. *Journal of Neuroscience*, *6*, 145–157.

Salin, P.-A., & Bullier, J. (1995). Corticocortical connections in the visual system: Structure and function. *Physiological Reviews*, *75*(1), 107–154.

Sakata, H., Shibutani, H., Ito, Y., & Tsurugai, K. (1986). Parietal cortical neurons responding to rotary movement of visual vtimulus in space. *Experimental Brain Research*, *61*, 658–663.

Salinas, E., & Abbott, L. F. (1997). Invariant visual responses from attentional gain fields. *Journal of Neurophysiology*, *77*(6), 3267–3272.

Sandon, P. (1990). Simulating visual attention. *Journal of Cognitive Neuroscience*, *2*, 213–231.

Scalf, P., & Beck, D. (2010). Competition in visual cortex impedes attention to multiple items. *Journal of Neuroscience*, *30*(1), 161–169.

Schall, J. D. (2001). Neural basis of deciding, choosing and acting. *Nature Reviews Neuroscience*, *2*, 33–42.

Schall, J. D., & Thompson, K. G. (1999). Neural selection and control of visually guided eye movements. *Annual Review of Neuroscience*, *22*, 241–259.

Schall, J. D., Sato, T., Thompson, K., Vaughn, A., & Chi-Hung, J. (2004). Effects of search efficiency on surround suppression during visual selection in frontal eye field. *Journal of Neurophysiology*, *91*, 2765–2769.

Sejnowksi, T., & Paulsen, O. (2006). Network oscillations: Emerging computational principles. *Journal of Neuroscience*, *26*(6), 1673–1676.

Serences, J. T., & Yantis, S. (2007). Representation of attentional priority in human occipital, parietal and frontal cortex. *Cerebral Cortex*, *17*, 284–293.

Shadlen, M., & Movshon, A. (1999). Synchrony unbound: A critical evaluation of the temporal binding hypothesis. *Neuron*, *24*, 67–77.

Shallice, T. (1988). *From neuropsychology to mental structure*. Cambridge, UK: Cambridge University Press.

Sheinberg, D. L., & Logothetis, N. K. (2001). Noticing familiar objects in real world scenes: the role of temporal cortical neurons in natural vision. *Journal of Neuroscience*, *21*(4), 1340–1350.

Sheliga, B. M., Riggio, L., Craighero, L., & Rizzolatti, G. (1995). Spatial attention-determined modifications in saccade trajectories. *Neuroreport*, *6*(3), 585–588.

Sherman, S. M., & Koch, C. (1986). The control of retinogeniculate transmission in the mammalian lateralgeniculate nucleus. *Experimental Brain Research*, *63*, 1–20.

Shiffrin, R. M., & Schneider, W. (1977). Controlled and automatic human information processing: II: Perceptual learning, automatic attending, and a general theory. *Psychological Review*, *84*, 127–190.

Shipp, S. (2003). The functional logic of cortico-pulvinar connections. *Philosophical Transactions of the Royal Society of London, Series B, Biological Sciences*, *358*(1438), 1605–1624.

Shipp, S. (2004). The brain circuitry of attention. *Trends in Cognitive Sciences*, *8*(5), 223–230.

Shubina, K., & Tsotsos, J. K. (2010). Visual search for an object in a 3D environment using a mobile robot. *Computer Vision and Image Understanding*, *114*(5), 535–547.

Shulman, G. L., Remington, R., & McLean, J. P. (1979). Moving attention through visual space. *Journal of Experimental Psychology*, *92*, 428–431.

Siegel, R. M., & Read, H. L. (1997). Analysis of optic flow in the monkey parietal area 7a. *Cerebral Cortex*, 7, 327–346.

Sillito, A., Cudiero, J., & Jones, H. (2006). Always returning: Feedback and sensory processing in visual cortex and thalamus. *Trends in Neurosciences*, 29(6), 307–316.

Simine, E. (2006). Motion Model: Extending and Improving Performance and Providing Biological Evidence for Motion Change Detectors. MSc Thesis, Department of Computer Science and Engineering, York University.

Simoncelli, E., & Heeger, D. (1988). A model of neuronal responses in visual area MT. *Vision Research*, 38(5), 743–761.

Singer, W. (1977). Control of thalamic transmission by corticofugal and ascending reticular pathways in the visual system. *Physiological Reviews*, 57, 386–420.

Singer, W. (1999). Neuronal synchrony: A versatile code for the definition of relations? *Neuron*, 24, 49–65.

Singer, W. (2007). Binding by synchrony. *Scholarpedia*, 2(12), 1657.

Singer, W., & Gray, C. M. (1995). Visual feature integration and the temporal correlation hypothesis. *Annual Review of Neuroscience*, 18, 555–586.

Slotnick, S. D., Hopfinger, J. B., Klein, S. A., & Sutter, E. E. (2002). Darkness beyond the light: attentional inhibition surrounding the classic spotlight. *Neuroreport*, 13(6), 773–778.

Smith, A. T., Singh, K. D., & Greenlee, M. W. (2000). Attentional suppression of activity in the human visual cortex. *Neuroreport*, 11, 271–277.

Sommer, M., & Wurtz, R. (2004a). What the brain stem tells the frontal cortex. I. Oculomotor signals sent from superior colliculus to frontal eye field via mediodorsal thalamus. *Journal of Neurophysiology*, 91, 1381–1402.

Sommer, M., & Wurtz, R. (2004b). What the brain stem tells the frontal cortex. II. Role of the SC-MD-FEF pathway in corollary discharge. *Journal of Neurophysiology*, 91, 1403–1423.

Spearman, C. E. (1937). *Psychology down the ages*. New York: MacMillan.

Sperling, G. (1960). The information available in brief visual presentations. *Psychological Monographs: General and Applied*, 74(498), 1–21.

Sperling, G., & Dosher, B. A. (1986). Strategy and optimization in human information processing. In K. Boff, L. Kaufman & J. Thomas (eds.), *Handbook of perception and human performance*. Vol. 1, *Sensory processes and perception* (pp. 2-1–2-65). New York: Wiley.

Sperling, G., & Melchner, M. J. (1978). Visual search, visual attention, and the attention operating characteristic. In J. Requin (ed.), *Attention and performance VII* (pp. 675–686). Hillsdale, NJ: Erlbaum.

Spratling, M., & Johnson, M. (2004). A feedback model of visual attention. *Journal of Cognitive Neuroscience*, 16(2), 219–237.

Stensaas, S. S., Eddington, D., & Dobelle, W. (1974). The topography and variability of the primary visual cortex in man. *Journal of Neurosurgery*, 40, 747–755.

Stockmeyer, L., & Chandra, A. (1988). Intrinsically difficult problems [Scientific American Inc., New York]. *Scientific American Trends in Computing*, 1, 88–97.

Styles, E. (1997). *The psychology of attention*. East Sussex, UK: Psychology Press Ltd.

Sunaert, E., Van Hecke, P., Marchal, G., & Orban, G. (1999). Motion-responsive regions of the human brain. *Experimental Brain Research*, 127(4), 355–370.

Sutherland, S. (1998). Book reviews. *Nature*, 392(26), 350.

Szczepanski, S., Konen, C., & Kastner, S. (2010). Mechanisms of spatial attention control in frontal and parietal cortex. *Journal of Neuuroscience*, 30(1), 148–160.

Tark, K., & Curtis, C. E. (2009). Persistent neural activity in the human frontal cortex when maintaining space that is off the map. *Nature Neuroscience*, 12(11), 1463–1468.

Taylor, J. G., & Rogers, M. (2002). A control model of the movement of attention. *Neural Networks*, 15, 309–326.

Thompson, K. G., Bichot, N. P., & Schall, J. D. (1997). Dissociation of visual discrimination from saccade programming in macaque frontal eye field. *Journal of Neurophysiology, 77*, 1046–1050.

Thompson, K. G., Biscoe, K. L., & Sato, T. R. (2005). Neuronal basis of covert spatial attention in the frontal eye field. *Journal of Neuroscience, 25*, 9479–9487.

Thornton, T., & Gilden, D. (2001). Attentional limitations in the sensing of motion direction. *Cognitive Psychology, 43*, 23–52.

Thorpe, S., & Imbert, M. (1989). Biological constraints on connectionist modelling. In R. Pfeifer, Z. Schreter, F. Fogelman-Soulié, & L. Steels (eds.), *Connectionism in perspective* (pp. 63–93). Amsterdam: Elsevier.

Thorpe, S., Fize, D., & Marlot, C. (1996). Speed of processing in the human visual system. *Nature, 381*, 520–522.

Tipper, S. P. (1985). The negative priming effect: inhibitory priming with to be ignored objects. *Quarterly Journal of Experimental Psychology, 37A*, 571–590.

Tishby, N., Pereira, F., & Bialek, W. (1999). The Information Bottleneck Method. Proc. 37th Allerton Conf. on Communication Control and Computing (pp. 368–377). September, Monticello, IL.

Titchener, E. B. (1908). *Lectures on the elementary psychology of feeling and attention.* New York: MacMillan.

Tombu, M., & Tsotsos, J. K. (2008). Attending to orientation results in an inhibitory surround in orientation space. *Perception & Psychophysics, 70*(1), 30–35.

Torralba, A. (2003). Modeling global scene factors in attention. *Journal of the Optical Society of America. A, Optics, Image Science, and Vision, 20*(7), 1407–1418.

Townsend, J. T. (1990). Serial vs. Parallel Processing: Sometimes they look like Tweedledum and Tweedledee but they can (and should) be distinguished. *Psychological Science, 1*, 46–54.

Traub, J. (1990). *Computation and science.* Computing Research News.

Triesch, J., Ballard, D., Hayhoe, M., & Sullivan, B. (2003). What you see is what you need. *Journal of Vision (Charlottesville, Va.), 3*, 86–94.

Triesch, J., Teuscher, C., Deak, G., & Carlson, E. (2006). Gaze following: Why (not) learn it? *Journal of Developmental Science, 9*(2), 125–147.

Treisman, A. (1964). The effect of irrelevant material on the efficiency of selective listening. *American Journal of Psychology, 77*, 533–546.

Treisman, A. (1996). The binding problem. *Current Opinion in Neurobiology, 6*(2), 171–178.

Treisman, A. (1999). Solutions to the binding problem: Progress through controversy and convergence. *Neuron, 24*(1), 105–125.

Treisman, A., & Gelade, G. (1980). A feature integration theory of attention. *Cognitive Psychology, 12*, 97–136.

Treisman, A., & Paterson, R. (1984). Emergent features, attention, and object perception. *Journal of Experimental Psychology: Human Perception and Performance, 10*, 12–31.

Treisman, A., & Schmidt, H. (1982). Illusory conjunctions in the perception of objects. *Cognitive Psychology, 14*, 107–141.

Treue, S., & Andersen, R. A. (1996). Neural responses to velocity gradients in macaque cortical area MT. *Visual Neuroscience, 13*, 797–804.

Treue, S., & Martinez-Trujillo, J. (1999). Feature-based attention influences motion processing gain in macaque visual cortex. *Nature, 399*(6736), 575–579.

Treue, S., & Maunsell, J. H. R. (1996). Attentional modulation of visual motion processing in cortical areas MT and MST. *Nature, 382*(6591), 539–541.

Trick, L. M., & Pylyshyn, Z. W. (1993). What enumeration studies can show us about spatial attention: evidence for limited capacity preattentive processing. *Journal of Experimental Psychology: Human Perception and Performance, 19*(2), 331–351.

Tsal, Y., Meiran, N., & Lamy, D. (1995). Towards a resolution theory of visual attention. *Visual Cognition, 2*(2), 313–330.

Tsotsos, J. K. (1980). A Framework for Visual Motion Understanding. PhD Thesis, Department of Computer Science, University of Toronto.

Tsotsos, J. K. (1987). A "Complexity Level" Analysis of Vision. In M. Brady and A. Rosenfeld (eds.), Proceedings of the 1st International Conference on Computer Vision (pp. 346–55). June 8–11, London, UK. Washington DC: IEEE Computer Society Press.

Tsotsos, J. K. (1988a). A "complexity level" analysis of immediate vision. *International Journal of Computer Vision* (Marr Prize Special Issue), *2*(1), 303–320.

Tsotsos, J. K. (1988b). How does human vision beat the computational complexity of visual perception? In Z. Pylyshyn (Ed.), *Computational processes in human vision: An interdisciplinary perspective*, (pp. 286–338). Norwood, NJ: Ablex Press,

Tsotsos, J. K. (1989). The Complexity of Perceptual Search Tasks. In N. Sridharan (ed.), Proc. 11th International Joint Conference on Artificial Intelligence (pp. 1571–1577). August 20–25, Detroit, MI. International Joint Conference on Artificial Intelligence.

Tsotsos, J. K. (1990a). Analyzing vision at the complexity level. *Behavioral and Brain Sciences*, *13*(3), 423–445.

Tsotsos, J. K. (1990b). A little complexity analysis goes a long way. *Behavioral and Brain Sciences*, *13*(3), 458–469.

Tsotsos, J. K. (1991a). Is complexity theory appropriate for analysing biological systems? *Behavioral and Brain Sciences*, *14*(4), 770–773.

Tsotsos, J. K. (1991b). Localizing Stimuli in a Sensory Field Using an Inhibitory Attentional Beam. RBCV-TR-91-37. University of Toronto.

Tsotsos, J. K. (1992a). On the relative complexity of passive vs active visual search. *International Journal of Computer Vision*, *7*(2), 127–141.

Tsotsos, J. K. (1992b). Image understanding. In S. Shapiro (ed.), *The encyclopedia of artificial intelligence* (2nd ed., pp. 641–663). New York: John Wiley & Sons.

Tsotsos, J. K. (1993). An inhibitory beam for attentional selection. In L. Harris & M. Jenkin (eds.), *Spatial vision in humans and robots* (pp. 313–331). Cambridge, UK: Cambridge University Press.

Tsotsos, J. K. (1995a). On behaviorist intelligence and the scaling problem. *Artificial Intelligence*, *75*, 135–160.

Tsotsos, J. K. (1995b). Towards a computational model of visual attention. In T. Papathomas, C., Chubb, A. Gorea, & E. Kowler (eds.). *Early vision and beyond* (pp. 207–218). Cambridge, MA: MIT Press.

Tsotsos, J. K. (1999). Triangles, pyramids, connections and attentive inhibition. *PSYCHE: An Interdisciplinary Journal of Research on Consciousness* 5(20).

Tsotsos, J. K., & Bruce, N. D. B. (2008). Computational foundations for attentive processes. *Scholarpedia*, *3*(12), 6545.

Tsotsos, J. K., Culhane, S., & Cutzu, F. (2001). From theoretical foundations to a hierarchical circuit for selective attention. In J. Braun, C. Koch, J. Davis (eds.), *Visual attention and cortical circuits* (pp. 285–306). Cambridge, MA: MIT Press.

Tsotsos, J. K., Culhane, S., Wai, W., Lai, Y., Davis, N., & Nuflo, F. (1995). Modeling visual attention via selective tuning. *Artificial Intelligence*, *78*(1–2), 507–547.

Tsotsos, J. K., Itti, L., & Rees, G. (2005). A brief and selective history of attention. In L. Itti, G. Rees, & J. K. Tsotsos (eds.), *Neurobiology of attention*. Amsterdam: Elsevier Press.

Tsotsos, J. K., Liu, Y., Martinez-Trujillo, J., Pomplun, M., Simine, E., & Zhou, K. (2005). Attending to visual motion. *Computer Vision and Image Understanding*, *100*(1–2), 3–40.

Tsotsos, J. K., Mylopoulos, J., Covvey, D., & Zucker, S. W. (1980). A framework for visual motion understanding. *IEEE Pattern Analysis Machine Intelligence*, *2*, 563–573.

Tsotsos, J. K., Rodríguez-Sánchez, A., Rothenstein, A., & Simine, E. (2008). Different binding strategies for the different stages of visual recognition. *Brain Research*, *1225*, 119–132.

Turing, A. M. (1936). On computable numbers, with an application to the Entscheidungsproblem. *Proceedings of the London Mathematical Society. Second Series*, *42*, 230–265.

Uhr, L. (1972). Layered "recognition cone" networks that preprocess, classify and describe. *IEEE Transactions on Computers*, C-21 (7), 758–768.

Ullman, S. (1984). Visual routines. *Cognition*, *18*, 97–159.

Ullman, S. (1995). Sequence seeking and counter streams: a computational model for bidirectional information flow in the visual cortex. *Cerebral Cortex*, *5*, 1–11.

Ullman, S. (2000). *High-level vision: Object recognition and visual cognition*. Cambridge, MA: MIT Press.

Ungerleider, L., & Mishkin, M. (1982). Two cortical visual systems. In D. Ingle, M. Goodale, & R. Mansfield (eds.), *Analysis of visual behavior* (pp. 549–586). Cambridge, MA: MIT Press.

Usher, M., & Niebur, E. (1996). Modeling the temporal dynamic of IT neurons in visual search: a mechanism for top-down selective attention. *Journal of Cognitive Neuroscience*, *8*(4), 311–327.

van der Wal, G., & Burt, P. (1992). A VLSI pyramid chip for multiresolution image analysis. *International Journal of Computer Vision*, *8*(3), 177–190.

Valdes-Sosa, M., Bobes, M., Rodriguez, V., & Pinilla, T. (1998). Switching attention without shifting the spotlight: object-based attentional modulation of brain potentials. *Journal of Cognitive Neuroscience*, *10*(1), 137–151.

Valiant, L. (1975). Parallelism in comparison problems. *SIAM Journal on Computing*, *4*(3), 348–355.

Vanduffel, W., Tootell, R. B. H., & Orban, G. A. (2000). Attention-dependent suppression of metabolic activity in early stages of the macaque visual system. *Cerebral Cortex*, *10*, 109–126.

Van Rullen, R., & Thorpe, S. J. (2001). The time course of visual processing: from early perception to decision making. *Journal of Cognitive Neuroscience*, *13*(4), 454–461.

Van Rullen, R., Carlson, T., & Cavanaugh, P. (2007). The blinking spotlight of attention. *Proceedings of the National Academy of Sciences of the United States of America*, *104*(49), 19204–19209.

Verghese, P., & Pelli, D. (1992). The information capacity of visual attention. *Vision Research*, *32*(5), 983–995.

von der Malsburg, C. (1981). The Correlation Theory of Brain Function. Internal Report. 81–2. Göttingen, Germany: Department of Neurobiology, Max-Planck-Institute for Biophysical Chemistry.

von der Malsburg, C. (1999). The what and why of binding: The modeler's perspective. *Neuron*, *24*, 95–104.

Wai, W., & Tsotsos, J. K. (1994). Directing Attention to Onset and Offset of Image Events for Eye-Head Movement Control. Proc. 12th IAPR Conf. on Pattern Recognition, Vol. A (pp. 274–279). October 9–13, Jerusalem. International Association for Pattern Recognition.

Walther, D., Itti, L., Riesenhuber, M., Poggio, T., & Koch, K. (2002). Attentional Selection for Object Recognition—A Gentle Way. In S-W. Lee, H. H. Buelthoff & T. Poggio (eds.), *Biologically Motivated Computer Vision* (pp. 472–479). Second IEEE International Workshop, BMCV 2002. December, Tuebingen, Germany.

Waltz, D. (1975). Understanding line-drawings of scenes with shadows. In P. H. Winston (ed.), *The psychology of computer vision* (pp. 19–91). New York: McGraw-Hill.

Wandell, B. & Silverstein, L. D. (1995). *Foundations of human vision*. Sunderland, MA: Sinauer.

Weber, C., & Triesch, J. (2006). A Possible Representation of Reward in the Learning of Saccades. In Proceedings of the Sixth International Workshop on Epigenetic Robotics "EpiRob" (pp. 153–160). September 20–22, 2006, Paris, France.

Weng, W., Jones, H., Andolina, I., Salt, T., & Sillito, S. (2006). Functional alignment of feedback effects from visual cortex to thalamus. *Nature Neuroscience*, *10*(9), 1330–1336.

Whittaker, S., & Cummings, R. (1990). Foveating saccades. *Vision Research*, *30*(9), 1363–1366.

Whitehead, S., & Ballard, D. (1990). Active perception and reinforcement learning. *Machine Learning*, *1990*, 179–188.

Wiesmeyer, M., & Laird, J. (1990). A Computer Model of 2D Visual Attention. In Proceedings of the Twelfth Annual Conference of the Cognitive Science Society (pp. 582–589). July 25–28, Cambridge, MA. Hillsdale NJ: Lawrence Erlbaum Associates.

Wilkes, D., & Tsotsos, J. K. (1992). Active Object Recognition. In N. Ahuja (ed.), Proc. Computer Vision and Pattern Recognition (pp. 136–141). June 15–18, Urbana, IL. Washington DC: IEEE Computer Society Press.

Wilson, H. R. (1999). *Spikes, decision and actions: The dynamical foundations of neuroscience.* New York: Oxford University Press.

Wolfe, J. M. (1994). Guided search 2.0: A revised model of visual search. *Psychonomic Bulletin & Review, 1*(2), 202–238.

Wolfe, J. (1998a). Visual search. In H. Pashler (ed.), *Attention* (pp. 13–74). London: University College London.

Wolfe, J. M. (1998b). What can 1,000,000 trials tell us about visual search? *Psychological Science, 9*(1), 33–39.

Wolfe, J. M. (2007). Guided search 4.0: Current progress with a model of visual search. In W. Gray (ed.), *Integrated models of cognitive systems* (pp. 99–119). New York: Oxford University Press.

Wolfe, J. M., & Gancarz, G. (1996). *Guided search 3.0: Basic and clinical applications of vision science* (pp. 189–192). Dordrecht, The Netherlands: Kluwer Academic.

Wolfe, J., Cave, K., & Franzel, S. (1989). Guided search: An alternative to the feature integration model for visual search. *Journal of Experimental Psychology. Human Perception and Performance, 15,* 419–433.

Wolfe, J., Klempen, N., & Dahlen, K. (2000). Postattentive vision. *Journal of Experimental Psychology. Human Perception and Performance, 26*(2), 693–716.

Wu, A., & Guo, A. (1999). Selective visual attention in a neurocomputational model of phase oscillators. *Biological Cybernetics, 80,* 205–214.

Wundt, W. (1874). *Grundzüge der Physiologischen Psychologie.* Leipzig: Engelmann.

Xiao, D. K., Marcar, V. L., Raiguel, S. E., & Orban, G. A. (1997). Selectivity of macaque MT/V5 neurons for surface orientation in depth specified by motion. *European Journal of Neuroscience, 9,* 956–964.

Yantis, S. (1998). Control of visual attention. In H. Pashler (ed.), *Attention* (pp. 223–256). East Sussex, UK: Psychology Press.

Yantis, S., & Jonides, J. (1984). Abrupt visual onsets and selective attention: evidence from visual search. *Journal of Experimental Psychology. Human Perception and* Performance, *10,* 601–621.

Yantis, S., & Serences, J. T. (2003). Cortical mechanisms of space-based and object-based attentional control. *Current Opinion in Neurobiology, 13,* 187–193.

Yarbus, A. L. (1967). *Eye movements and vision.* New York: Plenum Press.

Yashuhara, A. (1971). *Recursive function theory and logic.* New York: Academic Press.

Ye, Y., & Tsotsos, J. K. (1996). 3D Sensor Planning: Its Formulation and Complexity. In H. Kautz and B. Selman (eds.), Proc. 4th International Symposium on Artificial Intelligence and Mathematics. January 3–5, Fort Lauderdale, FL.

Ye, Y., & Tsotsos, J. K. (1999). Sensor planning for object search. *Computer Vision and Image Understanding, 73*(2), 145–168.

Ye, Y., & Tsotsos, J. K. (2001). A complexity level analysis of the sensor planning task for object search. *Computational Intelligence, 17*(4), 605–620.

Yuille, A., & Geiger, D. (1995). Winner-take-all mechanisms. In M. Arbib (ed.), *The handbook of brain theory and neural networks.* Cambridge, MA: MIT Press.

Zaharescu, A. (2004). A Neurally-Based Model of Active Visual Search. MSc Thesis, Department of Computer Science and Engineering, York University.

Zaharescu, A., Rothenstein, A. L., Tsotsos, J. K. (2005). Towards a biologically plausible active visual search model. In *Attention and performance in computational vision: Second International Workshop,* WAPCV 2004. Revised Selected Papers, Lecture Notes in Computer Science, Volume 3368/2005 (pp. 133–147). Heidelberg: Springer-Verlag.

Zelinsky, G., Rao, R., Hayhoe, M., & Ballard, D. (1997). Eye movements reveal the spatio-temporal dynamics of visual search. *Psychological Science, 8,* 448–453.

Zemel, R. S., & Sejnowski, T. J. (1998). A model for encoding multiple object motions and self-motion in area mst of primate visual cortex. *Journal of Neuroscience*, *18*(1), 531–547.

Zhang, L., Tong, M. H., Marks, T. K., Shan, H., Cottrell, G. W. (2008). SUN: A Bayesian framework for saliency using natural statistics. *Journal of Vision*, *8*(7): article 32, 1–20.

Zhou, K. (2004). Modeling Motion with the Selective Tuning Model. MSc Thesis, Department of Computer Science, York University.

Zoccolan, D., Cox, D., & DiCarlo, J. (2005). Multiple object response normalization in monkey inferotemporal cortex. *Journal of Neuroscience*, *25*(36), 8150–8164.

Zucker, S. W. (1981). Computer Vision and Human Perception: An Essay on the Discovery of Constraints. In P. Hayes and R. Schank (eds.), Proc. 7th Int. Conf. on Artificial Intelligence (pp. 1102–1116). August 24–28, Vancouver, BC.

Zucker, S. W., Leclerc, Y., & Mohammed, J. (1981). Continuous relaxation and local maxima selection—conditions for equivalence (in complex speech and vision understanding systems). *IEEE Transactions on Pattern Analysis and Machine Intelligence*, *3*, 117–127.

Zucker, S. W., Rosenfeld, A., & Davis, L. S. (1975). General Purpose Models: Expectations about the Unexpected. Fourth International Joint Conference on Artificial Intelligence, Vol. 2, Tblisi, USSR, September 1975. Reprinted in *SIGART Newsletter*, No. 54, October 1975, pp. 7–11.

Author Index

Subject Index

Abstract representation, 19, 242
Act psychology, 3, 63
Active vision, 3, 29–33, 58, 60, 63, 233
  active blackboard, 243
  active knowledge, 29
  active object recognition, 63
  active perception, 29
  active search, 182, 183
Adaptive Resonance Theory, 69–71, 74, 75
AIM (Attention via Information Maximization),
  73–75, 124, 125, 187, 189, 190, 203
Alerting, 55
Algebraic model, 2
Algorithm, 7, 15, 16, 18, 19–52, 59, 60
Algorithmic model, 69–71. *See also* Adaptive
  Resonance Theory (ART); Corollary Discharge
  of Attention Movement (CODAM); Not Overt
  Visual Attention (NOVA); Saliency Map
  Model; Shifter Circuits; SOAR-based model;
  Temporal Tagging Model; Visual Routines
Ambiguity Resolution Theory, 67
Animate Vision, 65, 66, 71
Area 7a, 152, 153, 161, 169, 186, 238, 242, 265, 271
At a glance (AG), 234, 235, 248
Attention (definition), 10, 51
Attentional footprint, 55
Attentional gain field, 77
Attention-Direction Theory, 3, 63
Attenuator Theory, 4, 64

Biased Competition, 5, 67, 68, 69, 71, 75, 95, 122,
  127, 128, 201, 204
Bias neuron, 109–110
Binding, 55, 56, 62, 96, 133–150
  convergence binding, 142–149, 160, 161, 164, 187,
    235, 242
  partial recurrence binding, 143, 145–148, 235
  full recurrence binding, 144, 145, 147, 148, 164,
    226, 235
  iterative recurrence binding, 144, 145, 147, 148,
    166, 168, 174, 186, 187, 202, 235
  type I, 144, 145, 147, 166, 168, 174

type II, 144, 145, 147, 186, 202
Blackboard, 240–243
Blurring problem, 43, 44, 84, 88
Bottleneck, 8, 11–13, 15, 16, 43, 52
  categorization bottleneck, 11
  iconic bottleneck, 12
  span of attention bottleneck, 11
Bottom-up, 22, 24, 39, 46, 47, 54, 55, 66–68, 72, 74,
  77, 87, 95, 257, 258, 261
Boundary problem, 39–42, 52, 54, 85, 88, 89, 119,
  124
Branch-and-bound, 83, 113, 147

Capacity, 7–12, 15, 16, 52, 58, 65, 81, 238
  limited, 8, 11, 12, 65
Cardinal cells, 140
Categorization, 11, 69, 82, 92, 135–137, 139, 142,
  146, 147, 169
Central attentional field, 89, 91
Classification, 134–137, 139, 142, 146, 147, 149, 168,
  190
Cocktail party effect, 11
Co-location (binding), 140
Combinatorics (combinatorial), 7, 8, 51, 62, 140
Computation
  principles, 15, 16
  computational model (definition), 59
  computational theory (Marr), 19
Computational complexity, 16, 21, 28, 33, 34, 41,
  51, 62, 64, 78, 81, 98, 233, 255
Computational model of visual attention
  (definition), 59
Cone (retinal), 40–42
Consciousness, 2, 3
Conspicuity. *See* Salience
Context, 44, 62, 66, 83–85, 113, 123, 124, 126, 189,
  244
  problem, 44, 46, 50, 88, 95, 115, 119, 196, 206, 208
Contour Detector (CODE) Theory of Visual
  Attention, 68
Contrast gain model, 68
Convergence (binding), 140

Printed in the United States
by Baker & Taylor Publisher Services